A Laboratory Guide to Clinical Diagnosis

R. D. Eastham

MD (Cantab) FRCP (Lond) FRCPath MRCPsych
DCP Dipl Path
*Consultant Pathologist to the Frenchay Group of Hospitals,
Bristol*

Fifth Edition

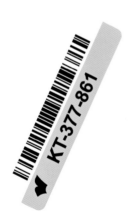

WRIGHT·PSG
Bristol London Boston
1983

©John Wright & Sons Ltd, 823–825 Bath Road, Bristol BS4 5NU. 1983

Published by
John Wright & Sons Ltd, 823–825 Bath Road, Bristol BS4 5NU, England
John Wright PSG Inc., 545 Great Road, Littleton, Massachusetts 01460, U.S.A.

First edition, 1964
Reprinted, 1966
Second edition, 1970
Third edition, 1973
Fourth edition, 1976
Fifth edition, 1983
Greek edition, 1973
Italian edition, 1976
Spanish edition, 1976

British Library Cataloguing in Publication Data

Eastham, R.D.
 A laboratory guide to clinical diagnosis. —.
 5th ed.
 1. Diagnosis, Laboratory 2. Medicine, Clinical
 —Laboratory manuals
 I. Title
 616.07'5'028 RB37

ISBN 0 7236 0653 6

Library of Congress Catalog Card Number: 83-42675

Typeset by Activity, Salisbury, Wilts
Printed in Great Britain by John Wright & Sons (Printing) Ltd at The Stonebridge Press, Bristol BS4 5NU.

A Laboratory Guide
to Clinical Diagnosis

Preface to the Fifth Edition

In this fifth edition of 'Laboratory Guide' the text has been extensively revised and rewritten. Rare disorders are marked with the symbol [R]. Since the fourth edition, many tests which could only be carried out in limited numbers and after often long delays in specialized centres, can now be rapidly and accurately performed as routine in most laboratories, improving the potential for rapid diagnosis in more conditions.

It is as important as ever that close consultation and cooperation between the clinician, the haematologist, microbiologist, chemical pathologist and clinical chemist are maintained.

R.D.E.

Preface to the First Edition

Following the success of *Biochemical Values in Clinical Medicine* and *Clinical Haematology*, many requests were received for a pocket-size book giving the relative merits of the laboratory tests used in the investigation and treatment of various diseases. This book is an attempt to answer such a need; it is set out in the usual order of a textbook of medicine and the text is deliberately kept brief and, in parts terse for reasons explained in the all-important Chapter 1.

It is hoped that this book will be of use not only in hospitals but also to general practitioners who have access to laboratory facilities in their practice area. Where more patients can be diagnosed and treated by their own doctors at home, the worry of admission to hospital is removed and the pressure on hospital beds is reduced. Also many patients can be more fully investigated pending examination by a specialist or while awaiting actual admission to hospital; such investigations could reduce the time spent by the patient in hospital and would enable the general practitioner to keep closer contact with his patient, with the opportunity for more detailed observation of diagnosis and treatment.

Finally, if the use of this book also brings about closer cooperation and understanding with mutual stimulation of interest between clinical specialists, general practitioners and clinical pathologists, it will have fulfilled its purpose.

R.D.E.
B.R.P.

Contents

Abbreviations

AA	Australia antigen
ABS	Fluorescent treponemal antibody test
ACTH	Adrenocorticotrophic hormone
ADH	Antidiuretic hormone
A/G ratio	Albumin/globulin ratio
AHG	Antihuman globulin
ASO	Antistreptolysin 'O'
ATP	Adenosine triphosphate
BAL	British anti-Lewisite
BCG	Bacille-Calmette-Guérin vaccine
BCR	British comparative ratio (prothrombin)
BFP	Bis-(monoisopropylamino)-fluorophosphine oxide
BFP	Biological false positive (syphilis)
BMR	Basal metabolic rate
BSP	Bromsulphthalein
cAMP	Cyclic-adenosine monophosphate
CRP	C-reactive protein
CSF	Cerebrospinal fluid
DFP	Di-isopropyl flurophosphate
DNA	Deoxyribonucleic acid
DOCA	Desoxycorticosterone acetate
EACA	Epsilon-aminocaproic acid
EBV	Epstein–Barr virus
ECF	Extracellular fluid
ECHO	Enteric cytopathic human orphan (virus)
EDTA	Ethylenediamine tetra-acetate
EHAA	Epidemic hepatitis-associated antigen
ELISA	Enzyme-linked immunosorbent assay
ERF	Effective renal blood-flow
ESR	Erythrocyte sedimentation rate
ESS	Erythrocyte sensitizing substance
FIGLU	Formimino-glutamic acid
FMDV	Foot and mouth disease virus
FSH	Follicle-stimulating hormone
FTA	Fluorescent treponema antibody test
GCFT	Gonococcal complement-fixation test
GFR	Glomerular filtration rate
Glucose T_m	Renal tubular excretory mass with reference to glucose
HAA	Hepatitis-associated antigen
HBD	Alpha-hydroxybutyric dehydrogenase
HCG	Human chorionic gonadotrophin
HDL	High-density lipoprotein
HGH	Human growth hormone
HI	Haemagglutination inhibition
5-HIAA	5-hydroxyindole acetic acid

HPG	Human pituitary gonadotrophin
5-HT	5-hydroxytryptamine
HVA	Homovanillic acid
ICDH	Isocitric dehydrogenase
IDL	Intermediate-density lipoprotein
LAP	Leucine aminopeptidase
LCM	Lymphocytic choriomeningitis (virus)
LDH	Lactate dehydrogenase
LDL	Low-density lipoprotein
LE	Lupus erythematosus
LGV	Lymphogranuloma venereum
LH	Luteinizing hormone
MCD	Mean cell diameter of erythrocyte
MCH	Mean corpuscular haemoglobin
MCHC	Mean corpuscular haemoglobin concentration
MCT	Mean cell thickness of erythrocyte
MCV	Mean cell volume of erythrocyte
MDH	Malate dehydrogenase
M/E	Myeloid/erythroid (ratio)
MIC	Minimum inhibitory concentration
MSH	Melanocyte-stimulating hormone
NAD	Coenzyme I
NADP	Coenzyme II
NBTZ	Nitroblue tetrazolium (test)
NEFA	Non-esterified fatty acid
NPN	Non-protein nitrogen
PAH	*Para*-aminohippuric acid
$PAHT_m$	Renal tubular excretory mass with reference to PAH
PAS	*Para*-aminosalicylic acid
PCV	Volume of packed red cells per 100 ml blood
PHI	Phosphohexose isomerase
PNH	Paroxysmal nocturnal haemoglobinuria
PTA	Plasma thromboplastin antecedent
PVP	Polyvinyl pyrrolidone
RA	Rheumatoid arthritis
RCFT	Reiter complement-fixation test
RNA	Ribonucleic acid
RPF	Renal plasma flow
SGOT	Serum glutamic oxalacetic transaminase (aspartate aminotransferase)
SGPT	Serum glutamic pyruvic transaminase (alanine aminotransferase)
SHA	Serum hepatitis antigen
SLE	Systemic lupus erythematosus
STA	Serum thrombotic activator
STS	Serological tests for syphilis
TGT	Thromboplastin generation test
TIBC	Serum total iron binding capacity

TPI	*Treponema pallidum* immobilization test
TPN	Triphosphopyridine nucleotide
TRH	Thyrotrophin-releasing hormone
TRIC	Trachoma inclusion conjunctivitis agent
TSH	Thyroid-stimulating hormone
TWBC	Total white blood-cell count
UIBC	Serum unsaturated iron-binding capacity
VCA	Virus capsid antigen
VDRL	Venereal Disease Research Laboratory
VLDL	Very low-density lipoprotein
VMA	Vanillylmandelic acid (4-hydroxy-3-methoxy-mandelic acid)
WR	Wassermann reaction
ZST	Zinc sulphate turbidity reaction

1 *Introductory*

The number and variety of laboratory tests available to assist clinicians in the diagnosis of disease increases each year. At the same time, with improvements in technology, tests, which a few years ago were difficult and expensive to perform, can now be carried out in routine working laboratories (e.g. detailed thyroid function tests). There is also a steady expansion in the number of defined and recognizable diseases or syndromes, with detailed reclassification of groups of diseases, and identification of specific enzyme deficiencies causing those diseases (e.g. mucopolysaccharidoses).

The range of diseases encountered in any country has been broadened by immigration of populations, and also by the great increase in world holiday travel. It is relatively commonplace for a citizen of the United Kingdom to be exposed to tropical diseases while on holiday abroad.

DIAGNOSIS

An indication of the value of particular tests in diagnosis is given in the first sentence of each disease section. While some tests enable a specific diagnosis to be made, other tests may only give support to clinical diagnosis. Further tests are given in the text to assist the clinician. Again in the first sentence in each section, a brief summary of clinical presentation is given as a thumbnail sketch, in the hope that this will be helpful.

TESTS OF PROGRESS

Following treatment, or during active progression of a disease process, laboratory tests are useful in assessing progress, and an indication of useful tests for this purpose is given.

TESTS PROVIDING USEFUL NEGATIVE RESULTS

These are self-explanatory. If a particular test is positive (or negative), then it is often possible to exclude a particular disease, saving unnecessary investigation. Sequential tests are of great value, both in diagnosis and in the assessment of the effects of continuing disease processes or response to treatment. A blood sample taken in the early stages of bacterial or viral infection, followed by a further blood sample taken 10–14 days later, may be very valuable for the demonstration of the development of specific antibodies against the infecting organism.

It is well worth while contacting the local laboratory to obtain a list of normal values for the tests performed, and also specimen collection requirements (e.g. clotted blood, heparinized blood, timing of collections etc.). It is also very useful to discuss complicated clinical problems with the local haematologist, microbiologist, chemical pathologist or clinical chemist, since some tests can be carried out together, or in a certain sequence, thus saving time and allowing more rigid, accurate diagnosis. This may help to avoid the so-called laboratory 'Friday afternoon syndrome' — specimens for analysis arriving with an urgent request for a complicated metabolic test, not having been collected into the correct containers, chilled or transported rapidly to the laboratory or, from the other side of the fence, the laboratory staff appearing to be unhelpful to the clinician. Prior discussion avoids this happening.

2 Infectious Diseases—I

VIRAL INFECTIONS

Viruses are obligate intracellular parasites which can cause:

1. Complete destruction of infected cells, e.g. anterior horn cells of spinal cord by poliovirus.
2. Cytopathic effects with formation of inclusion bodies and distortion of normal cell morphology, e.g. intranuclear inclusion bodies in herpes simplex virus infection, intracytoplasmic inclusion bodies in variola virus infection.
3. Syncytium or giant-cell formation, e.g. measles virus, varicella virus, cytomegalovirus infection.
4. Undetectable effects, e.g. latent infection with herpes simplex virus.
5. Proliferation, e.g. benign wart formation, malignancy in animals.

COLLECTION AND STORAGE OF SPECIMENS FOR VIRUS DETECTION AND DIAGNOSIS

Nasal-throat swabs—place in virus transport medium, keep cool (4 °C), transport to laboratory within 3 hours if possible.

Sputum—keep cool (water ice) and transport to laboratory within 3 hours if possible.

Blood—10 ml heparinized blood to be kept at 4 °C and delivered to the laboratory within 3 hours if possible.

Urine—mid-stream sample collected into sterile container, kept at 4 °C and transported to the laboratory within 3 hours if possible.

Faeces—collect into sterile container, keep at 4 °C and deliver to the laboratory within 3 hours if possible.

Cerebrospinal fluid—collect into sterile container, keep at 4 °C and deliver to laboratory within 3 hours if possible.

Biopsy and post-mortem material—place in sterile container. Do *not* add any formalin or other fixative. Keep cool at 4 °C and deliver to the laboratory within 3 hours if possible.

Viruses are destroyed if they are deep-frozen, e.g. −20 °C or less, otherwise there is the risk of serum samples becoming anticomplementary and making estimation of titres of antibodies impossible. It is very important that *two* samples be sent: the first as early as possible in the illness, and the second specimen taken at 10 days or later—this enables the rising titre to be detected.

Vesicle fluid or crusts can be examined by electron microscopy for the rapid diagnosis of orf, varicella-zoster virus, herpes simplex and vaccinia. Obviously this will only be performed following prior arrangement with the laboratory.

Whenever specimens of sputum, swabs, blood, CSF, faeces, etc., are sent to a laboratory for virological studies, it is vitally important that full relevant clinical information, including the duration of illness, should be sent with the

3

specimens, since it is on this information that the types of virological examinations will be decided.

Acute Non-bacterial Respiratory Disease

Culture of throat swabs and sputum samples may reveal the presence of influenza, parainfluenza, adenovirus, ECHO virus, reovirus, virus of specific fevers etc. Associated rise in titre of specific antibodies in the patient's serum helps to define the primary infection.

TESTS PROVIDING USEFUL NEGATIVE RESULTS

Cultures of throat swabs and sputum fail to grow known bacterial respiratory tract pathogens (e.g. haemolytic streptococci, *C. diphtheriae*).

RESPIRATORY VIRUS INFECTIONS

Clinical condition	Common causes	Less common causes
Epidemic influenza	Influenza A and B	Adenovirus Enterovirus Parainfluenza
'Influenza-like'	Adenovirus	Enterovirus Parainfluenza
Sore throat	Adenovirus (beta-haemolytic streptococcus)	Enterovirus Influenza A and B
'Common cold'	Rhinovirus	Parainfluenza Respiratory syncytial virus Enterovirus Adenovirus
Feverish 'cold'	Adenovirus Rhinovirus	Influenza A and B Parainfluenza Respiratory syncytial virus Enterovirus
Croup (infants)	Parainfluenza	Influenza A and B Enterovirus
Bronchiolitis (infants)	Respiratory syncytial virus	Parainfluenza Influenza A and B (*Mycoplasma pneumoniae*)
Pneumonia	Adenovirus (*Mycoplasma pneumoniae*) (secondary bacterial)	Respiratory syncytial virus (infants) Parainfluenza (infants) Psittacosis Q fever

The clinical picture following virus infection depends both on the nature of the virus and on the infected host.

NON-SPECIFIC VIRAL DISEASE

Primary Atypical Pneumonia

Diagnosis of this condition is confirmed by the finding of rising titres of cold agglutinins in many cases. Agglutinins against *Streptococcus MG* have been found in many cases. It would appear that with more sophisticated methods of culture of material for viruses this condition is probably a clinical condition caused by a variety of viruses, including:

Psittacosis-ornithosis virus
Adenovirus
Rhinovirus
Influenza B
Parainfluenza 1, 2, and 3
Enterovirus
Respiratory syncytial virus
Rickettsia burnetii
Eaton's agent

Neutropenia is common early in the condition, with a relative lymphocytosis, but following secondary bacterial invasion of the respiratory tract, neutrophilia develops with increases in the ESR and the plasma viscosity.

Chronic Non-specific Infectious Lymphocytosis in Children

Moderate leucocytosis with lymphocytosis lasting for months has been described, with low normal haemoglobin concentrations. The platelet count and ESR are normal, and the Paul–Bunnell heterophil antibody is negative.

Until tests for cytomegalovirus and toxoplasmosis have also been shown to be negative, this diagnosis must remain a very unsatisfactory one.

Acute Infective Lymphocytosis in Children

Diagnosis of this condition is confirmed by the finding of an absolute lymphocytosis persisting for 2–3 weeks in children. Eosinophilia is common. Although the condition is associated with abdominal pain, diarrhoea and vomiting, and although in one series an untyped enterovirus with neutralizing antibodies has been found, no single definite virus has been consistently associated with this disease yet.

TESTS PRODUCING USEFUL NEGATIVE RESULTS

The Paul–Bunnell heterophil antibody test is negative.

Aseptic Meningitis

Diagnosis of this condition is supported by the finding of moderately raised CSF protein, normal glucose and chloride concentrations, and, initially, normal cell counts. Later, there is a moderate rise in CSF lymphocytes, most commonly to about 100 per cmm (although counts can rise to 1000 per cmm rarely).

Identification of the infecting virus suggests the following pattern:

Seventy per cent unidentified (of which an unknown proportion will be due to LCM virus).

Thirty per cent identified: 50 per cent due to adenovirus
                            25 per cent due to mumps virus
Remainder:

Herpesvirus
LGV agent
Measles
Chickenpox
Varicella
Infective hepatitis
Sandfly fever
Infectious mononucleosis.

Lymphocytic choriomeningitis virus (LCM) may produce a 'flu-like illness or aseptic meningitis in man. This virus has rodents as its natural hosts.

Viral Encephalitis

Diagnosis of the virus infection causing encephalitis can be confirmed by isolation and culture of the virus from the patient's blood, throat swabs, and CSF. Immunofluorescent testing of brain biopsy material makes possible the rapid diagnosis of acute herpes simplex encephalitis, and hence its possible treatment with viricidal agents. The virus can be isolated on culture from brain tissue, especially from the brainstem and hippocampus in fatal cases.

Sera taken during the first few days of the infection and again after 3–4 weeks show rising titres of complement-fixing antibodies and neutralizing antibodies.

The CSF contains increased protein and there is an increase in the cell count (200–2000 per cmm) with 60–90 per cent of the cells neutrophils. There is a neutrophilia in the peripheral blood.

Various viruses may cause encephalitis:

Mumps	Coxsackie B
Measles	ECHO virus
Herpes simplex	Louping ill
Virus B	Japanese B virus
Vaccinia	Murray River encephalitis
Poliovirus	St Louis encephalitis
Coxsackie A	Russian spring–summer encephalitis

POXVIRUSES

The poxviruses are the largest of the true viruses, and possess a common nucleoprotein antigen demonstrable by complement fixation. Most of them invade the skin and produce vesiculopustular eruption, also disseminating widely in the susceptible host. They survive indefinitely at -75 °C, and are very resistant to drying. An infected room kept at room temperature remains infective for over a year.

Variola Major (Smallpox)

Although smallpox may apparently have been eliminated as a major disease, a description of laboratory diagnosis is retained.

Diagnosis of infection is confirmed by direct microscopy of prodromal or definitive rash, the lower epithelial cells containing elementary bodies (Guarnieri or Paschen bodies) in their cytoplasm. In the early stages, viral antigens are detectable in skin lesions by immuno-electrophoresis. In the early stages of severe smallpox, positive blood cultures of the virus on chorioallantoic membrane of embryo chicks is possible, and there may be enough virus in the blood to act as antigen in a complement-fixation test.

Material from vesicles can be cultured in chick embryo, the characteristic pocks growing by 60–72 hours (cf. vaccinia pocks growing by 36–48 hours). The material from smallpox vesicles can be used in complement-fixation tests with hyperimmune rabbit antivaccinial serum, or in a rapid immunodiffusion precipitation test in agar gel taking 2–6 hours.

By the third day of the illness complement-fixing antibodies, haemagglutination-inhibiting antibodies, and neutralizing antibodies have appeared in the serum, reaching peak values by the ninth day. (Recent vaccination in the past year produces similar serum titres.)

Where facilities are available and where the diagnosis is uncertain, electron microscopy is valuable in the diagnosis of vaccinia.

After initial neutropenia, neutrophilia occurs especially with secondary invasion of the skin lesions.

Variola Minor (Alastrim)

Diagnosis of this infection, which produces a disease resembling mild smallpox and which never gives rise to true smallpox, is essentially the same as for smallpox itself. Cross-immunity between the two diseases is complete.

Vaccination

Vaccinia virus is an artificially produced poxvirus maintained by dermal inoculation of sheep, cattle, or rabbits. The pustules produced on the animal skin are treated so that bacteria are killed without impairing the viral potency (poxviruses resists glycerol and weak phenol, which kills most bacteria).

PRIMARY VACCINATION

It is recommended that primary vaccination is not performed during the first year, but preferably in the second year of life. Primary vaccination should be avoided between the ages of 5 and 14 years, because of the increased risk of postvaccinial encephalitis between these ages.

In a non-immune subject immunity to smallpox is present by the tenth day, and smallpox infection at this time is mild, often with rash.

SECONDARY VACCINATION

The reaction is accelerated and is much milder. When no skin reaction is visible, either the subject is completely immune, or the lymph is an inactive specimen.

COMPLICATIONS OF VACCINATION

a. Secondary bacterial infection of vesicle and subsequent scabbed area.

b. Generalized vaccinia. This complication is rare, and is most likely to occur when the vaccinated subject is suffering from eczema or other chronic skin condition. Babies with eczema should never be vaccinated or exposed to recently vaccinated subjects. The condition varies from a few scattered vesicles to the appearance of typical smallpox.

The lesions of primary vaccination, secondary vaccination and vaccinia are essentially the same as the individual smallpox lesion, the lower layers of the epithelial cells at the margin of the lesion containing elementary bodies (Paschen bodies) in their cytoplasm.

c. Postvaccinial encephalitis. This very rare complication is a typical post-infection encephalitis (*see* p. 6). It is frequently fatal, and those who survive may suffer permanent damage to the central nervous system.

Cowpox

Diagnosis of this condition by the laboratory is very similar to that of *vaccinia* (*see above*). Guarnieri bodies, which are cytoplasmic inclusions, can be demonstrated in skin lesions. Serum tests are as for eruptive and healing stages of variola major (*see* p. 7).

Orf (Contagious Pustular Dermatitis)

Diagnosis of this virus infection, characterized by a single pustule developing into a granuloma following infection of a man by an infectious lamb, is usually made clinically, although the virus can be isolated from a lesion by inoculating a lamb. The virus cannot be grown on chick embryo, but has been grown in tissue culture.

Paravaccinia (Pseudo-cowpox; Milker's Nodes)

Diagnosis of this condition can be confirmed by examination of material from the smooth wart-like lesions found in infected man which become pustular. The virus, which produces a disease in cattle very similar to cowpox, is antigenically distinct from cowpox, and does not grow in chick embryo allantoic membrane.

Molluscum Contagiosum

Diagnosis of this condition is confirmed by histological examination of lesions. Infected epithelial cells contain many inclusion bodies typical of poxviruses— the inclusion body fills the cytoplasm and indents the nucleus.

Antigenically it is distinct from orf. The virus has shown limited growth in HeLa cells, but otherwise culture is not possible.

HERPES SIMPLEX INFECTION

CLINICAL PRESENTATION

1. Herpetic ulcerative stomatitis, especially in young children. The severity of the infection is increased by treatment with steroids.

2. Generalized infection of the newborn [R]. This condition is rapidly fatal. Infection of the infant is thought to occur during or shortly after birth.
3. Keratoconjunctivitis (usually unilateral).
4. Genital herpes—almost certainly sexually transmitted.
5. Herpetic whitlow.
6. Eczema herpeticum.
7. Herpes encephalitis.

Diagnosis of infection with herpes simplex virus is confirmed by the isolation of the virus from superficial lesions, and by rising specific serum antibody levels.

In generalized herpes infection of the newborn, caused by Type II herpes virus, intranuclear inclusion bodies are found in many organs at postmortem. Type I virus is more commonly found in the oral cavity.

In herpes encephalitis, the virus can be identified in brain biopsy material, and grown on culture. The CSF is sterile on bacterial culture, with a lymphocytic pleocytosis, and the serum/CSF antibody ratio 1:20 in sequential tests. Viral culture from lumbar CSF is rarely positive, whereas viral culture from ventricular CSF permits identification of the virus by immunofluorescence or electron microscopy.

Chickenpox (Varicella)

Diagnosis of infection with varicella-zoster virus causing chickenpox in children is usually not a problem, but can be confirmed by microscopy of material from vesicles, in which large multinucleate cells with typical Cowdry type A inclusion bodies are present in nuclei. The lesions are also found in the respiratory tract, gastrointestinal tract, myocardium, spleen, kidneys, pancreas, adrenals and ovaries. These elementary bodies agglutinate with convalescent serum.

Infection during pregnancy has a 20 per cent fetal mortality-rate. Pneumonia occasionally develops, especially in adults, and this is viral in origin and not due to secondary bacterial invasion. Rarely, post-infection encephalitis occurs. Any patient infected who is on treatment with steroids is at serious risk, and steroids should be discontinued if at all possible.

In cases in which the differential diagnosis is between chickenpox and smallpox, vesicle fluid or crusts can be examined by electron microscopy and the different viruses distinguished.

Complement-fixing antibody tests can be carried out on paired serum samples.

TESTS PROVIDING USEFUL NEGATIVE RESULTS

Vesicle fluid does not fix complement when antivaccinial serum is added.

Herpes Zoster (Shingles)

Diagnosis of infection with varicella-zoster virus in adults causing typical shingles is not usually a problem. Susceptibility to infection is increased during immunosuppressive therapy, lymphoreticular malignancies, irradiation therapy, local tumour invasion and with increasing age. The virus spreads to neurons or stellate cells in sensory ganglion during an attack of chickenpox, and becomes latent. Activation of virus replication with waning cell-mediated immunity results in shingles, usually affecting a sensory ganglion and one dermatome.

Intranuclear inclusions may be demonstrated in degenerating epithelial cells, the microscopic appearances being identical with those of chickenpox. The virus can be grown from swabs from lesions or from crusts from skin lesions. In tissue culture it produces typical Cowdry type A intranuclear inclusion bodies, but in artificial culture the virus cannot break out of cells.

TESTS PROVIDING USEFUL NEGATIVE RESULTS

The organism cannot be grown on chick embryo, unlike herpes simplex and variola viruses.

CYTOMEGALOVIRUS INFECTION

1. Congenital Cytomegalovirus Infection

Diagnosis of this condition, characterized by systemic illness, hepatospleno-megaly, jaundice, petechial rash, chorioretinitis, cerebral calcification and microcephaly, is confirmed by isolation of the virus and demonstration of large inclusion-bearing cells in tissues and urine. The cord serum cytomegalovirus IgM antibody is also increased. Thrombocytopenia may persist for weeks to months. Probably less than 10 per cent of congenitally infected neonates show damage; the majority are symptom-free. Infection in the first trimester is associated with microcephaly and mental retardation.

TESTS OF PROGRESS

The infant remains infected and infectious for months to years, and the virus is excreted in saliva, gastric juice and urine.

At post-mortem, typical cytomegalic changes can be demonstrated in salivary glands, adenoids, kidneys, liver and lymph glands.

2. Acquired Cytomegalic Inclusion Disease

Diagnosis of cytomegalovirus infection acquired after birth is confirmed by growth of the virus on culture from tissues or from excretions (saliva, urine, throat swabs). In primary infection, 'glandular fever-type mononuclear' cells are found in the peripheral blood. Complement-fixing antibodies appear in the serum, and a rising titre may be demonstrated using early and late samples. Immediately after birth, an acquired infection may be covered by maternal antibodies, since up to 50 per cent of mothers carry cytomegalovirus antibodies. In older children and others, malaise, sore throat, adenopathy, frequently abnormal liver function tests and atypical lymphocytes are found. The infection is not serious, but like infectious mononucleosis, ampicillin given during the acute stages is associated with a maculopapular rash. After several months, complement-fixing antibodies and IgG and IgM antibodies, detectable using fluorescent antibody, develop.

In biopsy material, histological examination reveals intranuclear inclusion bodies, and the virus can be seen on electron microscopy.

Complement-forming antibodies may not develop in immunosuppressed patients, a clinical group especially susceptible to cytomegalovirus infection.

TESTS PROVIDING USEFUL NEGATIVE RESULTS

The Paul–Bunnell test is negative.

B Virus Infection

Herpes B virus of monkeys can occasionally produce a fatal encephalitis and ascending paralysis in man.

ADENOVIRUS

Since most of this group do not produce overt infection in the laboratory animals, they have only fairly recently been discovered as a cause of disease in man. They produce a soluble antigen common to the whole group, and can cause pharyngitis and regional lymph-gland enlargement in man. By 5 years of age, 60 per cent of children have developed antibodies against adenovirus.

CLINICAL MANIFESTATIONS

1. *Pharyngoconjunctival Fever*. Most commonly found in children.
2. *Follicular Conjunctivitis*. Occurs in adults.
3. *Epidemic Keratoconjunctivitis*. This condition has occurred in widespread epidemics associated with swimming baths, and is caused by adenovirus type 8.
4. *Acute Respiratory Disease*. This condition has occurred in military training camps, and severity has ranged from 'common cold' to pneumonia.
5. *Aseptic Meningitis*. Virus can be isolated from the CSF (*see* p. 18).
6. *Mesenteric Adenitis*. Virus can be isolated from enlarged mesenteric lymph glands removed at surgical laparotomy for suspected appendicitis in children.

Diagnosis of these conditions can be confirmed by isolation of the virus from nasopharyngeal swabs or conjunctival scrapings during the acute stage, and from faeces later.

The diagnosis can also be confirmed by the demonstration of rising titres of complement-fixing antibodies between the acute and convalescent serum samples.

PAPOVAVIRUSES

(Include papilloma virus, polyoma virus, and vacuolating monkey virus.) They have no common antigenic relationship, although they have a similar structure and develop in cell nuclei.

Verruca (Warts)

Human warts occur most commonly on the hands and feet of children or about the genitalia of adults. They may also occur as laryngeal warts.

Diagnosis is confirmed by the demonstration of inclusion bodies in cell nuclei in the upper layers of epithelium. The virus content reaches a maximum by 6 months, and the wart then gradually regresses. The virus is difficult to culture.

MYXOVIRUSES

With the exception of influenza virus, each of these diseases represents a single antigenic type, and immunity to infection is lifelong.

Influenza

Parainfluenza: $\left\{ \begin{array}{l} \text{Parainfluenza} \\ \text{Mumps} \end{array} \right.$

Measles

Respiratory syncytial virus

Rabies

Influenza

Diagnosis is made by isolation and culture on chick embryo of influenza virus A or B from throat swab, garglings, post-mortem lung material, and tracheobronchial mucosa. Sera taken within the first 72 hours of onset and again 2–3 weeks later show a rise in titre of haemagglutination-inhibiting or complement-fixing antibodies. Prophylactic vaccination may complicate the interpretation of results.

Blood counts in the early stages reveal lymphocytosis (relative or absolute) with neutropenia. Later, secondary bacterial invasion of the respiratory tract is accompanied by neutrophilia plus evidence of bacterial infection.

Epidemics are due to either influenza virus A or virus B, and major antigenic changes in the virus occur at approximately 10-year intervals, with minor antigenic drift occurring from year to year. Influenza vaccines contain contemporary influenza A component and lesser amounts of influenza B antigen.

Croup or Acute Laryngotracheobronchitis

Diagnosis of the causative organism in croup is by isolation from throat swabs or nasal washings on culture in chick embryo, yielding parainfluenza virus, types 1, 2, or 3, or influenza A virus. The severity of infection with these organisms in children can range from a mild 'cold' through acute laryngotracheobronchitis to pneumonia.

Further confirmation can be shown with rising antibody titres from the acute stage to convalescence.

(Parainfluenza virus types 1 and 3 can also cause acute bronchopneumonia and bronchiolitis in infants under 6 months, although respiratory syncytial virus is a commoner cause.)

Mumps (Epidemic Parotitis)

Diagnosis of infection with mumps virus is frequently made on clinical grounds. Confirmation is possible by isolation of the virus from saliva, urine, or from CSF in mumps meningitis. Comparison of acute and convalescent sera give rising titres of complement-fixing antibodies against virus particle antigen (V) and soluble virus antigen (S), and haemagglutination-inhibiting antibody to mumps virus. All these antibodies appear in the first few days of illness, the V titre being higher and lasting longer than the S titres. Serum amylase is raised whether the pancreas is involved or not. Histology of parotid gland biopsy material (taken if the diagnosis is not suspected) reveals duct cell degeneration. Similarly, destruction of the epithelium of the seminiferous tubules may be seen in testicular biopsy material. Perhaps up to 40 per cent of males have orchitis, but subsequent sterility is rare.

TESTS OF PROGRESS

It is recommended that boys approaching puberty, with no history of mumps infection, should be immunized.

Measles (Morbilli)

1. CLASSIC MEASLES

Diagnosis of measles is usually clinical. Virological confirmation of diagnosis may be required from autopsy material in cases of:
    a. Patients who have died before the typical rash has developed.
    b. Patients suffering from encephalitis following an earlier ill-defined illness.
    c. Patients with giant-cell pneumonia.
Measles virus can be cultured from nasal and throat secretions, sputum, blood and urine. Measles antigen can be demonstrated in the skin by immunofluorescence, and the virus can be demonstrated by electron microscopy. Complement-fixing antibodies disappear rapidly from the serum, and if complement-fixing antibodies are present, especially with a rising titre, the diagnosis is confirmed.

Haemagglutination-inhibiting and neutralizing antibodies persist in the serum for a very long time, and their presence in the absence of rising titres indicates infection with measles at some time.

TESTS OF PROGRESS

At the height of the illness neutropenia is common, with thrombocytopenia. Secondary bacterial invasion can cause bronchopneumonia, but in severe cases there may be pure virus pneumonia.

In leukaemia, mucoviscidosis, Letterer–Siwe disease and patients with reduced immune responses, infection with measles may cause giant-cell pneumonia, a prolonged and usually fatal condition.

Attenuated measles virus may be given to produce active immunity. This should not be given to infants less than 9 months, and should not be given to any patient being treated with steroids or immunosuppressive drugs.

2. SUBACUTE SCLEROSING PANENCEPHALITIS (Van Bogaert's disease) [R]

Diagnosis of this progressive fatal disease is confirmed by the isolation of measles virus from brain biopsy material. There are inclusion bodies in neuronal and glial cells, with neurone loss. Measles antigen can be demonstrated in the brain tissue using immunofluoresence. Serum complement-fixing antibodies and haemagglutination-inhibiting antibodies reach very high titres, and very high titres are also present in the CSF (unlike classic measles). Virus-specific IgM antibodies in the CSF indicate the persistence of the measles virus in the central nervous system.

TESTS OF PROGRESS

This rare condition may develop in the second year after an attack of measles. The risk of development of this panencephalitis is ten times greater after measles than after attenuated measles virus vaccination.

Respiratory Syncytial Virus Infection

Diagnosis of respiratory syncytial virus infection, a major cause of bronchiolitis and pneumonia in infants under 1 year of age, is confirmed by isolation of the virus from throat swabs or tissue cultures taken during the first 4–5 days of illness. Aspirated nasopharyngeal washings can also be used, and culture on human cancer cell lines produces giant cells and syncytia. The virus can be identified using fluorescent antibody techniques. Complement-fixing antibodies or neutralizing antibody to respiratory syncytial virus in sera taken in the acute illness and 14–21 days later, show a significant rise in titre (the rise in titre may not be marked in infants).

The virus can cause 'colds' in adults.

TESTS OF PROGRESS

Placentally transmitted antibody (universal) has little or no protective effect. Possibly the antibody present in breast milk is protective. The virus is shed for 1 week (up to 3 weeks) of the infection.

TESTS PROVIDING USEFUL NEGATIVE RESULTS

Parainfluenza virus Type 3 also attacks infants during their first few months of life.

Rabies (Hydrophobia)

Diagnosis of this viral encephalitis can be confirmed during the patient's life by demonstration of the virus by animal inoculation or immunofluorescent techniques, of saliva, throat or tracheal secretions, tears, CSF, corneal smears, urine sediment, or skin biopsy near bite site with peripheral nerve fibrils.

Serum antibody levels rise rapidly, but the effects of serovaccine therapy must be taken into account.

After death, typical Negri bodies are found in the cytoplasm of nerve cells in the hippocampus, and the virus can be demonstrated by immunofluorescence. Suspensions of brain can be inoculated into mice intracerebrally, again producing typical changes. Virus can also be demonstrated in the human salivary glands. Infection can follow dog, fox, wolf, skunk or some bat bites. Infection of a human by a human case is very rare.

If a dog is caught after biting a man, and it is not obviously rabid, then if it survives more than ten days it is not rabid. Negri bodies can be demonstrated in the nerve cells of a rabid dog. Animals suffer from either a dumb form or furious form of rabies, and their saliva is highly infectious.

The incubation in man averages 2–3 months from an infected bite (9 days–19 years has been quoted). The incubation period is shorter in young children, severe bites, and bites nearer to the central nervous system.

ARBOVIRUSES

These viruses have avian or mammalian hosts and a blood-sucking arthropod as vector. Infection of a host by an infected vector (e.g. tick) results in symptom-free viraemia which will infect further biting vectors. Man is infected by the bite of an infected vector, and in most instances does not develop sufficient viraemia to act as a source of infection of further blood-sucking arthropods.

Epidemics of arbovirus infections in man can occur all the year round in the tropics, whereas in temperate climates the diseases occur in the summer months when arthropods are active.

By means of chick red-cell agglutination properties, it is possible to divide arboviruses into three antigenically distinct groups—Group A, Group B and Group C.

GROUP A ARBOVIRUSES

Group A: Equine encephalitis, comprising three distinct viruses:
1. Western United States of America.
2. Eastern parts of North and South America.
3. Northern parts of South America.

The vectors are mosquitoes, with primary hosts in birds in (1)+(2), the primary hosts in (3) being unknown as yet.

Group A Arbovirus Encephalitis

Diagnosis can be made by taking serum samples within a few days of the onset of illness and again during convalescence. There is a rise in titre of haemagglutination-inhibiting antibodies, neutralizing antibodies, and complement-fixing antibodies.

There is much antigenic overlapping.

GROUP B ARBOVIRUSES

Yellow Fever
St Louis Encephalitis:
  Indonesia
  Japan and Eastern Russia
    (Japanese B encephalitis)　　　Antigenically related viruses,
  Australia　　　with birds as hosts and
    (Murray Valley fever)　　　mosquitoes as vectors.
  Central Africa
    (West Nile encephalitis)

Tick-borne Encephalitis:
Louping ill in Anglo-Scottish border
India
Malaya
Japan
North America
Dengue: Four related serotypes of virus. Man is the primary host, with the urban mosquito the vector.

Yellow Fever

Diagnosis can be confirmed by isolation of the virus by the intracerebral inoculation of the patient's blood into mice in the first few days of the disease, and subsequent specific neutralization tests to identify the virus.

Serological diagnosis is made using paired acute and convalescent sera. Neutralizing antibodies, complement-fixing antibodies, and haemagglutination-inhibiting antibodies increase during the disease. Unfortunately if the patient has had yellow fever vaccine, or has previously been infected with any group B arbovirus, serological diagnosis is impossible because of cross-reactions.

The virus can be isolated from post-mortem cerebral material by intracerebral inoculation into mice. The mice die as a result of the virus infection, and the virus can then be identified by complement-fixation tests, haemagglutination-inhibition tests, or neutralizing antibody tests.

The patient during an attack develops severe jaundice, with raised serum bilirubin, proteinuria, neutropenia, and anaemia. In fatal cases, the liver shows mid-zonal necrosis. The parenchymal cells are severely damaged, and 'Councilman bodies' may be seen, consisting of globular cells containing punched-out acidophilic hyaline bodies.

The virus is carried in monkeys in the jungle, with mosquitoes as the vector, and in consequence this form of the disease in man, jungle yellow fever, can only be protected against by vaccine. By contrast, if mosquitoes are eliminated from inhabited areas, then urban yellow fever is eliminated.

Group B Arbovirus Encephalitis

Diagnosis can be made by taking serum samples within a few days of the onset of illness and again during convalescence. There is a rise in titre of haemagglutination-inhibiting antibodies, neutralizing antibodies, and complement-fixing antibodies. Neutralizing antibodies appear a few days after onset, and persist for life. Complement-fixing antibodies appear after 10–14 days or even later.

There is much antigenic overlapping.

Dengue

Diagnosis of this infection caused by an arthropod-borne arbovirus can be confirmed by isolation of the virus from the patient's blood by inoculation of

blood into a laboratory animal during the first few days of illness. Patient's sera taken early in the disease and again in convalescence give a rising titre of antibodies, which are diagnostic.
Neutropenia and often thrombocytopenia occur during the active disease.

TESTS PROVIDING USEFUL NEGATIVE RESULTS
If necessary, tests may be used to exclude measles, scarlet fever, malaria, typhus, yellow fever and smallpox.

GROUP C ARBOVIRUSES

Sandfly Fever (Phlebotomus Fever)
Diagnosis may be confirmed by sera taken during the acute and convalescent stages of the illness which show a rising antibody titre, which may persist for a further 2 years.
In sandfly fever man is the primary host, and the sandfly, *Phlebotomus papatasi*, is the vector.

Epidemic Haemorrhagic Fever
Diagnosis of the many varieties of viral epidemic haemorrhagic fever is still debated, since specific viruses have not been demonstrated in large series of cases. Patients suffer from renal damage, showing as progressive renal failure with rising blood urea, proteinuria, fluid and electrolyte imbalance, and with thrombocytopenia in some cases.

Encephalitis Lethargica
The encephalitis lethargica which occurred in epidemics about the 1920s was characterized by ocular palsies and drowsiness, which was often followed by Parkinson's disease and mental deterioration. Japanese type A virus, von Economo, has been thought to be the cause of such epidemics.

REOVIRUSES
Reoviruses (respiratory-enteric orphan) appear to be the most widespread group of viruses in nature, being found in animals, plants and even algae. Occasional definite outbreaks of fever, rhinitis, pharyngitis and diarrhoea, with or without rashes, have been described in association with these viruses in children, and occasional cases of aseptic meningitis due to reovirus have been diagnosed; otherwise they appear to be mainly non-pathogenic in man.

PICORNAVIRUS INFECTIONS
These very small viruses replicate in the cytoplasm of cells.
Picornaviruses include
    Enteroviruses—(multiplying in the alimentary tract)

Polioviruses
Coxsackie A virus
Coxsackie B virus
ECHO virus (Enteric Cytopathic
    Human Orphan)
Rhinoviruses—(multiplying in the nose)
    Unclassified
    Non-human picornavirus—FMDV (Foot and Mouth Disease Virus)
    Manifestations of Picornavirus Infections
        Aseptic meningitis (non-paralytic polio)
        Paralytic poliomyelitis
        Encephalitis (see Viral Encephalitis, p. 6)
        Herpangina
        Epidemic pleurodynia (Bornholm disease)
        Viral pericarditis
        Viral myocarditis
        Epidemic viral diarrhoea
        Upper respiratory tract infections (see Respiratory Infections, p. 206)
            Hand, foot and mouth disease in man.

Aseptic Meningitis (Non-paralytic Polio)

Diagnosis of the causal virus may be determined by isolation of the infecting virus from CSF. Such cultures may yield:

Poliovirus
Coxsackie A virus   Any of these viruses may be isolated
Coxsackie B virus   from throat swabs or faeces.
ECHO virus

Serological diagnosis alone is not possible, as there is no common antigen for any of the subgroups. A rise in titre of antibody between acute and convalescent sera to a virus isolated from the nasopharynx or faeces indicates that the virus is probably the cause of the illness.

The CSF shows a moderate pleocytosis, the total cell count rarely exceeding 500/cmm. The protein content of the CSF is normal or slightly raised.

Paralytic Poliomyelitis

Diagnosis of this condition is confirmed by the isolation of the virus (which may be poliovirus in widespread outbreaks, Coxsackie A, Coxsackie B, or ECHO virus in sporadic cases) from the CSF in tissue culture. The CSF shows a slight increase in cells and protein in the preparalytic stage, pleocytosis is at its maximum in the first week of the paralytic stage (up to 200/cmm, rarely higher), persisting for about 3 weeks from the onset of paralysis, with protein concentrations of up to 80 mg/100 ml.

For epidemiological studies, the virus can be isolated from the faeces.

Serological diagnosis is difficult, since so many of the population have been immunized against poliovirus. If the initial serum sample taken in the acute stages contains low antibody titres against poliovirus, then a rise in antibody titre in the convalescent serum sample confirms the diagnosis.

In the majority of cases the virus multiplies in the tonsillopharyngeal and ileal regions, invading the bloodstream and causing slight fever and malaise, neutralizing antibodies appearing in the blood after 7 days. These patients, with no further symptoms, continue to excrete the virus in the pharyngeal secretion for the next 3 to 4 months.

In probably less than 1 per cent of cases, invasion of the central nervous system occurs, with signs of viral meningitis. Again, some of these patients recover without further trouble, while other cases then progress to paralytic poliomyelitis.

It is worth remembering that:

Primary infection with poliovirus in adults more often leads to serious disease.

Pregnant women are particularly at risk in a primary infection.

Physical activity in the preparalytic phase increases the likelihood of paralysis.

Tonsillectomy. If a child develops poliomyelitis within a month of tonsillectomy, the severe bulbar variety of poliomyelitis is more likely.

Following intramuscular inoculation of alum-precipiated diphtheria, pertussis, or tetanus prophylactics, paralysis in the inoculated limb is more likely. Immunization should not be performed when poliomyelitis is epidemic. Subcutaneous immunization is safer.

Herpangina

Diagnosis of this condition of painful lesions of the palate and tonsillar pillars is confirmed by isolation of Coxsackie A virus from swabs from the lesions, and by the demonstration of rising antibody titres to the virus between sera taken in the acute stages and again in convalescence.

Epidemic Pleurodynia (Bornholm Disease)

Diagnosis of infection with Coxsackie B virus causing pleurodynia can be confirmed by the isolation and culture of the virus from the pharynx or faeces during or shortly after the acute phase of the illness. The virus may be isolated and cultured from the CSF meningo-encephalitis.

Sera taken early in the illness and again about 14 days later show a rising antibody titre.

TESTS PROVIDING USEFUL NEGATIVE RESULTS

Biochemical tests for evidence of recent myocardial infarction are negative, the severe chest pain in some cases strongly suggesting acute myocardial infarction.

There is no neutrophilia, as might be expected in developing acute appendicitis, the severe pain localized in abdominal muscles in some cases suggesting this condition.

Viral Pericarditis

Diagnosis of this condition, which occurs sporadically during outbreaks of epidemic pleurodynia or aseptic meningitis, can be confirmed by the demonstration of a rise in antibody titre to either Coxsackie A virus or Coxsackie B virus, from sera taken in the early stages of the illness to convalescence.

Viral Myocarditis

Diagnosis of this condition, which mainly occurs in newborn babies in nurseries, is confirmed by the isolation of Coxsackie B virus from faeces. The infants develop loose stools, followed 3–8 days later by fever, tachycardia and ECG changes of myocarditis.

The condition is very serious in young babies, but is much less severe when it occurs in older children.

Epidemic Viral Diarrhoea

Diagnosis of this condition, which affects young children in closed communities, but which can affect adults, can be confirmed by the isolation from faeces of many patients of poliovirus type 2 and 3, Coxsackie B type 3, and ECHO types 7, 9, 11, 14 and 18. Obviously in any given outbreak the same single type of virus will be found in cases.

Virus Gastroenteritis

1. PARVOVIRUS-LIKE VIRUS

Electron microscopy of stools in the acute phase, with peak excretion of virus at 36 hours, reveals large numbers of the virus. Radioimmunoassay can be used to detect antibodies.

2. ROTAVIRUSES

Electron microscopy of stools in the acute phase reveals large numbers of the virus. Multiple serotypes exist, and ELISA can be used to detect the rotavirus, compare antigenicity and detect any immune response.

3. OTHER VIRUSES

Identifiable using electron microscopy of stools, in acute diarrhoea in infants.
  a. Astroviruses.
  b. Coronavirus enteritis.
  c. Caliciviruses—of animal origin may be associated with outbreaks of 'winter vomiting disease'.

Hand, Foot and Mouth Disease

Diagnosis of the highly contagious infection with vesicular eruptions in the mouth and on the hands and feet can be confirmed by direct inoculation of vesicle fluid into laboratory mice, or indirectly by neutralization tests or complement-fixation tests. The virus causing this disease is Coxsackie A 16.

Foot and Mouth Disease of Cattle

The slaughter policy is a consequence of the fact that animals who recover from this devastating illness excrete the virus for several months afterwards. It has recently been shown that the virus can be carried in the human nose for days, a potent source for further spread of the disease, e.g. a veterinary inspector travelling from dealing with infected animals to inspect animals suspected of being in the early stages of the disease could infect these latter animals.

UNGROUPED VIRUSES

Infectious Mononucleosis (Glandular Fever)

Diagnosis of this acute infective disease, occurring most commonly in adolescents and young adults and also children, characterized by signs and symptoms including fever, sore throat, lymphadenopathy, splenomegaly and abnormal lymphocytes in the peripheral blood, is confirmed by the demonstration of increasing antibody titre to Epstein–Barr virus (EBV), using complement-fixation, immunodiffusion, ELISA or neutralization techniques. The virus can be identified using specific EBV antibody and immunofluorescence. Routinely, the Paul–Bunnell test is used; this test becomes positive at two weeks and persists for months (using sheep cell agglutination after adsorption of serum on guinea pig kidney—the antibody being adsorbed on ox red cells).

Many patients have raised serum aspartate and alanine aminotransferase activities, and some may become jaundiced with increasing liver damage. If benign lymphocytic meningitis develops, the CSF protein and lymphocyte count are abnormally increased. In the early stages of the disease neutropenia and thrombocytopenia are often found, followed by lymphocytosis with persisting neutropenia, and numerous atypical mononuclear cells (the EBV replicates on the B-lymphocyte).

TESTS OF PROGRESS

In EBV infection, virus capsid antigen (VCA) develops rapidly in the blood (indicating recent infection), while complement-fixing antibodies develop more slowly (and may be used to indicate past infection). The RA test and tests for syphilis may temporarily become positive.

Treatment with ampicillin is followed by a secondary rash, and if a streptococcal infection is superimposed, erythromycin should be given instead.

TESTS PROVIDING USEFUL NEGATIVE RESULTS

Atypical mononuclear cells appear during toxoplasmosis, cytomegalovirus infection, and during other virus infections, but the Paul–Bunnell test is usually negative. Glandular fever can superficially resemble acute leukaemia, with thrombocytopenia, bizarre white blood cells in the peripheral blood, but only very unusually when acute haemolytic anaemia develops, does the haemoglobin level fall. Bone marrow aspirate examination is indicated if sequential blood counts are equivocal.

Rubella (German Measles)

Diagnosis of rubella infection is confirmed by serological tests. Isolation of the virus is unreliable, e.g. in possible infection of the mother during pregnancy. Sera should be taken as soon after contact with infection as possible and repeated in 3–4 weeks. Haemagglutination-inhibition (HI) is initially negative, becoming positive by 3–4 weeks, rubella-specific IgM antibody increasing at the same time. IgM antibody indicates recent infection. IgG antibody and HI titres remain raised for months after infection.

TESTS OF PROGRESS

HI test can be used to detect susceptible subjects in need of vaccination, e.g. young girls. Attenuated rubella vaccine can cross the placenta and cause damage to the fetus. Therefore vaccination of a susceptible woman should not take place until after 2 months of effective contraception (where indicated). After rubella vaccination, after some years, the subjects become seronegative. It is not known how susceptible these subjects are to subsequent exposure to rubella infection.

ANTENATAL SUSPECTED CASES

1. *Within one week of illness suspected of being due to rubella*
   a. No Hi titre in first specimen, with raised HI titre in the second serum sample = rubella infection.
   b. Low titre positive HI antibody in first specimen with:
      i. Rising HI titre indicates recent rubella infection.
      ii. No change in HI titre indicates rubella infection in the remote past.
   c. High HI titre in first specimen, with raised IgM rubella-specific antibody titre indicates recent infection.

2. *After contact with known rubella case (first serum sample taken 7–10 days later*
   a. No detectable HI antibody in first specimen, with seroconversion indicates rubella infection.
   b. Low HI titre in first specimen, rising in second specimen, indicates rubella infection.
   c. Static antibody levels in two sera, indicates IgM antibody tests. If there is a rising IgM rubella-specific antibody titre, then this indicates recent rubella infection.

If the IgM levels do not show any increase in the second specimen, the HI antibodies found could indicate rubella infection earlier in the current pregnancy.

Detection of active rubella infection during pregnancy is very important in the prevention of the birth of severely damaged infants (*see* Congenital Rubella).

Tests for haemolytic streptococci, scarlet fever and infectious mononucleosis are negative.

Congenital Rubella

Rubella infection of the fetus may cause the pregnancy to terminate in abortion or stillbirth, or the neonate may survive, to be born with abnormalities due to congenital rubella infection. Fifty per cent of such infants are infected during the first month of pregnancy; 22 per cent of infants infected in the second month are malformed, the percentage falling to 6 per cent when infected in the third month of pregnancy.

Diagnosis is confirmed by isolation of the virus from the urine and from nasopharyngeal swabs. The infants are a source of large numbers of virus, excretion of virus falling to low levels by 6 months after birth. Neonatal serum contains a high titre of rubella-specific IgM and HI antibodies. Maternal-derived rubella-specific IgG detectable by HI test (half-life 21 days) declines progressively over 6 months after birth, whereas in the infected infant HI titres persist.

Acquired rubella infection is uncommon under 1 year of age. Infected infants, apart from showing congenital damage, such as cataract, mental retardation, heart defects, etc. often have anaemia, with many 'bur' red-cells and persistent thrombocytopenia. The CSF protein is increased and there is pleocytosis.

Detection of maternal rubella infection early in pregnancy is very important, so that therapeutic abortion can be offered, to prevent the risk of birth of virus-damaged infants.

HEPATITIS

For details of haematological and biochemical changes *see* pp. 181–4.

Hepatitis A (Infective Hepatitis)

Diagnosis of hepatitis due to picornavirus hepatitis A virus (HAV), which replicates in the gut and the liver, is confirmed by demonstration of the virus in faeces. A single blood sample taken within 10–12 weeks of onset can be used to demonstrate a significant increase in IgM antibody against HAV in the serum. Alternatively, using two consecutive spaced serum samples, a rise in antibody titre against HAV, using complement fixation, immune adherence, haemagglutination or radioimmunoassay, also enables confirmation of the diagnosis.

The incubation period of the disease is 15–50 days.

Human normal immunoglobulin protects exposed subjects for up to 5 months (e.g. subjects entering an environment with a high incidence of hepatitis A). IgM antibodies disappear during the first 6 months, but IgG antibodies against HAV persist for many years.

Hepatitis B (Serum Jaundice)

Diagnosis of infection with hepatitis B virus (HBV) is confirmed by electron microscopy of serum particles. Serum may contain empty spheres and tubules (virus coat material) and mature virus particles (Dane particles). Surface antigen (HBsAg) may be detected on the surface of all these three particles. HbcAg is the core antigen of the virus, and HbeAg is an internal component of core antigen.

1. *Before symptoms appear.* One month before symptoms appear, HbsAg and HBeAg are present in the serum.

2. *Symptoms.* HBsAg is increased for about 6 weeks, during the acute stage. A rising titre of HBcAg indicates acute infection, and HBeAg also is a marker for infectivity.

3. *Convalescence.* Anti-HBsAg antibodies appear in convalescence and recovery. HBeAg is rapidly cleared from the blood and anti-HBe antibodies appear with low infectivity and only minor changes in the liver.

Early appearance of anti-HBcAg with increased aminotransferase activities indicates recent infection.

4. *Persistence and carriers.* The sex ratio of carriers of hepatitis B is 2 males to 1 female. Carrier mothers infect their babies during the perinatal period, and such babies become chronic carriers. HBcAg and HBeAg are markers of infectivity.

TESTS OF PROGRESS

Immunoglobulin should be given as soon after exposure to infection as possible, and within 24 hours at least, for protection.

Active immunization will soon become possible.

Hepatitis Non-A, Non-B

Hepatitis non-A, non-B, occurs as a sporadic or epidemic disease. It may occur following blood transfusion. There are no tests for its direct diagnosis.

TESTS PROVIDING USEFUL NEGATIVE RESULTS

Tests for the presence of infection with hepatitis A virus, hepatitis B virus, cytomegalovirus and Epstein–Barr virus are all negative.

Lassa Fever [R]

Diagnosis of this very dangerous and potentially lethal infection can be made by growth of the virus in tissue culture after isolation from CNS material.

Complement-fixing antibodies rarely appear in the serum before 14 days.

The infection is due to an arenovirus, and one animal reservoir is known to be a rat, *Mastomys natalensis*.

Marburg Virus Disease and Ebola Fever

Diagnosis of these conditions, characterized by haemorrhagic fever with intestinal bleeding, is confirmed by the demonstration of virus particles by electron microscopy in liver and kidney. The mortality rate is about 20 per cent. The virus persists in semen, and can be transmitted sexually.

PRESUMED VIRAL INFECTIONS

1. *Kuru*. Occurring in Eastern Highlands of New Guinea.
2. *Creutzfeldt–Jakob disease*.

In both diseases the nature and morphology of a causative agent has not yet been described, and no demonstrable immune response has been detected.

Creutzfeldt–Jakob Disease [R]

This rare condition, characterized by progressive degeneration of the brain and spinal cord, appears to be due to a transmissible slow virus. Primates, mice, cats and guinea pigs are susceptible to intracerebral, subcutaneous or intravenous inoculation of the virus which can be isolated from lymph node, liver, kidney, spleen, lung, cornea, CSF and brain. Since the virus is dangerous, special precautions must be taken at any post-mortem.

There is a 10 per cent family history of presenile dementia in families of a case, and the patients have a high incidence of eye or brain operations during the previous two years before death.

PSITTACOSIS-LGV-TRACHOMA-PLT GROUP

The organisms in this group are much closer to the rickettsias and bacteria, as they contain both RNA and DNA; their cell walls contain muramic acid, they divide by binary fission, and are susceptible to certain antibiotics.

Inclusion Conjunctivitis (Swimming-pool Conjunctivitis, Paratrachoma)

Diagnosis of infection of the newborn infant's conjunctiva with this organism which may be harboured in the adult female genital tract can be confirmed by the finding of typical inclusion bodies on microscopy of scrapings from the conjunctiva.

In adults, this organism can cause conjunctivitis following infection via non-chlorinated swimming-pool water.

Epithelial scrapings from the lower fornix contain basophilic cytoplasmic inclusion bodies. The infecting agent is a *Bedsonia*.

TESTS OF PROGRESS

Treatment with sulphonamides results in rapid cure (cf. trachoma which requires prolonged treatment).

Inclusion Blenorrhoea

Diagnosis of infection can be confirmed by demonstration of typical inclusion bodies on microscopy of urethral discharge or cervical scrapings. The organism causing inclusion conjunctivitis in newborn infants is also a cause of non-specific urethritis in adults and of non-specific cervicitis in adult females.

Lymphogranuloma Venereum

Diagnosis of infection with this organism, (chlamydia Group A) a common venereal disease in warm climates, is confirmed by microscopy of smears of pus or biopsy material from ulcers, when elementary bodies may be seen. The organism can be isolated after inoculation into chick embryo yolk sac or brain of laboratory mouse. It has also been isolated from the blood, and from the CSF in cases of meningitis.

Using formolized yolk-sac cultures of the organism (lygranum) as antigen, a skin test (intradermal Frei test) can be carried out. The test becomes positive by 2–6 weeks after infection, but is positive in psittacosis infection also.

Complement-fixing antibodies develop and rising titres in early and late serum samples are diagnostic, although again there is cross-reaction with psittacosis.

Both the skin test and complement-fixing antibodies are positive as long as the organism is in the body (which can be for many years).

TESTS PROVIDING USEFUL NEGATIVE RESULTS

Dark ground examination of material from ulcers to exclude syphilis. Negative tests for chancroid caused by *Haemophilus ducreyi*. Absence of acid-fast bacilli.

Trachoma

Diagnosis of trachomal infection (perhaps 400 000 000 people are suffering from it now) is confirmed by the demonstration of the presence of the characteristic inclusion bodies (Halberstaedter–Prowazek) in scrapings of conjunctiva, especially from the upper tarsus.

Positive complement-fixing antibodies occur in the serum, but there is cross-reaction with antigens of the lymphogranuloma-psittacosis group.

TESTS OF PROGRESS

Secondary bacterial infection may occur. Following apparently successful treatment of trachoma, the administration of cortisone may be useful, since any trachoma agent still present is reactivated.

Psittacosis

Diagnosis of infection with the psittacosis organism (chlamydia Group B) can be confirmed by isolation of the organism following intraperitoneal inoculation of mice with blood from a patient, or following intranasal inoculation of mice with sputum from a patient during the first few days of the disease before treatment. The organism can be isolated from the patient's blood during the first 2 weeks of the disease, and from sputum during the first month. The organism may be excreted in the sputum for years in a few cases.

Serum samples tested during the first week of the disease and again 3 weeks later show a diagnostic rise in complement-fixing antibodies. The complement-fixing antibodies are only group-specific and there is cross-reaction with the lymphogranuloma venereum group. The titre remains high in carriers of the disease, and bird fanciers and others who handle infected birds frequently may have a moderately raised antibody titre with no history of disease. The whole-blood white-cell count is not markedly altered during the illness.

Psittacosis is an endemic and epidemic disease of the parrot family of birds. Young birds excrete the organism in their droppings and nasal secretions. Adult female birds excrete the organism in their droppings when sitting on their eggs. The dust of dried bird droppings is therefore a dangerous source of infection in man, infection being by inhalation.

Parrot and turkey strains appear to be the most virulent. Pigeon strains are probably not very virulent, and budgerigars apparently rarely are associated with human disease. The organism can be isolated from lung or spleen in fatal cases (although antibiotics may make this difficult).

Cat-scratch Disease (Sterile Regional Lymphadenitis; Benign Inoculation Lymphoreticulosis)

TESTS SUPPORTING CLINICAL DIAGNOSIS

a. Intradermal Test. A skin test can be made, using treated pus from lesions of a known case. Positive result occurs in 48 hours showing a papule 0·5–1·6 mm in diameter and surrounding erythema 1–6 mm in diameter. Negative results are found in some cases.

b. Microscopy of lymph-node biopsy may show 'granular corpuscles' which are regarded as non-specific by some workers.

c. Thirty-three per cent of cases may show antibodies in the serum to the lymphogranuloma venereum-psittacosis group of antigens.

NON-SPECIFIC TESTS

The whole-blood white-cell count is usually normal, but may be increased in some cases.

The ESR may be normal or increased.

TESTS PROVIDING USEFUL NEGATIVE RESULTS

Cultures of primary lesion and affected lymph glands are sterile. No virus presumed to be the infectious agent has yet been isolated from known cases.

Pasteurellosis, infection with *Pasteurella multocida*, may follow cat bites. Sterile cultures from lesions exclude this.

RICKETTSIAL INFECTIONS

The rickettsiae are visible under the light microscope, and contain both DNA and RNA, unlike the viruses. Dividing by simple binary fission like bacteria, they are much nearer to bacteria than viruses. All the species of the genus *Rickettsia* are vectored by arthropods, and most share antigens with one or more strains of *Proteus* species.

An exception in this group is *Coxiella burnetii*, which is probably not arthropod vectored, and which does not contain *Proteus* spp. antigens.

Unlike virus diseases, rickettsial infections and Q fever (caused by *C. burnetii*) respond to treatment with broad-spectrum antibiotics.

Epidemic Typhus (Epidemic Louse-borne Typhus; Brill-Zinsser Disease)

Diagnosis of infection with *Rickettsia prowazekii* can be confirmed by isolation of the organism following animal inoculation with blood taken from a patient during the first 10 days of illness. *R. prowazeki* can be isolated from laboratory lice after they have fed on patients. Lice become infected after feeding on a patient and excrete rickettsia after 3–5 days. When they bite, and feed, they also defaecate on the skin. The infected louse dies after 7–10 days.

The organisms can be grown on yolk-sac membranes; fluorescent antibody staining is possible for identification of the specific organism.

Patient's serum taken early in the disease and again 3 weeks later reveals a significant rise in complement-fixing antibodies (both group-specific and type-specific occur), which persists for years.

Sheep or human Group-O erythrocytes can be sensitized by treatment with rickettsiae and are then agglutinated by antisera developed against most members (ESS or erythrocyte sensitizing substance).

Similarly the Weil–Felix reaction can be used. This is a non-specific agglutination test for various rickettsial antibodies of the typhus group against strains of *Proteus* spp. The O, or somatic, antigens of *Proteus* strains X2, X19, and XK are agglutinated by convalescent sera from cases of rickettsial infection.

Previous vaccination against rickettsial disease may make the interpretation of results difficult.

During the second and third week of infection, anaemia develops and the urine contains protein and red cell.

BRILL–ZINSSER DISEASE

Louse-borne typhus fever can recur several years after the original disease. The condition is less severe, and there are low or absent titres of OX agglutinins in the Weil–Felix reaction, with a very rapid rise in specific antibodies in the serum. It is believed that the rickettsiae remain dormant in the lymph nodes until some unknown factor stimulates their release and multiplication. Such cases may well start a new epidemic if lice are infected.

Murine Typhus (Flea-borne)

Diagnosis of infection with *Rickettsia typhi* (also known as *Rickettsia mooseri*), which is transmitted to man from rats and mice by the rat flea, is essentially the same as for epidemic typhus.

Antigenically infection with *Rickettsia prowazekii* can be distinguished from infection with *Rickettsia typhi* by tests for complement-fixing antibodies using washed suspensions of specific organisms.

An attack of either murine or epidemic typhus renders the patient immune to subsequent attacks of both, whereas vaccination with suspensions of inactivated rickettsiae only protects the subject against the type incorporated in the vaccine.

Scrub Typhus

Diagnosis of infection with *Rickettsia tsutsugamushi*, which is transmitted to man from small rodents by the larvae of mites left in the skin ('chiggers'), is essentially the same as for epidemic typhus. Specific complement-fixing antibodies appear in the same manner. The Weil–Felix reaction is chiefly against *Proteus* spp. OX-K. Considerable antigenic variation exists between the strains of *R. tsutsugamushi* and immunity to heterologous strains only lasts for 1 or 2 years, so that further infections may occur.

Rocky Mountain Spotted Fever

Diagnosis of infection with *Rickettsia rickettsi*, which is transmitted to man from small rodents by ticks, is essentially the same as for epidemic typhus.

Tick-borne Typhus

Diagnosis of infection with *Rickettsia conorii* (in Europe, India, and Africa), *Rickettsia australis* (in Australia), and *Rickettsia sibericus* (in Russia) are essentially the same as for epidemic typhus.

Rickettsialpox

Diagnosis of infection with *Rickettsia akari*, which is transmitted to man from house mice via the mouse mite, is essentially the same as for epidemic typhus.

Trench Fever

Diagnosis of infection with *Rickettsia quintana*, which is transmitted to man by body lice, which are not killed by the infection, is essentially the same as for epidemic typhus.

Q Fever

Diagnosis of infection with *Coxiella burnetii* is confirmed by isolation of the organism on culture on chorio-allantoic membrane or in the yolk sac of the developing chick embryo. The organism can be isolated from the patient's blood in the febrile phase of the illness, following inoculation into a guinea pig, or from the patient's urine early in convalescence.

Following intraperitoneal inoculation of the patient's blood the organism can be isolated from the mouse spleen, but the risk of infection of laboratory workers is very great with this procedure.

With sera taken in the early days of illness and again 3 weeks later, rising titres of both specific complement-fixing antibodies and specific agglutinins can be demonstrated.

The organism appears to lie quiescent in the tissues of domestic animals, multiplying during pregnancy in the placenta, which is probably the major source of infection in man, although the organism is also excreted in the animal's milk. Great care must be taken when working with this organism.

TESTS PROVIDING USEFUL NEGATIVE RESULTS

The Weil–Felix reaction is negative (unlike rickettsial infection) and cold-agglutinin titres are not raised.

BACTERIAL INFECTIONS

Anthrax

In man infection presents as:

MALIGNANT PUSTULE

The patient develops an ulcer (malignant pustule) and may subsequently develop fatal septicaemia.

WOOL-SORTER'S DISEASE (PULMONARY ANTHRAX)

Following inhalation of anthrax spores from hides of infected animals a very severe pneumonia and rapidly fatal septicaemia develop.

Diagnosis of anthrax infection in man can be confirmed by microscopy of smears from the exudate or from an unbroken vesicle on the edge of the pustule when large gram-positive bacilli are seen. In pulmonary anthrax sputum, pleural fluid, and vomit and faeces in intestinal cases should be examined microscopically. All material is cultured.

In septicaemia, blood cultures for the organism are positive. In fatal cases, post-mortem material can be cultured for the organism. Special precautions must be taken as the organism is dangerous.

Following isolation of the organism, subcutaneous inoculation of a 24-hour broth culture into a mouse or guinea-pig protected by antitoxins against Clostridia, is made, and with true *Bacillus anthracis* the animal is dead in 2 days. The organism can be identified by immunofluorescence.

A high or rising titre of antibodies in the patient's serum can be demonstrated by a specific precipitin test.

It is important to remember that it is illegal to perform a post-mortem examination on an animal suspected of anthrax. It is sufficient to obtain blood from an ear for microscopy and culture.

Bacillary Dysentery

Causative organism: Shigella.

Diagnosis of infection is confirmed by the isolation of *Shigella sonnei, Shigella shigae,* or *Shigella flexneri* on culture of blood, pus, or mucus in faeces. Rectal swabs can be used for sampling in acute cases. Immunofluorescent staining techniques make rapid diagnosis possible from direct microscopy of fresh stools.

Neutrophilia is common, with evidence in severe cases of loss of body water and dehydration (both in haematocrit readings and plasma sodium, potassium, chloride and urea).

Serum agglutination tests may on rare occasions assist diagnosis after the first week, but by then the organism should have been isolated on culture and identified, whereas serum antibodies may not develop.

Following recovery from the infection, it is important to check whether the patient is still excreting the organism, especially if the patient comes into close contact with the general public, e.g. food handler.

TESTS PROVIDING USEFUL NEGATIVE RESULTS

Absence of pathogenic amoebae on microscopy of fresh preparations of blood and mucus in faeces.

Bartonellosis, Oroya Fever

Causative organism: Bartonella bacilliformis.

Diagnosis of infection, which follows the bite of infected sandflies in Peru, Colombia and Ecuador, is confirmed by the development of severe haemolytic anaemia, in which the organisms can be seen on microscopy in the erythrocytes. Blood cultures are positive.

The haemolytic anaemia is acute and severe.

VERRUGA PERUANA

The acute condition may be followed by chronic granulomatous lesions of the skin, and the organisms can be seen on microscopy in the endothelial cells in the lesions. Blood cultures are positive.

TESTS PROVIDING USEFUL NEGATIVE RESULTS

Attempts to exclude other forms of haemolytic anaemia are probably not useful (e.g., negative Coombs' test) as the organisms should be seen in up to 90 per cent of red cells in the acute haemolytic attack.

Brucellosis (Undulant Fever; Malta Fever; Abortus Fever)

Diagnosis of infection with *Brucella* sp., characterized by febrile illness with variable constitutional upset, is confirmed by isolation of the organism from blood cultures (frequent samples taken during periods of pyrexia with prolonged incubation, as organisms are usually only scanty in the blood). At autopsy, cultures should be made from spleen, liver, kidney and mesenteric glands in a suspected case.

Diagnosis can also be confirmed by the demonstration of specific antibody titre rise. Serum agglutinins appear within 5–7 days of infection. IgM antibodies indicate an acute infection, whereas IgG antibodies and positive complement-fixation tests confirm chronic infection. A brucella agglutination titre of more than 1:160 is diagnostic of infection. Unfortunately the brucellin skin test, and brucella antigen present in some contaminated foods, can cause an anamnestic reaction. Prozones of inhibition by blocking antibodies can obscure the serum agglutination test. The Coombs' antiglobulin method avoids this snag. There is considerable antigenic overlapping between *Br. abortus* (from cattle), *Br. melitensis* (from goats, sheep and pigs) and *Br. suis*

Enzyme linked Immunosorbent Assay

(from pigs). There is also a common H antigen present in brucella, *F. tularensis* and *Vibrio cholerae*. It is recommended that the brucellin skin test should not be used in diagnosis, as it can cause an anamnestic reaction, and cause the appearance of brucella antibodies.

TESTS OF PROGRESS

The leucocyte count is variable, with often an absolute lymphocytosis. Moderate anaemia may develop, especially in severe infections, and the plasma viscosity rises with the increase in serum globulin.

Treatment with co-trimoxazole 1–2 g b.d. for 8 weeks, or tetracycline, results in persistently negative blood cultures. During a severe infection, myocarditis and endocarditis may develop, and when antibiotic treatment is started, there may be a Herxheimer reaction.

Pasteurization of milk and dairy products reduces the risk of brucellosis.

ELISA is useful for screening large populations for antibodies, and for differentiating between acute (IgM) and chronic (IgG) phases.

Chancroid (Soft Chancre due to Haemophilus ducreyi)

Diagnosis of this infection can be confirmed by isolation of the organism by microscopy and culture of material from a sore or from affected lymph glands.

An intradermal skin test, using suspensions of killed organisms, gives a further method of detection, but there is some cross-reaction with the antigen used in the Frei test for lymphogranuloma inguinale (*see* p. 26). Also, positive results may result in the absence of clinical history or signs of infection. The skin test remains positive for many years after infection. In some cases, biopsy of the edge of a sore may be necessary.

TESTS PROVIDING USEFUL NEGATIVE RESULTS

In the absence of complicating infections, tests for the presence also of syphilis, granuloma inguinale, granuloma venereum and herpes are negative.

Cholera

Diagnosis of infection by the classic non-haemolytic *Vibrio cholerae* or the haemolytic El Tor vibrio (on laboratory culture), characterized by diarrhoea ranging from mild to very severe watery diarrhoea with circulatory collapse, dehydration and severe salt loss, with eventual death (in the absence of intense intravenous salt and fluid replacement), is confirmed by the isolation on culture of the organism from vomit or stool. Cultures at post-mortem should be taken from the duodenum and small intestine.

A high proportion of people in an epidemic are asymptomatic (especially with *Vibrio El Tor*). The mobile case with mild diarrhoea is most dangerous to the community.

TESTS OF PROGRESS

While the vibrio is excreted in the stools for 1–2 weeks in classic cholera, the El Tor strain may continue to be excreted for up to 3 months (or even 3 years), the patients becoming healthy carriers.

The efficacy of antibiotic therapy is still uncertain. Both organisms survive in water with a low saline content, El Tor surviving longer, and surviving in prepared food. The bacterial dose to cause infection has to be high, as the gastric juice acid protects by killing the organism eaten with food or contaminated water. Achlorhydria or previous partial gastrectomy increases the risk of infection.

The enterotoxin produced by the vibrio fixes to intestinal cells, and releasing cAMP results in a massive outpouring of sodium chloride and water into the intestinal lumen.

Following inoculation against cholera, antibodies, including agglutinating antibody, a vibriocidal antibody, coproantibody (IgA), and an antitoxin antibody, produce only 50 per cent protection, lasting for only 3 months.

Conjunctivitis

Identification of the infecting organism can be made by microscopy and culture of pus or mucus or scrapings from the conjunctiva. Organisms which may be found include:

Haemophilus influenzae
Streptococcus pneumoniae
Streptococci
Staphylococcus pyogenes
Moraxella lacunata
Escherichia coli
Neisseria gonorrhoeae
Viruses (*see* p. 3 et seq.)
    (Sensitivity reaction mimicking infection)

It is important before eye operations to exclude the presence of any pathogens in the conjunctival sac.

Cysts (Infected)

Identification of the infecting organism or organisms can be determined by microscopy and culture of material from the cyst.

Diphtheria

Diagnosis of this infection, characterized by infection of the nasopharynx, larynx, less commonly conjunctiva and other sites (e.g. skin ulcers), with respiratory and circulatory collapse in severe toxin-producing cases, is confirmed by isolation of *Corynebacterium diphtheria* from swabs taken from infected sites. Rapid identification is possible, using fluorescent-antibody techniques. Demonstration of toxin production by the isolated strain of the organism should be carried out. In severe cases, neutrophilia and heavy proteinuria are found.

TESTS OF PROGRESS

Antitoxin should be given as early as possible, depending on the site of any membrane, degree of toxicity and duration of illness. Penicillin (or erythromycin) is effective against most strains of diphtheria and reduces toxin production. Positive carriers of the organism should be treated with erythromycin, and repeat swabs taken until they are negative.

Ideally, early immunization of all children should enable elimination of the disease. Sensitivity to diphtheria toxoid increases with increasing age, so that late primary immunization (after 10 years of age) must be carried out carefully. In the past, the Moloney test was used to detect subjects likely to suffer constitutional reactions to diphtheria toxoid (negative reactors require immunization, and positive reactors do not require immunization).

The Schick test detects susceptibility to diphtheria toxin, positive reactors requiring immunization.

Typhoid and Paratyphoid Fever (Enteric Fever)

1. TYPHOID FEVER

Characterized by a brief attack of gastroenteritis, followed, after a variable incubation period, by severe systemic illness, with intestinal haemorrhage or perforation in severe cases.

Diagnosis of infection with *Salmonella typhi* can be confirmed by isolation of the organism:

a. From blood cultures during the first 7–10 days (50 per cent of blood cultures taken during the 2nd and 3rd weeks may be positive).

b. From faecal cultures during the 2nd and 3rd weeks (50 per cent of cultures taken in the 1st week are positive). Faeces contain *S.typhi* for over 2 months after treatment with antibiotics.

c. Isolation of the organism from urine cultures are positive in 25–33 per cent of cases at some time, but there is no regular excretion of the organism.

d. Bile cultures are always positive.

e. Bone marrow aspirate cultures give a high percentage of positive cultures.

f. Cultures from rose spots in the skin give more than 50 per cent positive results.

Antibodies appear in the serum during the infection, and serum samples taken more than 5 days apart show a significant increase in O and H antibodies. In areas where enteric fever is rare, the diagnosis may be suspected when both the O and H antibody titres exceed 1:40.

Following recent antityphoid vaccination, both O and H titres are high, O titres falling below 1:100 by one year.

Vi antigen is thought to protect O antigen against agglutination by O antibody. In many patients Vi-antibody disappears when the organism is no longer being secreted (but this is not always reliable). Using Vi phage at least 50 different types of *S. typhi* can be identified, and thus Vi phage typing is very useful in epidemiological studies.

During the acute illness, anaemia develops, which may become hypochromic following intestinal bleeding. Neutropenia is found during the third and fourth weeks, although neutrophilia follows intestinal perforation. With severe diarrhoea, dehydration with sodium, potassium and chloride imbalance develops.

2. PARATYPHOID A

The condition is common in Asia and in Western Europe.

3. PARATYPHOID B

This milder disease is fairly common in Europe.

4. PARATYPHOID C

Often associated with pneumonia, arthritis, meningitis and endocarditis due to *S. paratyphi C* or *S. cholerae-suis*.

Paratyphoid A, B and C—blood cultures are positive within 10 days, and agglutinins appear by the end of the 1st week. *S. paratyphi A* and *B*, have no Vi antigen, whereas with *S. paratyphi C* the Vi antigen is constant.

TYPHOID AND PARATYPHOID CARRIERS

Faecal carriers—bile always contains *S.typhi*, or *S.paratyphi B*.

Urine carriers—urine contains *S.typhi* and *S. paratyphi B* in the first 2 months.

Carriers should therefore be screened with urine and faecal cultures.

VACCINATION

S.typhi vaccination is very effective and systemically less disturbing if given intradermally.

Vaccination against paratyphoid A, B and C is not very effective.

Erysipelas

Diagnosis of this acute non-suppurating inflammation of the skin caused by *Streptococcus pyogenes* can be confirmed by isolation of the organism from cultures of swabs taken from the primary lesion (e.g. throat, wound) or from fluid from skin blebs. In severe and deteriorating cases blood cultures may be positive for the organism (i.e. streptococcal septicaemia).

Neutrophilia occurs in most cases.

Erysipeloid

Diagnosis of infection with *Erysipelothrix rhusiopathiae,* most often seen in butchers and cooks, etc., handling animals, fish and their products, can be confirmed by culture of material obtained from under the skin over the inflammatory swelling, or by culture of saline injected into the lesion and then reaspirated.

The organism *E. rhusiopathiae* is a very unusual cause of bacterial endocarditis.

Campylobacter Diarrhoea

Infection with this vibrio-like gram-negative thermophilic organism is a frequent cause of bacterial diarrhoea in the United Kingdom, especially in the summer months.

Diagnosis is confirmed by isolation of the organism from faeces, grown on antibiotic-reinforced medium at 43 °C in a special atmosphere.

Increase in complement-fixing antibodies of 1:8 or more indicates a recent infection. Specific agglutinins develop after infection also. Bacteraemia is rare except in the very debilitated or the immunosuppressed.

TESTS OF PROGRESS

The stools are clear of the organism within 2–5 weeks with or without treatment with erythromycin.

Reiter's syndrome can develop, and arthropathy may develop in HLA 27 subjects after infection.

Pseudomembranous colitis

Pseudomembranous colitis due to infection with *Clostridium difficile* is predisposed to by treatment with: penicillin, ampicillin, lincomycin, or clindamycin.

Normally *Cl. difficile* represents less than 2 per cent of the gut flora. In pseudomembranous colitis, the numbers are greatly increased, and it is possible to demonstrate the presence of toxins from the organism.

TESTS OF PROGRESS

Treatment with vancomycin, 125–500 mg 6-hourly orally.

TESTS PROVIDING USEFUL NEGATIVE RESULTS

There is no evidence of staphylococcal enteritis. In ischaemic colitis there is no proliferation of *Cl. difficile*.

Food Poisoning

1. SALMONELLA TYPE

Diagnosis of infection with a salmonella other than *Salmonella typhi, Salmonella paratyphi A, B,* or *C,* for example, *Salmonella typhimurium, Salmonella enteritidis, Salmonella newport*, etc. can be confirmed by isolation of the infecting organism on culture from faeces, vomit and suspected food (if this is available) consumed during the previous 24 hours.

Infection may be derived from infected animals or poultry (or their eggs), or from fouling of food by infected mice and rats, or from symptomless human carriers.

The source of the infection can be detected by suitable sampling of materials and their culture.

2. *TOXIN TYPE*

Diagnosis of toxin-induced food poisoning is supported by an incubation period between the eating of the suspected food and violent vomiting, diarrhoea and prostration of rarely more than 6 hours and never more than 12 hours (i.e. the toxin is in the food and acts as soon as it is absorbed).

There are no satisfactory tests for enterotoxins in food. The diagnosis is supported if cultures of suspected food yield very rich growths of bacteria:

Heat-resistant strains of *Clostridium welchii* type A
Staphylococcus pyogenes
Proteus spp.
Other coliform organisms

See Chapter 9.

Furunculosis

Identification of the organism (almost always *Staphylococcus pyogenes*) can be obtained by microscopy and culture of pus obtained from the lesion. Phage typing can be carried out to identify the staphylococcus further, in relation to other infected patients, and the pattern of antibiotic sensitivities and resistances can be determined for thorough treatment and eradication. Swabbing of sites, such as upper respiratory tract and perineum, which are acting as reservoirs for the infecting organism, should also be undertaken and cultured before and after treatment.

Gas Gangrene

Diagnosis of gas gangrene is essentially clinical. Laboratory confirmation of the presence of clostridia can be confirmed by culture of swabs from deep in necrotic tissue. Smears made from this material reveal predominantly gram-positive bacilli with few pus cells. In severe cases, blood cultures for *Clostridium welchii, Clostridium septicum*, or *Clostridium oedematiens* may be positive.

Clostridial Cellulitis

Infection in the depths of a wound with clostridia without gross tissue necrosis, following trauma, is commoner than true gas gangrene.

Glanders and Melioidosis

1. *GLANDERS*

Diagnosis of this infection, primarily of horses, mules and asses, characterized in many by cellulitis, necrosis, abscess formation and septic thrombophlebitis in man, is confirmed by the isolation of *Pseudomonas mallei* from discharges from lesions (or from internal nodules after death).

Microscopy of pus reveals beaded gram-negative bacilli. Guinea pig inoculation is often useful in isolation of the organism.

Complement-fixing antibodies develop and show a significant increase in paired serum samples. The agglutination test is unreliable.

The mallein-intradermal skin test should not be used in man, as it causes severe reactions.

2. MELIOIDOSIS

Diagnosis of this rare infection, primarily occurring in rats, and sometimes dogs, horses and pigs, occurring in India, the Far East, Northern Australia and the USA, and characterized by (*a*) the commoner pyaemic form with abscesses and local adenitis, or (*b*) the less common, rapidly fatal septicaemic form in man, is confirmed by the isolation on culture of *Pseudomonas pseudomallei* from pus or blood. Microscopy of pus reveals the organism.

Serum agglutination tests are of little value in the diagnosis.

Gonococcal Infection

Diagnosis is confirmed by the examination of material obtained from infected sites—cervix and vagina in females, urethra and prostatic massage material from prostate, seminal vesicles and epididymis in males, urethra, oropharynx, oesophagus, rectum, aspirates from infected joints, and skin scrapings.

Direct microscopy reveals intracellular gram-negative diplococci in early acute infections, later many organisms are extracellular. The 'direct' fluorescent antibody test is useful only if highly specific antigonococcal sera are available. Culture on special media must follow.

In neonates, transfer from the infected maternal pudenda causes gonococcal conjunctivitis. Microscopy and culture of eye swabs enables the diagnosis to be confirmed.

In complicated cases, e.g. salpingitis, arthritis, meningitis, endocarditis, abscess, or septic dermatitis, culture from the appropriate site enables isolation and identification of the organism.

TESTS OF PROGRESS

Following determination of the sensitivity of the isolated organism to penicillin, and if penicillin-resistant, to kanamycin, streptomycin and tetracycline, suitable treatment can be given. Epidemiological studies can be made using the organism as a marker.

The gonococcal complement-fixation test (GCFT) is useful in complicated cases (e.g. arthritis), as the test becomes negative following successful treatment.

Impetigo

Diagnosis can be confirmed by isolation on culture from swabs, from active lesions or from decrusted lesions, of either *Staphylococcus pyogenes* with subsequent phage typing for epidemiological studies or of *Streptococcus pyogenes*.

Nasal swabs are useful in the detection of symptom-free carriers of the infecting organism in an outbreak (in a school or other closed community).

Legionnaires' Disease

Diagnosis of infection with *Legionella pneumophila*, characterized by malaise, aching muscles, headaches, high fever and non-productive cough, is confirmed by the demonstration of rising titre of serum antibodies—a single titre of more than 1:128, or two results showing significant increase, are diagnostic of this infection.

L. pneumophila can be grown from tracheal aspirate, pleural fluids, or from post-mortem lung samples (the disease has a 15 per cent mortality rate), and its identity confirmed using fluorescent antibody techniques.

Direct visualization of the organism from infected samples is difficult. The organism also disappears when serum antibodies appear in the patient. Serum lactate dehydrogenase, aspartate aminotransferase and creatine phosphokinase activities are all increased. Plasma sodium concentration falls below 130 mmol/l, and plasma inorganic phosphate falls below 2·5 mmol/l. There is microscopic haematuria with proteinuria and azotaemia.

TESTS OF PROGRESS

Rising titres of antibodies are found in convalescence. Following treatment with erythromycin, the organism disappears.

The organism may be found in air conditioning and water heating systems in communal buildings, e.g. hotels, hospitals.

TESTS WHICH PROVIDE USEFUL NEGATIVE RESULTS

Tests for pneumococci, staphylococci, mycoplasma, Q fever and psittacosis are negative.

Leprosy

Diagnosis of chronic infection with *Mycobacterium leprae*, which can cause:
1. Lepromatous leprosy (nodular)—multiple lesions scattered over the skin, and affecting nasal mucosa, with negative lepromin test.
2. Tuberculoid leprosy (cutaneous and neural)—skin lesions and nerve involvement with sequelae, with positive lepromin test.
3. Dimorphic (intermediate) leprosy—the skin lesions may appear to be lepromatous or tuberculoid, with marked nerve involvement.
4. Indeterminate—hypopigmented macular lesions, not anaesthetic and often single. Diagnosis is confirmed by the demonstration of *M. leprae* in nasal scrapings and skin or nerve biopsy material. When the diagnosis is in doubt, material from lesions can be inoculated to produce lepromatous infection in the mouse foot pad. *M. leprae* may be found in bone marrow histiocytes (using Fite's special stain), otherwise bacillus-stained ghosts are seen in the cells.

TESTS OF PROGRESS

Skin smears and biopsy material are examined for the bacillus during therapy. Moderate anaemia develops during the disease, with increased globulin and falling serum albumin. Amyloidosis may develop in the absence of treatment, and false positive results of tests for syphilis occur.

Otitis Externa

Identification of the organism causing the infection can be determined by microscopy and culture of swabs taken from the lesion. Culture of nasal swabs may reveal the source of the infecting organism.

It is important to remember to culture for fungi as well as bacteria, and to investigate the possibility of allergy to substances such as dyes, etc. causing a dermatitis.

Otitis Media (Acute and Chronic)

Identification of the organism causing otitis media may be determined by isolation of the organism on culture from material from discharge or secretions. In acute cases, culture of throat swab may indicate persistence of the infecting organism.

Paronychia

Identification of the infecting organism can be determined by microscopy and culture of pus from the lesion. In recurrent lesions, it is important to culture swabs from sites possibly acting as reservoirs for the infecting organism (e.g. nose, perineum).

Pertussis (Whooping Cough)

Diagnosis of infection with *Bordetella pertussis*, causing whooping cough, is essentially clinical in the acute stages. The organism can be grown and identified from pernasal swabs or cough plates during the first and second weeks of infection.

Agglutinating antibodies and complement-fixing antibodies can be shown to increase significantly with paired serum samples, but antibody titres do not assist in the diagnosis of the acute disease.

During the early stages there is neutropenia, following by a marked lymphocytosis which may be high enough to be described as a leukaemoid reaction.

TESTS PROVIDING USEFUL NEGATIVE RESULTS

Absence of positive cultures from pernasal swabs or cough plates do not exclude the diagnosis.

Plague

RAT PLAGUE

Infection with *Yersinia pestis* passes from rat to rat via the rat fleas. When an infected rat dies, its fleas seek a new host, bite it, and infect it. When an epidemic of plague develops in the grey rat (*Rattus norvegicus*) the black rat (*Rattus rattus*) which inhabits houses becomes infected, and when a black rat dies, its fleas seek a new host, man or rat.

Diagnosis of human infection with *Y.pestis*, characterized by sudden onset of fever, headache, general body aches and prostration, with pain in groins or other sites of developing buboes, is confirmed by isolation of the organism from blood cultures (the finding of the organism in direct stained blood films is a bad sign), aspiration from buboes (painful), sputum in pulmonary plague, or CSF in plague meningitis. Cultures should be made from spleen and obvious buboes at post-mortem. Fluorescent microscopy enables rapid diagnosis to be made. Paired serum samples for complement fixation and haemagglutination tests show a rising titre of antibodies, antibodies appearing by 8–14 days. Serological results may be useful in retrospect.

In outbreaks of plague, dead rats and associated insects should be examined and cultures taken from dead rat liver, spleen and enlarged lymph glands.

TESTS OF PROGRESS

In severe cases, plague meningitis may develop. Disseminated intravascular coagulation also occurs in severe cases.

Plague vaccination with attenuated organisms gives temporary immunity lasting only a few months, but this may be useful in an epidemic.

'SYLVATIC' PLAGUE

Plague also affects rodents which inhabit the steppes and prairies (rather than the woods), and the insects associated with these rodents can bite hunters and trappers to produce infection with *Y. pestis*. The disease is severe, and usually pneumonic.

Diagnosis can be confirmed by microscopy and culture of sputum, and isolation of the infecting organism.

Prostatitis (including Seminal Vesiculitis)

Diagnosis of this condition, with identification of the infecting organism, can be confirmed by microscopy and culture of material obtained from the urethra, following prostatic massage, if necessary. Examination of urine samples may reveal traces of protein, mucus and increased numbers of neutrophils.

Neutrophilia is found in acute prostatitis.

TESTS PROVIDING USEFUL NEGATIVE RESULTS

Following prostatic massage to obtain material for examination, the serum acid phosphatase activity is raised above normal for a day or more, in the absence of prostatic carcinoma.

Suppurative Mastitis

Identification of the organism (most commonly *Staph. pyogenes*) can be confirmed by microscopy and culture of pus from the lesion. Phage typing can be carried out to identify the particular type of the staphylococcus, which can be very useful in cross-infection studies in closed communities (e.g. maternity hospitals). The pattern of sensitivity and resistance to various antibiotics should also be determined. The upper respiratory tract and the perineum should be swabbed and cultured to determine whether these sites are acting as a reservoir for the infecting organism, before and after suitable treatment for the eradication of the infecting staphylococcus.

Reiter's Syndrome (Non-specific Urethritis, Polyarthritis and Conjunctivitis or Iritis)

TESTS SUPPORTING CLINICAL DIAGNOSIS

The urethral smear contains neutrophils and epithelial cells, but is sterile on culture.

Synovial fluid from an affected joint is turbid, containing less than 20 000 neutrophils/ml with a glucose concentration of about 4·4 mmol/l (80 mg/100 ml).

NON-SPECIFIC TESTS

Moderate anaemia develops in some cases, with a moderate neutrophilia.

The ESR and plasma viscosity may be increased.

TEST PROVIDING USEFUL NEGATIVE RESULTS

Rose–Waaler and latex globulin tests for evidence of active rheumatoid arthritis are negative.

Scarlet Fever

Diagnosis of scarlet fever, a general erythematous rash which appears in some children in association with infection with *Strep. pyogenes*, is confirmed by the isolation of the organism on culture from nose and throat swabs. Additional evidence is provided by the demonstration of blanching of reddened skin 8–12 hours after intradermal injection of scarlet-fever antitoxin.

There is a moderate neutrophilia during the infection. Following successful treatment, nose and throat swabs should give negative cultures for the *Strep. pyogenes*.

Only a small proportion of patients infected with *Strep. pyogenes* develop scarlet fever, which is said to be due to the erythrogenic toxin produced by the organism. The most susceptible patients are children aged between 6 months and 3 years.

Staphylococcal Infections

Diagnosis of infection with *Staph. pyogenes* depends on isolation of the organism from the infected lesion. Apart from determination of the antibiotic sensitivites of the organism for successful treatment, typing of the organism for epidemiology, especially in hospitals and institutions, is important.

The organism can be classified by:

a. Phage typing.

b. Pattern of antibiotic sensitivity and resistance. The incidence of penicillin-resistant strains tends to be low in the general population, but high in hospitals, and a careful watch should be kept for methicillin-resistant strains (which are multiresistant).

c. (Serotyping into Types I, II, III. Technically difficult.)

Such typing is useful in the detection of the spread of staphylococcal infection via patients and healthy carriers.

Streptobacillary Fever, Haverhill Fever (a variety of Rat-bite Fever)

Diagnosis of infection with *Streptobacillus moniliformis* (also called *Haverhillia multiformis* or *Actinomyces muris*) can be confirmed by microscopy and culture of pus from the bite site, metastatic abscess, infected joint, or blood culture.

The organism can be inoculated into mice, on isolation, since the organism is a normal commensal of the rat's nasopharynx but gives rise to epizootics in mice. Infected mice may contaminate milk, and humans may be infected by drinking the milk.

Rising titres of agglutinins against the organism developing in the patient's serum are also diagnostic.

The infection is accompanied by marked neutrophilia.

Stye

Identification of the organism causing a stye (usually *Staph. pyogenes*) can be made by microscopy and culture of pus from the lesion. Phage typing for cross-infection studies and the antibiotic pattern of resistance and sensitivity for thorough treatment can be carried out, and swabbing of other sites including the nasopharynx and perineum can be carried out so that reservoirs of the organism can be cleared.

Sycosis Barbae

Identification of the organism causing sycosis barbae can be made by microscopy and culture of swabs taken from the infected area. The organism most commonly found is *Staph. pyogenes*. Phage typing, antibiotic sensitivity pattern, and swabbing of other sites acting as reservoirs for the organism should be carried out.

Tetanus

Diagnosis of tetanus is essentially clinical. Confirmation by isolation of the organism on culture of pus or tissue scrapings is difficult, and bacteriological confirmation that the organism isolated is in fact *Clostridium tetani* takes time. Negative results do not affect the clinical diagnosis or the treatment.

TESTS OF PROGRESS

Once tetanus toxoid has fixed to nerve cells, it cannot be neutralized by antitoxin. Active immunization results in prolonged immunity, which can be boosted by further injections of tetanus toxoid every few years. Maternal tetanus antitoxin does cross the placenta.

Tuberculosis

Diagnosis of infection with *Mycobacterium tuberculosis* can be confirmed by isolation of the organism by microscopy and culture of material from tuberculosis lesions. Due to the scantiness of the bacilli in some of these lesions and to the intermittent excretion of tubercle bacilli in some cases according to the type and stage of the lesion, repeated sampling is necessary. It is vital to isolate the organism and test its sensitivity to antituberculous drugs as soon as possible. Resistance can develop to a single drug in 1–3 months, if given alone. Treatment should therefore consist of a combination of agents to which the particular strain is sensitive.

Some affected sites are best suited for biopsy techniques, since biopsy material can be examined both by microscopy and culture. Animal inoculation can be used to supplement culture, for isolation of scanty organisms, virulence testing, and typing of strains of *Mycobacterium tuberculosis* (human, bovine and, rarely, avian).

a. Pulmonary tuberculosis: Sputum, laryngeal swab or aspirate, bronchial swab, or lavage, gastric lavage or faeces (where sputum is swallowed, e.g. children), pleural fluid or pus.

b. Urinary tract tuberculosis: Overnight urine sample or 24-hour sample is collected for examination and culture. It is important to avoid contamination with saprophytic acid-fast bacilli, which may occur in watertaps.

c. Male genital tract tuberculosis: Pus, biopsy sample and sometimes urine.

d. Female genital tract tuberculosis: Endometrial curettings or biopsy from other sites. Less satisfactorily, the menstruum may be examined.

e. Tuberculosis of alimentary tract: Material for examination may be obtained from mouth ulcers, or, indirectly, from faeces, or from biopsy material.

f. Tuberculous adenitis, osteomyelitis, arthritis, abscesses, ulcers, otitis and infections of serous cavities: Fluid, pus, or biopsy material from the specific lesion.

g. Tuberculous meningitis: CSF.

Hypersensitivity develops in an individual 4–6 weeks after a primary infection or 1–3 months after BCG vaccination and a positive skin tuberculin test demonstrates this (Mantoux test, Heaf test). A positive-test result is interpreted with the patient's history, and clinical state, plus the immunity of the population. A negative-test result excludes a past or present tuberculous infection, but sensitivity may be reduced in certain circumstances:

a. Small children may become negative (revert) with healing of the lesion.

b. The test may have been performed too early, before there has been time for sensitivity to develop.

c. During acute miliary tuberculosis, tuberculous meningitis, measles, scarlet fever, influenza, Hodgkin's disease and other reticuloses, Boeck's sarcoidosis.

d. Late pregnancy and puerperium.

e. Old age, and occasionally in middle age, for some unexplained reason.

f. With ultraviolet light therapy and sunbathing.

g. In individuals with low sensitivity.

It is recommended that pre- and post-BCG testing should be performed on different arms, and that no test be done until 3 weeks after any vaccination with living material (e.g. smallpox, poliomyelitis, yellow fever).

Complement-fixation tests and haemagglutination tests have not been found useful in practice.

Anaemia develops, which increases with increasing severity of the disease. Acute haemolytic anaemia may occur in acute miliary tuberculosis. The ESR and the plasma viscosity increase, as plasma fibrinogen and alpha- and gammaglobulins increase. Serum albumin falls as the globulins increase. In terminal cases, the total serum proteins fall, and the plasma viscosity falls below the lower limit of normal.

Neutrophilia occurs in acute exacerbations, and in acute disseminated tuberculosis the blood count may be leukaemoid, with either gross neutrophilia or lymphocytosis. There tends to be relative monocytosis during healing of tuberculous lesions.

In non-urinary tract tuberculosis, the urine contains protein, which increases grossly in the rare development of amyloides. In urinary-tract tuberculosis, the urine contains red cells, neutrophils and variable numbers of tubercle bacilli.

In tuberculous meningitis, there are usually increased numbers of lymphocytes, but there may also be increased numbers of neutrophils. The CSF glucose concentration may be diminished in gross infection.

Pleural fluid and ascitic fluid, if present, contain increased numbers of lymphocytes and raised protein content, but there may be increased neutrophil counts if there is secondary infection.

TESTS OF PROGRESS

With healing and recovery the ESR and the more sensitive plasma viscosity return to normal.

TESTS PROVIDING USEFUL NEGATIVE RESULTS

Subject to the exceptions already listed earlier, negative skin tuberculin tests indicate no present or previous tuberculous infection.

Other Mycobacterium Infections (Tuberculoid Mycobacteria)

These organisms have a lower infectivity that *M. tuberculosis*, are much less sensitive to antibiotics, and when acting as the infective agent, result in a positive tuberculin skin test.

1. *M. kansasii*—causes benign lung disease in elderly men. There may be anaemia, neutropenia and thrombocytopenia.

2. *M. marrinum* (*balnei*)—mild ulceration of the skin following abrasions caused in swimming pools. The organism should be cultured at 31 °C.

3. *M. scrofulaceum*—causes lymphadenitis in children.

4. *M. intracellulare* (battery bacillus)—causes a disease resembling pulmonary tuberculosis in elderly men.

5. *M. ulcerans*—causes slowly spreading indolent ulcers in people living in the country in Australia.

6. *M. burali*—causes skin ulcers in Uganda.
7. *M. fortuitum*—causes suppurative lesions in men and cattle.

Tularaemia

Diagnosis of this infection, which is a natural infection of many rodents with *Brucella tularensis*, can be confirmed in man by culture of the organism from nodules, pustules, ulcers, blood, pleural exudate, or sputum, on special media.

Lymph-gland biopsy material or material from ulcers may be injected into guinea pigs as a means of isolating the organism.

A skin test with antigen made from detoxified *Br. tularensis* becomes positive by the third day of illness.

Serum agglutinins and complement-fixing antibodies develop during the second week of illness, so that infection can be confirmed by a rising titre of antibodies from the acute stage of the illness to convalescence. There is some crossing with *Brucella abortus*, but at a lower titre. Up to a third of patients with antibodies in their sera appear to have had subclinical infection.

In outbreaks an examination of infected rodents and the insects found on them should be made. The organism is found in vole faeces and in contaminated hay.

Neutrophilia is found in the acute stages, with thrombocytopenia. If a pleural exudate develops, it is found to have a high protein content with a relatively low white-cell count (2000–3000 per cmm).

(The cross-reaction with antigens of *Br. abortus* supports the inclusion of the organism in the brucella group. Some authorities include it with pasteurella organisms.)

Urethritis (Non-specific)

Diagnosis of the cause of non-specific urethritis can be made by examination of smears from material from the urethra, and culture of this material. Organisms which may cause non-specific urethritis include:
> *Mycoplasma hominis*
> Trachoma inclusion conjunctivitis agent (TRIC)
> *Trichomonas vaginalis*
> *Candida albicans*

TESTS PROVIDING USEFUL NEGATIVE RESULTS

Patients with this complaint should be shown to be free both of gonorrhoea and syphilis.

Vaginitis (including Cervicitis (Non-gonococcal))

Diagnosis of the cause of vaginitis and cervicitis can be made by microscopy and culture of material from upper vaginal and cervical swabs. Organisms which may cause vaginitis and cervicitis include:
> *Mycoplasma hominis*
> Trachoma inclusion conjunctivitis agent (TRIC)

Trichomonas vaginalis
Candida albicans

Yeasts and trichomonas are often found on routine microscopy of urine samples.

3 Infectious Diseases—II

SPIROCHAETAL INFECTIONS

Bejel

Diagnosis of infection with this cutaneous spirochaetal disease of the Middle East is confirmed by the demonstration of the presence of an organism indistinguishable in appearance from *Treponema pallidum* in local lesions by dark-ground microscopy. Serological tests for syphilis and the *T. pallidum* immobilization test (TPI) are positive.

The infection is regarded either as a modification of syphilis or as a separate entity.

Leptospirosis

Diagnosis of leptospirosis can be confirmed by demonstration of the organism in fresh blood by dark-ground microscopy (difficult, using triple centrifugation) or by inoculation of blood into guinea pigs during the first week of illness. It is important that blood for inoculation should be obtained before treatment with antibiotics is started. In cases of meningitis, inoculation of CSF into a guinea pig may also reveal the organism.

During the second and third weeks of the illness, the organism may be recovered by inoculation of fresh urine into guinea pigs, or by demonstration of the leptospira by dark-ground microscopy of urine deposits (the leptospira rapidly disintegrates in acid urine).

Serum antibodies appear after the first week and rise to peak values by the third week. These may be demonstrated by complement-fixation or agglutination techniques. A rising titre of antibodies from the early stages of the disease to the fourth to seventh weeks is diagnostic.

For dark-ground microscopy of blood, blood samples should be taken before meals to avoid complicating lipaemia.

Normochromic anaemia with marked neutrophilia, raised ESR, and proteinuria are found in the early stages. In cases in which liver damage occurs, biochemical findings of hepatitis with haemolysis are found. Some cases develop severe renal damage, with raised blood urea, oliguria and production of urinary casts.

The CSF protein is increased in most cases during the first 2 weeks. With actual meningitis, the cell count in the CSF rises (up to 300, rarely up to 2000 per cmm), predominantly neutrophils at first and predominantly lymphocytes later.

Leptospira are divided into:

a. Leptospira biflexa complex—consisting of leptospira which are saprophytic and which have no known hosts.

b. Leptospira interrogans complex, which include about 130 serotypes occurring throughout the world, arranged in 16 serogroups (World Health Organization, 1967):

i. *Leptospira icterohaemorrhagiae*—affecting man, rats, dogs, cattle, causing Weil's disease.

ii. *Leptospira canicola*—affecting man, dogs, pigs, causing canicola fever.

Pinta

Diagnosis of infection with this cutaneous spirochaetal disease of South America is confirmed by the demonstration of the presence of *Treponema carateum* and *Treponema herrejoni* by dark-ground microscopy in material from the initial and the generalized papules, and in material from affected regional lymph glands. The treponemata are not found in depigmented spots.

Treponemata can also be demonstrated in pintids in the secondary stage and may persist in these lesions for a long time.

Serological tests for syphilis and the treponema immobilization (TPI) test become positive 5–12 months after infection. There is much weaker cross-immunity with syphilis than is the case with yaws.

The signs of chronic infection are found in the blood. This infection is regarded either as a modification of syphilis or as a separate entity. Coincidental infection with syphilis is common.

Rat-bite Fever (Sodoka)
(See also Streptobacillary Fever)

Diagnosis of infection with *Spirillum minus* is confirmed by demonstration of the organism on dark-ground microscopy in fresh exudate from the wound, oedema fluid near a bite, or in aspirate from an infected lymph gland. The organism is also isolated by inoculation of fresh exudate from the wound, lymph gland aspirate, or blood into a guinea pig.

Neutrophilia is frequently found. Serological tests for syphilis give false-positive results.

Relapsing Fever

LOUSE-BORNE RELAPSING FEVER

The louse, *Pediculus humanus*, becomes infective 3–5 days after feeding on an infected man. Infection follows crushing of the louse on the human skin; organisms being liberated from the body cavity of the louse to enter through minute abrasions in the skin.

Diagnosis of infection with *Treponema recurrentis obermeieri* (also known as *Borrelia*) can be confirmed by demonstration of the organisms in the peripheral blood by dark-ground microscopy or in stained blood films, in blood taken during the acute phase of the disease.

Between attacks, when there are only scanty organisms in the blood, the organism can be isolated by inoculating fresh blood intraperitoneally into a mouse. Blood samples taken from the mouse tail daily will show the organism.

The urine may contain protein, red blood cells and casts, and there is a marked neutrophilia in the blood. Serological tests for syphilis are often positive. Jaundice may develop.

TICK-BORNE RELAPSING FEVER

Many mammals in Africa, especially rodents, act as reservoirs of infection. Infection is transmitted to man from infected ticks while they are feeding on him.

Diagnosis of infection with *Treponema duttoni* (also known as *Borrelia*) is confirmed by demonstration of the organism in the same manner as in louse-borne relapsing fever.

Syphilis

TESTS AVAILABLE

1. Direct dark-ground microscopy of material from primary chancre or from moist secondary lesions, with demonstration of *Treponema pallidum*.
2. Reagin tests (including cardiolipin, Wassermann reaction, Kahn test, Venereal Disease Research Laboratory (VDRL) slide test), are not completely specific.
3. Reiter complement-fixation test is more specific.
4. *T. pallidum* fluorescent antibody test (FTA) ⎫ all specific but
   T. pallidum immobilization test   ⎬ require specialized
   T. pallidum haemagglutination test   ⎭ laboratory

Diagnosis
1. *Primary*
   Demonstration of *T. pallidum* by dark-ground microscopy of material from chancre. Reagin serological tests may be negative, and repeat negatives should be obtained regularly for 2–3 months before syphilis is excluded. After identification of the organism, treatment can be started, and serological tests may not become positive.
2. *Secondary*
   Dark-ground microscopy of moist surfaces of lesions reveal the presence of *T. pallidum*. Serological tests are strongly positive. (False positive reagin test results may occur with other diseases, including rubella and infectious mononucleosis, but the FTA, immobilization and haemagglutination tests do not give false positive results.)
3. *Tertiary*
   All serological tests are positive. In meningovascular syphilis all tests in serum and CSF are positive, with increased CSF pressure, protein and cell count.
4. *Congenital syphilis*
   The neonate serum gives positive test results, either from passive transfer

of maternal antibody, the titre falling rapidly in the first 2–3 months, or from active infection, in which case the titre remains high and rises. After a mother acquires a syphilitic infection in late pregnancy, the infant gives negative serological results at first, but develops clinical syphilis at 1–2 months after birth.

5. *Following treatment*

If treatment is early, serological tests may remain negative. Following treatment, positive tests become negative—the longer the delay before treatment is started, the slower the return to negativity. If treatment is started in the late stages of syphilis, serological tests may never become negative, but their titre falls progressively. Following this slow fall, a sudden rise in titre suggests reinfection.

The FTA titre rises first and falls last. VDRL tests increase more slowly and fall rapidly, being a useful indicator of response to treatment; if the titre is greater than 1:8 the disease is still active.

During treatment of neurosyphilis, the cell count in the CSF falls to normal by 3 months, the protein content to normal by 4 months, but antibody tests remain positive in the CSF. Serological tests should become negative by 1 year. Retreatment is indicated if the CSF cell count fails to fall.

6. *Biological false positive results*

These may occur with reagin rests, but not with FTA and the other two specific tests.

True positive tests for syphilis occur in diseases caused by morphologically similar organisms, such as trepanomatosis, yaws, bejel, pinta.

Yaws

Diagnosis of infection with *Treponema pertenue* is confirmed by demonstration of the organism in fluid from skin granulomas, frambesia and plantar papules. It is important to distinguish it from the commensal *Borrelia refringens*.

Serological tests for syphilis and the treponema immobilization (TPI) test becomes positive a few weeks after the appearance of the primary lesion, and remain positive as long as the infection is active.

TESTS PROVIDING USEFUL NEGATIVE RESULTS

Tests for syphilis and treponema immobilization tests on CSF remain negative, in the absence of syphilis.

MYCOTIC INFECTIONS

Actinomycosis (Streptothricosis; Leptothricosis)

Diagnosis of infection with *Actinomycosis israeli* can be confirmed by microscopy and examination of pus for 'sulphur granules' and by culture. The organism grows anaerobically, and the so-called 'sulphur granules' are found to consist of gram-positive branching filaments. Microscopy and culture of material taken at tissue biopsy (especially from the wall of an abscess) may be very useful.

Although agglutinins and complement-fixing antibodies may be present in the serum, they have not proved to be useful.

Neutrophilia and raised ESR are usually found.

Aspergillosis

Diagnosis of infection with *Aspergillus* species can be confirmed by microscopy and culture of material from infected sites. It is important to avoid contamination of samples, as the *Aspergillus* sp. is very common (*see also* 'Pulmonary Aspergilloma', p. 207). *Aspergillus fumigatus* can be isolated from 10 per cent of bronchitic sputums, i.e. 'ubiquitous'. Sputum 'casts' may contain fungi (visible on section) and eosinophils.

DIAGNOSIS OF ALLERGIC ASPERGILLOSIS

Apart from infection of bronchiectatic or old tuberculosis cavities in the lungs, sensitivity to the organism may develop in patients, resulting in asthma. In these latter patients, sputum culture for *Aspergillus* sp. is positive, and, in addition, serum precipitins are present, with skin sensitivity to extracts of aspergilli and eosinophilia. Of patients with allergic aspergillosis 70 per cent have positive serum precipitins. Treatment with prednisolone results in relief of signs and symptoms, with falling eosinophil counts and reduced sputum volume.

Bagassosis

Diagnosis may be supported by the finding of serum precipitins against *Thermosporapolyspora vulgaris*.

Blastomycosis (North American) (Gilchrist's Disease)

Diagnosis of infection with *Blastomyces dermatitidis* is confirmed by microscopy and isolation on culture of the organism from scrapings from cutaneous lesions and from pus from abscesses on the periphery of the lesion. In systemic infection, the organism is isolated from sputum, urine and CSF.

Complement-fixation tests show crossing with histoplasmin but with lower titres. Complement-fixation tests may be negative with localized infection, but become positive in systemic disease, with high titres. A positive result justifies a presumptive positive diagnosis.

Similarly a positive skin test (tuberculin type) in parallel with negative coccidioidin and histoplasmin tests justifies a presumptive positive diagnosis. Four per cent of normal people may have positive skin tests to *Blastomyces*.

Hypochromic anaemia with neutrophilia and raised ESR are found.

TESTS OF PROGRESS

A fatal outcome is to be expected in patients with a high antibody titre (indicating extensive disease) and a negative or weakly positive skin test (indicating anergy). The best prognosis is in patients with hypersensitivity and without complement-fixing antibodies.

Blastomycosis (South American) (Paracoccidiodal Granuloma; Lutz–Splendore–De Almeida's Disease)

Diagnosis is confirmed by the microscopy and isolation on culture of *Blastomyces brasiliensis* from scrapings from affected skin and mucous membranes, from pus from fluctuant nodules, and sputum in cases with systemic infection.

Complement-fixing antibodies may be absent in localized disease, and are present in systemic disease.

Skin reactions (tuberculin type) may be absent in localized disease or in anergic cases with overwhelming infection.

Iron-deficient anaemia develops with neutrophilia and raised ESR. Hypersensitivity is accompanied by eosinophilia.

Candidiasis (Moniliasis; Thrush; Mycotic Vulvovaginitis; Bronchomycosis)

Diagnosis of infection with *Candida* sp. (most commonly *Candida albicans*) is confirmed by isolation of the organism on culture from vaginal, oral and skin swabs, sputum and faeces.

Certain conditions, such as debility, diabetes, antibiotic and steroid therapy predispose to candidiasis. Pregnant women and infants are liable to infection.

Serum-antibody tests are not of use, as many normal people have raised titres. Similarly, skin tests are not helpful.

In infection, only moderate increases in neutrophil counts are found.

Chromoblastomycosis (Verrucous Dermatitis)

Diagnosis of this condition is confirmed by the isolation on culture of crusts and pus from lesions of any of *Hormodendrum pedrosoi*, *Hormodendrum compacta*, or *Phialophora verrucosa*.

As in North American blastomycosis, serum complement-fixing antibodies titres correlate with clinical condition, falling with improvement.

Cryptococcosis (European Blastomycosis; Torulosis)

Diagnosis of infection with *Cryptococcus neoformans (Torula histolytica)* is confirmed by the isolation on culture from pus, sputum, or CSF. Infected material from a patient, and saline suspensions of pure cultures should be injected into mice, to produce budding encapsulated fungus in 3–4 weeks.

Bentonite flocculation tests for antibodies to cryptococci in the serum are possible, but up to 2 per cent of tests are false positives, and there is cross-reaction with other systemic fungal diseases. Cryptococcal antibodies persist for years in the serum.

In suspected infection of the CSF apart from direct culture and inoculation in laboratory mice, direct microscopy of the fluid is useful. The CSF protein is increased, with pleocytosis and moderate reduction of fluid glucose concentration.

Coccidioidomycosis (Coccidioidal Granuloma; Valley Fever; Desert Rheumatism; San Joaquin Fever; Posada–Wernicke's Disease)

Diagnosis of infection with *Coccidioides immitis* can be confirmed by microscopic examination of sputum, gastric contents, CSF, exudates, pus and scrapings from cutaneous lesions, followed by culture. Suspensions from cultures can be inoculated into mice (peritoneum) or guinea pigs (testicles). Infection develops within 7–10 days. The arthrospores from cultures develop directly into spherules which can be demonstrated after 4–6 days in the pus from the orchitis in the guinea pig or from the peritonitis in the mouse.

Similarly, biopsy material from cutaneous lesions or abscesses, or obtained at post-mortem, should be cultured.

In asymptomatic and mild primary infections, the precipitin and complement-fixation tests are negative. In severe primary infection the pricipitin test becomes positive, but usually reverts to negative by 30–60 days. Complement-fixing antibodies appear later in a primary severe infection and persist for a few weeks. The persistence of antibodies, especially with a rising titre, indicates a change to the disseminated form of the disease.

Skin tests become positive in 87 per cent of patients during the first week, and in 99 per cent of patients after the second week of the illness. There is a cross-reaction with histoplasmin and blastomycin, but the results are less strongly positive. A positive skin test to coccidioidin injection merely indicates infection with *C. immitis* at some time in the patient's life.

Hypochromic anaemia develops, with slight neutrophilia or leucopenia.

TESTS OF PROGRESS

The ESR is increased throughout the disease, and a raised ESR with rising antibody titre indicates a grave prognosis.

Erythrasma

Diagnosis of infection with *Nocardia minutissima* can be confirmed by microscopy of skin scrapings from affected areas, especially from those areas which fluoresce under a Wood's light. Culture of the fungus is not a routine procedure, and diagnosis depends on identification of short, delicate, branching filaments in the affected skin.

Farmer's Lung

Diagnosis is supported by the finding of precipitating antibodies in the serum to various organisms and fungi associated with mouldy hay, mouldy sugar cane, mushroom compost:

Micropolyspora faeni (Thermopolyspora polyspora) (the most common)
Aspergillus clavatus
Penicillium
Coniosporium corticale

Mucor
Candida
Intradermal skin tests may be positive to various fungal antigens and hay extracts.
(Avian protein and porcine pituitary snuff can cause a similar disorder.)

TESTS PROVIDING USEFUL NEGATIVE RESULTS

Tests for the presence of tuberculosis, sarcoidosis, histoplasmosis and blastomycoses are negative.

Geotrichosis

Diagnosis of infection with *Geotrichum* sp. is confirmed by direct microscopic examination of sputum, pus from oral lesions, and faeces. Cultures should be made from these materials. *Geotrichum* spores may be present in normal stools.
Skin tests with a *Geotrichum* vaccine are of no value.

Histoplasmosis

Diagnosis of infection with *Histoplasma capsulatum* can be confirmed by microscopy and culture of material from cutaneous and mucosal lesions, sputum, and gastric washings. Biopsy materials obtained from oronasopharyngeal lesions, lymph glands, and bone marrow are examined by microscopy for the presence of intracellular, oval, yeast-like fungi in mononuclear cells and by subsequent culture. All laboratory animals are susceptible to the infection. Intracerebral, intraperitoneal and intravenous injections of the yeast phase of cultures into mice produce infection and death.

Histoplasmin skin tests become positive in infected cases a few weeks after infection but can stimulate humoral antibodies with 'false-positive' results 2 days later, in histoplasmin-hypersensitive subjects. Precipitins appear early in the serum. Complement-fixing antibodies appear in the serum and reach peak values by 2–3 weeks, falling during the next 4–8 months. Cross-reactions with *Blastomyces* antigen may occur. Colloidin agglutinin tests become positive by the end of the second week.

Hypochromic anaemia develops with leucopenia. In children there may develop lymphocytosis with atypical mononuclear cells present.

Maduromycosis (Madura Foot; Mycetoma)

Diagnosis of a chronic infection of the feet (or less commonly of the hands) with swellings and sinuses caused by a variety of different fungi can be confirmed by microscopic examination of pus and curettings from sinuses, followed by culture of the material. Organisms isolated include: *Allescheria; Aspergillus; Sterigmatocystis; Penicillium; Madurella; Indiella; Glenospora; Monosporium; Cephalosporium; Phialophora.*

Mucormycosis

Diagnosis of infection by *Mucor* sp. causing a rapidly fatal inflammatory disease with vascular thrombosis and invasion of walls and lumina of blood vessels can be made by microscopy and culture of material from sites of infection during life or at post-mortem. Careful identification of cultured fungi is important after noting the presence of mycelium in the tissues, since the true identity of the aetiological agent has not yet been established.

Nocardiosis (Nocardial Mycetoma; Actinomycotic Madura Foot; Actinomycosis; Streptorhicosis)

Diagnosis of a chronic suppurative and granulomatous disease of the subcutaneous tissues with *Nocardia* sp. can be confirmed by microscopy of pus from an abscess or draining sinus. Opaque flecks or granules appear as lobulated, tangled masses of delicate filaments, the ends of which are not usually club-shaped. Cultures should be made from this material. Various *Nocardia* sp. have been isolated: *Nocardia asteroides; Nocardia brasiliensis; Nocardia madurae; Nocardia pelletieri; Nocardia paraguayensis; Nocardia caprae.*

Guinea pigs inoculated intraperitoneally with large amounts of inoculum die within 7–10 days.

Tissue from nocardial mycetoma shows granules in miliary abscesses. The nature of antibodies in this condition is not known. Nor do skin tests appear to be useful.

Nocardial mycetoma does not alter the TWBC or the ESR until secondary bacterial infection has taken place. Systemic nocardiosis causes neutrophilia with increased ESR.

Otomycosis (Fungous Infection of the Ear)

Diagnosis of fungous infection of the external ear can be confirmed by microscopy and culture of epithelial material and debris from the ear. A wide variety of fungi have been isolated from cases.

TESTS PROVIDING USEFUL NEGATIVE RESULTS

Absence of growth of haemolytic streptococci on suitable media. Absence of fungi on microscopy of material from seborrhoeic dermatitis or allergic dermatitis.

Penicilliosis

Diagnosis of infection of lungs, skin, or urinary tract with *Penicillium* sp. or closely related *Scopulariopsis* sp. can be confirmed by microscopy of material from infected sites and subsequent culture.

Piedra (Black Piedra; White Piedra; Tinea Nodosa; Trichomycosis Nodosa)

Diagnosis of fungous infection characterized by the presence of stony hard nodules along the hair shafts can be confirmed by direct microscopy of infected hairs, followed by culture.

Pityriasis Versicolor (Tinea versicolor; Chromophytosis; Dermatomycosis Furfuracea; Liver Spots; Tinea Flava; Pityriasis Versicolor Tropica)

Diagnosis of this chronic asymptomatic superficial fungous disease caused by *Malassezia furfur* can be confirmed by microscopy of skin scrapings from macules, especially from those areas fluorescing under Wood's light. Culture of skin material is not effective. Skin-biopsy specimens reveal the organisms present in abundance in the middle and deeper layers of the stratum corneum.

Rhinosporidiosis

Diagnosis of infection with *Rhinosporidium seeberi* can be confirmed by direct examination and microscopy of infected material from nose, pharynx, larynx, eye, lacrimal sac and skin. Culture has not been successful. On biopsy, the polyps consist of granulomatous material with large sporangia containing large number of spores, and ruptured sporangia.

Sporotrichosis

Diagnosis of infection with *Sporotrichum schenckii* can be confirmed by microscopy of pus, followed by culture of pus and material from infected sites taken at biopsy. Pus for culture can be taken by sterile aspiration from unopened subcutaneous nodules. The material can be injected intraperitoneally into white mice or rats. Smears of pus from the subsequent peritonitis reveal numerous gram-positive, cigar-shaped, intracellular organisms.

It is important to note that the causative organism cannot usually be demonstrated in sections of tissue.

Complement-fixing antibodies, agglutinins and precipitins develop in the sera of infected patients. Pathogenic *Sporotrichum* isolated from man in North and South America, South Africa, and Europe, from horses, and from timbers in South African gold mines have been shown antigenically to be identical.

Skin tests using a heat-killed vaccine become positive as early as the fifth day following infection.

TESTS PROVIDING USEFUL NEGATIVE RESULTS

Tests for the presence of syphilis, tuberculosis, glanders, leprosy, tularaemia and blastomycosis are negative.

Tinea (Ringworm)

Diagnosis of infection of skin, nails, or scalp can be confirmed by microscopy and culture of:

    a. Skin scrapings from the active periphery of the lesion.

    b. Nail clippings, nail scrapings, and subungual debris.

    c. Hairs, especially those which fluoresce under a Wood's light or appear lustreless or broken. Skin scrapings from areas where the hairs are affected are useful.

    d. Domes of vesicles should be snipped off for microscopy and culture.

Contacts, both human and animal, and infected fomites, should also be investigated.

Skin tests may be of value in obscure cases.

Trichomycosis Axillaris (Trichonocardiosis)

Diagnosis of infection of axillary and pubic hair, with the development of yellow (flava), red (rubra), or black (nigra) concretions around the hair shaft, can be confirmed by microscopy of the infected hair and subsequent culture.

PROTOZOAN INFECTIONS

Amoebiasis

Diagnosis of amoebiasis can be confirmed by the identification of vegetative forms, cysts, or precysts of *Entamoeba histolytica* in fresh, warm, liquid faeces, especially in blood-streaked exudate, in which mobile trophozoites should be looked for. Formol-ether concentration specimens of faeces can be examined for cysts.

Scrapings of lesions at sigmoidoscopy can also be examined for trophozoites. If there is severe inflammation, scrapings should not be attempted beyond the rectal ampulla, to avoid perforation. In the absence of obvious lesions, blood-streaked exudate or liquid faeces should be examined directly, and samples can be fixed in Schaudinn's solution and stained for examination. Ingestion of red cells by the parasites is useful in detection, as other entamoeba do not ingest red cells.

Stools should be examined for the parasite in cases of amoebic hepatitis and abscess. Aspirate from an abscess does not have a foul odour, and does not yield bacteria on anaerobic culture, and perhaps 50 per cent of the aspirates contain trophozoites on examination. The last pus aspirated should be examined. Neutrophilia, with increased serum alkaline phosphatase activity and bilirubin, occurs. The patient becomes anaemic. In cutaneous amoebiasis, perianal scrapings yield numerous trophozoites (differential diagnosis includes syphilis, tuberculosis, neoplasm). Pulmonary amoebiasis may develop from liver abscess.

Brain amoebic abscess is rare, and in most cases derive from liver abscess. Serological tests include indirect haemagglutination, immunofluorescence, and complement fixation, which are sensitive tests, but which are performed in specialized laboratories. Countercurrent electrophoresis and immunodiffusion are less sensitive, but are suitable for routine laboratories. Serological tests remain positive for varying times after cure (up to 5 years), and indicate amoebic invasion at some time. The degree of positivity does not differentiate between extra-intestinal and intestinal disease. In a small number of invasive cases, including extra-intestinal disease, serological tests can be completely negative. Serological tests are useful in critically ill patients when adequate parasitological examination is impossible because an interfering substance has been given—the serological tests are 85–95 per cent positive in such cases of amoebiasis.

TESTS OF PROGRESS

Disappearance of parasites from the stools and improvement in anaemia follow specific treatment. During treatment of amoebic hepatic disease with emetine, serum creatine phosphokinase activity increases.

Primary Amoebic Meningo-encephalitis [R]

1. Rare systemic complication of *E. histolytica* infection.
2. *Acanthamoeba*—presents as chronic illness in a compromised host.
3. *Naegleri Fowleri*

Presents as acute infection in healthy young adults, from natural and thermally polluted fresh water. The organisms normally feed on bacteria, and can be cultured on suspensions of *E. coli* or *K. aerogenes* at 37–45 °C. In distilled water at 37 °C the organism reverts to biflagellate form and then reverts back again.

Babesiosis

1. UNITED STATES OF AMERICA

Babesia microti is carried by deer ticks, and humans with intact spleens are infected via tick bites on islands off the New England coast. The disease is relatively avirulent.

2. EUROPE

Infection with *Babesia divergans* and *Babesia bovis* from cattle is especially fatal in splenectomized subjects or patients with impaired immune defences, and it is usually fatal.

Diagnosis of babesiosis is confirmed by the demonstration of 'Maltese-cross-type organisms in the erythrocytes in stained blood films.

Balantidiasis

Diagnosis of this condition, presenting with symptoms similar to those of invasive amoebiasis, but with a greater tendency in severe cases to proceed to perforation of the bowel, with intermittent diarrhoea in mild cases, is confirmed by the demonstration of trophozoites in unformed or dysentery stools, or cysts and trophozoites in formed stools. The organism can be cultured in vitro. The animal reservoir is the pig.

Coccidiosis, Isosporiasis

Diagnosis of infection with *Isospora belli* and *Isospora hominis*, characterized by colicky abdominal pain, flatulence and diarrhoea rarely lasting more than 2–3 weeks, a mild and self-limiting condition, is confirmed by the identification of immature or mature oocysts in fresh stools, facilitated by concentration using zinc sulphate flotation.

Giardiasis

Giardia lamblia is a common inhabitant of the human intestine and often has no pathogenic effect, but may be associated with attacks of diarrhoea, or possibly duodenitis or, less probably, cholangitis.

Diagnosis of the presence of this parasite is confirmed by identification of trophozoites in loose stools (direct examination, as attempts to concentrate destroy them). Live trophozoites can also the obtained from duodenal aspiration or from swallowed recoverable nylon yarn.

Diagnosis can also be confirmed by demonstration of the parasites in duodenal and jejunal mucosal biopsy material. *In vitro* culture of the organism is difficult.

Granuloma Venereum (Granuloma Inguinale)

Diagnosis of infection with *Donovania granulomatosis* can be confirmed by microscopy of tissue scrapings from granuloma or aspirate from neighbouring enlarged lymph glands. Small rod-shaped organisms may be seen, with pink capsules and more heavily stained bodies, producing the so-called 'safety-pin' appearance. Culture can be performed on special media.

Intradermal skin tests using antigen prepared from the causative organism, when positive, produce reaction maximal at 24 hours and fading in 2 days.

Precipitin and complement-fixing antibody tests are available.

TESTS PROVIDING USEFUL NEGATIVE RESULTS

Tests for syphilis (suggested by the venereal sore) are negative unless there is also syphilitic infection.

Leishmaniasis

A. CUTANEOUS LEISHMANIASIS *(Oriental Sore; American Mucocutaneous Leishmaniasis; Espundia)*

Diagnosis of cutaneous leishmaniasis and mucocutaneous leishmaniasis can be confirmed by the demonstration of *Leishmania tropica* in the cutaneous form and *Leishmania braziliensis* in the mucocutaneous form in stained films made from serum from the indurated edge of ulcers, culture of biopsy material from the margin of an ulcer. In the mucocutaneous type, mucosal scrapings can be inoculated into laboratory animals for culture.

Serological tests are probably of value in the mucocutaneous variety.

TESTS PROVIDING USEFUL NEGATIVE RESULTS

Negative tests for syphilis, yaws, tuberculosis, leprosy and various mycoses may be useful.

B. VISCERAL LEISHMANIASIS *(Kala-azar)*

Diagnosis of this condition can be confirmed by demonstration of the parasite (*Leishmania Donovani*) in blood films (in which there may be very few parasites), aspirates of lymph nodes or lymph-node biopsy, nasal scrapings (in the Sudan), aspiration biopsy of liver or spleen.

Anaemia develops and is progressive, with leucopenia and thrombocytopenia. Serum albumin falls progressively and serum globulin levels are greatly increased, with raised ESR and plasma viscosity. Later, serum bilirubin may rise.

Complement-fixing antibody and agglutination tests are not reliable. Biopsy material can be inoculated into hamsters for growth of the parasite.

Malaria

Diagnosis of malarial infection can be confirmed by microscopy of blood films stained at pH 7·0–7·4. If the solutions are more acid, then parasites may not take up stain properly. The maximum number of parasites are circulating following the 'cold stage' for about 6 hours as the body temperature is rising. Microscopy of bone-marrow aspirate may show parasitized red cells and macrophages containing pigment.

Incubation periods for mosquito-transmitted malaria:

Plasmodium falciparum	12 days
Plasmodium vivax	13–15 days
Plasmodium ovale	13–15 days
Plasmodium malariae	up to 1 month.

Antibodies to malaria appear after 1 week, reaching maximal titres after several months, and declining slowly during the next year. Both the indirect haemagglutination test and indirect fluorescent antibody test can be used in screening populations for the prevalence of malaria, and for screening blood donors in malarial areas. In chronic cases, the complement-fixation test is positive in 80 per cent.

In the acute stage biological false-positive tests for syphilis occur in over a quarter of cases. Anaemia develops with basophilic stippling of red cells, plus poikilocytosis and anisocytosis. There is frequently leucopenia with increased monocytes. Urinary urobilinogen output is increased, following the haemolytic anaemia. Transient jaundice may occur.

In Blackwater Fever oxyhaemoglobin and methaemoglobin appear in the urine, whilst in the extremely dangerous cerebral malaria fibrinogen and fibrin degradation products appear in the plasma (i.e. intravascular coagulation syndrome).

TESTS OF PROGRESS

Prophylactic treatment should start before entry into a malarial area. Primaquine should be taken prophylactically for 14 days after leaving, after taking prophylactic chloroquine, to eradicate the hepatic stages of plasmodial infection.

Subsequently, blood films should be examined during pyrexial attacks, should they occur.

Pneumocystis Pneumonii (Pneumocystosis Carinii)

Diagnosis of this condition, characterized by insidious onset of chest infection with respiratory distress with a subacute course, is confirmed by the demonstration of the organism in sputum, pharyngeal washings, tracheal aspirate, or by direct lung biopsy or needle biopsy of lung. Cysts, sporozoites and trophozoites may be seen after staining.

High titres of humoral antibodies may be detected in serum using complement fixation or immunofluorescence, but malnourished infants, infants with hypogammaglobulinaemia and immunosuppressed patients do not produce high diagnostic titres.

It is possible that the organism is a latent opportunistic organism. In the peripheral blood the white blood cell count is normal or slightly raised, and eosinophilia is common.

TESTS OF PROGRESS

The condition may be associated with cytomegalovirus infection in infants and adults, and with cryptococcosis in adults.

Pneumocystis carinii can be isolated from post-mortem material.

Sarcosporidiosis

Diagnosis of this uncommon condition in man can be confirmed by histological examination of cysts causing swelling in muscles, with identification of cysts of *Sarcocystis lindemanni* (Miescher's tube) which contain large numbers of so-called Rainey's corpuscles ($14 \times 6\,\mu$).

Toxoplasmosis

IN INFANTS

Transplacental infection can occur, and rarely congenital fetal disease develops, with varying degrees of brain damage, myocarditis and/or chorioretinitis. The risk of such infection is greatest between the 2nd and 6th months of pregnancy. The infected mother can be treated with a course of spiramycin.

Diagnosis of the infection can be confirmed by animal inoculation of CSF, blood, tissue extracts, but isolation of the organism is not easy. Positive results indicate the presence of invasive trophozoites.

IN CHILDREN AND ADULTS

Recent infection can be detected using the Sabin–Feldman dye test, which demonstrates specific IgG antibody in serum. Recent infection results in at least a fourfold increase in titre in paired sera, with titres reaching up to 1:1000 within 1–2 months. After 2 months, this test is unreliable. Using immunofluorescence, an increase in IgM antibody can be demonstrated. Positive results indicate a recently acquired infection, or reactivation of infection. A negative result indicates no infection during the previous three weeks—although compromised hosts, with defective immunity, have a high risk of central nervous system toxoplasmosis, and serological tests are falsely negative.

Positive haemagglutination tests should be confirmed by specific IgM tests. Animal inoculation with blood, CSF or tissue extracts, can be used to demonstrate the organism, but the technique is difficult.

In children and adults, during a febrile attack, many atypical mononuclear cells may be seen in the peripheral blood.

TESTS PROVIDING USEFUL NEGATIVE RESULTS

In acute febrile attacks, the Paul–Bunnell test is negative (cf. infectious mononucleosis). Positive histological diagnosis can only be made if a cyst is found.

Trichomoniasis

a. Trichomonas hominis is an inhabitant of the human intestines. Although it may be found in faeces in diarrhoea, it is not known to be a pathogen.

b. Trichomonas vaginalis may be isolated in non-specific urethritis in males and in vaginitis in females. It can be identified in wet fresh films, or stained with Giemsa, acridine orange, or Papanicolaou stains. The organism can be culture on Feinberg–Whittington medium.

Trypanosomiasis

AFRICAN TYPE (SLEEPING SICKNESS) (IN GAMBIA AND RHODESIA)

Diagnosis of this condition can be confirmed by the demonstration of the parasites *Trypanosoma gambiense* (chronic sleeping sickness) or *Trypanosoma rhodesiense* (acute sleeping sickness) in stained blood films, sternal marrow aspirate, lymph-node fluid aspirate, or CSF preferably obtained by cisternal puncture obtained at the stage of cerebral involvement.

Culture of the parasite is possible but difficult. Laboratory animal inoculation should be carried out.

A highly specific complement-fixation test for *T. gambiense* is now available. The Paul–Bunnell test for heterophile antibodies may also be positive.

In acute sleeping sickness, there is anaemia, purpura and increased monocytes. In chronic sleeping sickness, anaemia and monocytosis develop later.

When the cerebral stage develops, the CSF contains increased numbers of lymphocytes and parasites, with increased protein content. The CSF IgM concentration is greatly increased.

SOUTH AMERICAN TYPE (CHAGAS'S DISEASE)

Diagnosis of this condition can be confirmed by the demonstration of the parasite *Trypanosoma cruzi* in stained blood films, lymph-node fluid aspirate, and blood and lymph-node aspirate can be inoculated into laboratory animals. Clean-bred triatomid bugs are fed on patient or his blood, and trypanosomes develop in the bugs' hind-guts in about 2 weeks.

A specific complement-fixation test is now available for the diagnosis of this condition.

Histological identification of the infection can be made on biopsy material or at post-mortem.

As in the African varieties, anaemia develops with monocytosis.

METAZOAN INFECTIONS

NEMATODES

Ascariasis

Diagnosis of infection can be confirmed by the demonstration of ova of *Ascaris lumbricoides* in the stools. These ova are mature within 1–2 weeks after shedding and remain viable in suitable conditions for months or even years. In 5 per cent of cases only male worms are present in the gut, and in these cases no ova will be found; therefore the diagnosis will be made by the identification of the worms in the faeces after therapy. Rarely, embryos may be coughed up in the sputum when the larvae migrate from intestines to lungs, and hence to be reswallowed down the oesophagus, during their 2-month cycle of maturation.

The intestinal bleeding causes hypochromic anaemia with moderate neutrophilia and often marked eosinophilia.

Maturation cycle in man lasts 2 months.

Seventy five per cent of patients given piperazine citrate 75 mg/kg body weight up to a maximum single dose of 5 g, are cleared.

Capillariasis

1. CAPILLARIA HEPATICA INFECTION [R]

Diagnosis of this condition, characterized by hepatomegaly with pneumonitis and fever, possibly also with ascites, is confirmed by the demonstration of the specific ova in liver biopsy material. The condition is accompanied by a leucocytosis with eosinophilia.

TESTS PROVIDING USEFUL NEGATIVE RESULTS

Tests for the presence of toxocariasis, or the invasive stages of ascariasis or schistosomiasis are negative.

2. CAPILLARIASIS PHILIPPINENSIS INFECTION

Diagnosis of this condition, caused by ingestion of raw or inadequately cooked Apogon fish in the Philippines and Far East (fish infected from human sewage), and characterized by intermittent diarrhoea and malabsorption, is confirmed by the demonstration of the ova in patients' stools.

Dracunculosis (Dracontiasis)

Diagnosis of infection with *Dracunculus medinensis* can be confirmed by applying a drop of water to a fresh cutaneous ulcer, and after a few minutes aspirating the fluid and examining it for larvae. The body of the worm is visible and palpable under the skin, and the head of the worm can be identified in an uncomplicated ulcer. The life span of this organism in man is 12 months.

During migration of the gravid female, eosinophilia indicates an allergic reaction.

Enterobiasis (Oxyuriasis; Pinworm Infection)

Diagnosis of infection with *Oxyuris vermicularis* can be confirmed by the demonstration of ova in perianal scrapings (taken early in the morning, as the gravid female lays her eggs in that area during the night). Ova may also be found in finger-nail scrapings, as the infection is associated with pruritus ani.

Adult worms may occasionally be found in appendices removed at operation.

There may be neutrophilia. Eosinophilia is fairly common.

Maturation cycle in man lasts 15–26 days.

Filariasas

Wucheria bancrofti and Brugia malayi
Diagnosis of infection can be confirmed by demonstration of microfilaria in blood films taken at night and by histological examination of biopsy material. Maturation time in man is 2–3 weeks. Calcified worms can be seen on x-ray in glands or elephantoid tissue.

Loa loa
Diagnosis of infection can be confirmed by the demonstration of microfilaria in blood films taken about midday. Occasionally adult filaria can be seen under the conjunctiva or in biopsy material of a swelling. Maturation time is 10–12 days in man.

Onchocerca volvulus
Diagnosis of infection can be confirmed by the demonstration of adult filaria in excised nodules, or of microfilaria in shavings of skin. Maturation time in man is 6 days or more.

Intradermal and complement-fixation tests may be useful in filarial infections other than those due to *Onchocerca*. The tests are group specific, not species specific.

Eosinophilia may be found, with allergic reaction.

Hookworm Infection (Ancylostomiasis)

Diagnosis of infection with either *Ancylostoma duodenale* (Europe, N Africa, India, SE Asia) or *Necator americanus* (USA, Central America, Central and SW Africa, Oceania, SE Asia) can be confirmed by the finding of ova in the stools. Iron-deficient anaemia develops following continuing bloodloss, and eosinophilia is common.

Maturation cycle in man takes 35 days.

Strongyloidiasis (Strongyloidosis)

Diagnosis of infection with *Strongyloides stercoralis* can be confirmed by the finding of rhabditiform and occasionally filariform larvae in fresh stools and occasionally in sputum. Larvae will develop, if specimen of faeces is left to stand.

In cases with pneumonitis, sputum may be tinged with blood. Leucopenia may follow an initial neutrophilia. Eosinophilia up to 40 per cent may be found, an expression of the severe general allergic state set up.

Maturation cycle in man lasts 17 days.

Hyperinfection with *Strongyloides stercoralis* with invasive filariform larvae, producing lesions in the colon, lungs and liver, have been described in patients being treated with immunosuppressive drugs.

Toxocara Infections

In the United Kingdom over 20 per cent of all cats and dogs are infected with *Toxocara catis* or *Toxocara canis* respectively. Puppies are infective about 3 weeks after birth, and contact between children and puppies before they have been dewormed, and nursing bitches should be avoided. Soil in public parks is often infected with viable *T. canis* eggs. Perhaps 2 per cent of the United Kingdom population have been infected and most infections are subclinical.

The disease is characterized by respiratory symptoms, enlarged liver and abdominal pain, splenomegaly, lymphadenopathy, ocular lesions, and, rarely, encephalopathy or myocarditis. There is marked eosinophilia with increased serum IgM and IgE levels. Positive diagnosis can be confirmed using ELISA and fluorescent antibody tests in the acute stage, when rising antibody titres may be demonstrated. The larvae of the nematodes are surrounded by fibrous tissue and fail to develop in the human.

Trichinosis (Trichiniasis; Trichinelliasis)

Diagnosis of infection with *Trichinella spiralis* can be confirmed by the finding of adult worms and larvae during the period 7–14 days after ingestion of infected meat, during the phase of enteritis and invasion.

Later, the diagnosis can be confirmed by histological investigation of cysts in muscles. At this stage, examination of the stools for ova is of no value.

Using trichinal cyst extract as antigen, the Bachman intradermal skin test can be used. The skin test becomes positive at the end of the third week after infection, and remains positive for up to 7 years. Some cross-reactions occur with members of the same genus (e.g., *Trichuris* infections). Precipitin tests on the patient's serum also become positive by the end of the third week, and remain positive for a year. Flocculation tests, or better, fluorescent antibody tests are also positive.

Neutrophilia with eosinophilia may occur by the tenth day after infection. By the third or fourth week very high eosinophil counts may be found. Serum aminotransferase activities are increased.

Encysted larvae may be demonstrated in infected meat.

Trichocephaliasis (Trichuriasis; Whipworm Infection)

Diagnosis of infection with *Trichuris trichiura* can be confirmed by the demonstration of ova in faeces—concentration methods may be needed. Surgical specimens of the appendix and caecum may contain larvae and adult worms.

The maturation cycle in man is about 3 months, and the ova mature in moist soil after shedding in 3–5 weeks.

Eosinophilia occurs in about a quarter of cases.

CESTODES

Beef Tape-worm Infection

Diagnosis of infection with *Taenia saginata* can be confirmed by the demonstration of gravid segments, ova, and scolices in stools. Ova can be demonstrated on cellophane swabs of the perianal skin.

Cysticercosis is unknown with *Taenia saginata* infection. Eosinophilia occurs in perhaps 10 per cent of cases. Maturation time in man is 8–10 weeks, and its life span is apparently up to 25 years.

Fish Tape-worm Infection

Diagnosis of infection with *Dibothriocephalus latus* can be confirmed by the demonstration of ova in the stools and by identification of the adult worm after treatment. In patients in whom the adult worms have attached high up in the small intestines, segments of adult worms may be vomited, and these patients are also liable to develop megaloblastic anaemia with low serum B_{12} levels, as the worms appear to be able to extract the vitamin from the patient's diet.

The maturation time of the worm in man is about 3 weeks, and it has a life span of several years.

Pork Tape-worm Infection

Diagnosis of infection with *Taenia solium* can be confirmed by the demonstration of gravid segments of the worm, ova and scolices in faeces. Histological examination of cysticeri (infection with larvae) which may occur in any site also confirms infection. Eosinophilia is commoner when worms are present in the intestines than when cysticercosis has developed.

The maturation time in man in 3 months, and apparently its life span can be up to 25 years.

Hydatid Disease

Diagnosis of hydatid disease can be confirmed by a complement-fixation test, which is positive in up to 80 per cent of cases. Titres of more than 1:8 suggest hydatid infection. The complement-fixation test is best performed using optimal dilution of hydatid cyst fluid.

Using serum, the haemagglutination and indirect fluorescent antibody tests are more frequently used.

The Casoni skin test is no longer used.

Histological examination of a resected cyst can confirm the diagnosis, as the cyst contains brood capsules and scolices, enabling the identification of *Echinococcus granulosus* and *Echinococcus multilocularis*. At operation it is very important that the cyst should be removed totally and intact, as leakage or rupture can lead to severe allergic reaction, anaphylactic shock, and secondary implantation (e.g. in peritoneal cavity).

TESTS OF PROGRESS

The complement-fixation test, using serum, falls after surgical removal, to normal by 3 months. The haemagglutination and indirect fluorescent antibody tests are very sensitive, and are useful in the detection of recurrence after apparent complete surgical removal.

Hymenolepis Nana Infection

Diagnosis of infection with *Hymenolepis nana* can be confirmed by the demonstration of ova in the faeces. With heavy infection it can be associated with enteritis and anaemia, with eosinophilia. Ova are passed in the stools 30 days after infection.

TREMATODES

Schistosomiasis

INTESTINAL AND VISCERAL TYPES

Diagnosis of infection with *Schistosoma mansoni* or *Schistosoma japonicum* can be confirmed by the finding of ova in the faeces in the acute stage. Later, ova may be found in scrapings of rectal and colonic granulomas.

VESICAL TYPE

Diagnosis of infection with *Schistosoma haematobium* can be confirmed by the finding of ova in urine in the acute stage. Later, ova may be found in scrapings of lesions in the bladder wall. Ova may also appear in the faeces, following rectal involvement. The skin test, using antigen prepared from infected snail liver, is reliable, but the test, once positive, remains positive for years. Complement-fixing antibody (group antigen) may be positive in the early stages of the disease. It is less specific in the later stages of the disease.

In both types of the disease, liver biopsy may show ova with localized granulomatous reaction, portal tract infiltration, or diffuse fibrosis in up to 40 per cent of cases.

Severe iron-deficiency anaemia, eosinophilia, and raised ESR are found in both types. Haematuria, pyuria and chyluria occur in the vesical type in addition.

Sheep Liver-fluke Infection

Diagnosis of infection with *Fasciola hepatica* can be confirmed by the demonstration of ova in faeces. Eosinophilia is common. With increase in serum gammaglobulin, the ESR is increased. Liver biopsy may show focal granulomas, with eosinophilic infiltration of necrotic foci.

The fasciola complement-fixation test is positive, as is the double-diffusion precipitin test.

TESTS PROVIDING USEFUL NEGATIVE RESULTS

The Casoni and hydatid complement-fixation tests are negative.

Clonorchis Infection

Diagnosis of infection with *Clonorchis sinensis* following ingestion of infected, raw or undercooked fish can be confirmed by the demonstration of ova in the stools or in bile aspirate.

Eosinophilia occurs, and later changes due to cirrhosis, portal hypertension, and occasionally pancreatic duct obstruction occur.

Infection with Fasciolopsis buski

Diagnosis of infection with *Fasciolopsis buski* can be confirmed by the demonstration of ova, and sometimes adult trematodes in the faeces. Anaemia may develop following bleeding and eosinophilia is common.

The complement-fixation test available, gives cross-reaction with *Fasciola hepatica*.

Larvae mature in man in 3–4 weeks.

Lung-fluke Infection

Diagnosis of infection with *Paragonimus westermani* can be confirmed by demonstration of ova in sputum or faeces. Using extract of adult flukes as antigen a complement-fixation test is useful in confirming the diagnosis.

Eosinophilia occurs. Later, with development of lung damage, changes due to bronchiectasis or lung abscess may be found.

ANIMAL VECTORS OF HUMAN DISEASE

Domestic Dog (Domestic Cat—but much less risk, as the cat is cleaner in its habits)
Rabies
Tick typhus (Mediterranean)
Toxoplasma gondii
Kala-azar
Leptospirosis
Toxocara
Microsporum canis (Ringworm)
Echinococcus

Ancylostoma caninum and *Ancylostoma braziliense* (creeping eruption)
Birds
Ornithosis/psittacosis
Domestic Animals
Brucellosis (cattle, goats, pigs)
Anthrax (cattle and sheep)
Tuberculosis (bovine)
Leptospirosis (pig)
Salmonella (especially battery farmer)
Erysipeloid
Tetanus
Encephalitis (Russian spring/summer, and louping ill)
Cow-pox
Hand-foot-mouth (distinct from foot-and-mouth disease)
Orf (from lambs)
Q-fever
Trichophyton infection
Actinomycosis (?)
Taenia saginata (cattle)
Taenia solium (pigs)
Fasciola hepatica (sheep)
Trichinella (pigs)
Wild Animals
Plague (rats)
Salmonella (rats in granaries)
Rat-bite fever
Leptospirosis (rats)
Tick-fevers (via rodents)
Murine typhus ⎫
Entamoeba histolytica ⎪
Giardia lamblia ⎬ monkeys
Schistosomiasis ⎪
Virus-B encephalomyelitis ⎭
Yellow fever
Fish tape-worm
Salmonella in many wild animals
Virus encephalitis virus carried by birds
Cryptococcus ⎫
Histoplasma ⎬ in pigeon droppings

ARTHROPODS AND HUMAN DISEASE

Myiasis (Maggot Infestation)
Diagnosis can be confirmed by the finding of eggs of flies, or maggots in wounds.

Jigger Fleas (Tunga Penetrans)
Diagnosis of burrowing into the skin by this flea is confirmed by removal and identification of the adult female. The adult female burrows into the skin,

usually of the toes, laying her eggs and then dying. Intense itching and secondary infection occur.

Pediculosis

Diagnosis can be confirmed by the finding of lice, concretions and eggs of lice on affected hairs.

Pneumocystosis

Diagnosis can be confirmed by the finding of mites or cysts in sputum or at post-mortem in alveolar exudate in lung sections. Complement-fixing antibodies can be detected, and many cases have a marked eosinophilia.

Scabies

Diagnosis can be confirmed by the removal and identification of mites from the inner end of epidermal tunnels, especially found between the fingers and the toes.

Scorpion Sting

Following being stung by a scorpion there is marked neutrophilia. Serum creatine phosphokinase activity is often increased. In severe reaction (e.g. in young children), acute pancreatitis, acute haemolytic anaemia and defibrination syndrome may develop.

Spider Bite

Following a spider's bite (by a poisonous variety), neutrophilia occurs, and an acute haemolytic anaemia with thrombocytopenia may develop.

Hornet Sting (Vespa Affinis)

If a large volume of venom is injected into the patient (i.e. multiple stings), toxic muscle damage results, with myoglobinaemia and myoglobinuria present in severe cases. Serum alanine and aspartate aminotransferase activities, creatine phosphokinase activity and lactate dehydrogenase activity are increased (i.e. released from damaged muscle).

There may be nephrotoxic effects with developing renal failure also.

Bee Sting

Reactions to bee stings, when they occur, are usually acute anaphylactic. Specific IgE (allergic) antibody to bee venom and IgG (blocking) antibody to bee venom can be measured in patients clinically sensitive to bee stings. A rising titre of IgG antibody indicates a decline in the degree of hypersensitivity, either occurring naturally or following immunization.

Bee keepers who have a rising IgE antibody titre should be offered immunization.

Wasp Sting

Reactions to wasp stings, when they occur, are usually acute anaphylactic. Radioimmunoassay test (RAST) is available for the detection of IgE (allergic) and IgG (blocking) antibodies, as with bee venom.

Tick Paralysis

Various hard ticks can attach themselves to the human skin, especially of children, and inject neurotoxin present in their saliva. Varying degrees of paralysis and unconsciousness may develop 5–10 days after attachment.

Diagnosis of the condition can be confirmed by discovery and removal of the tick, with recovery of the patient (unless there is a second tick still attached).

TESTS PROVIDING USEFUL NEGATIVE RESULTS

The CSF protein content and cell count remain normal.

4 Physical Injury, Malignancy, Dermatological Conditions

PHYSICAL INJURY

Asbestosis

Diagnosis is supported by the finding of evidence of progressive lung function impairment with the presence of 'asbestos bodies' in the sputum. 'Asbestos bodies' are long golden-yellow or brown structures, consisting of asbestos fibres coated with iron-containing protein, usually segmented along their length and bulbar at their ends. These 'bodies' indicate exposure to asbestos, and are not proof of disease due to inhaled asbestos.

Pyrexia

With each increase of 1 °C above normal the BMR increases by approximately +13 per cent. Urine urobilinogen output may be increased. Iron absorption is profoundly depressed. There may be achlorhydria or hypochlorhydria, which recovers with return of the body temperature to normal.

Heat Stroke

Diagnosis is confirmed by measurement of the body temperature. Sweating ceases even though the body temperature exceeds 40·6 °C. Progressive haemoconcentration, hypernatraemia and increasing plasma osmolality, is accompanied by oliguria (eventually anuria) and rising blood urea.

Disseminated intravascular coagulopathy may develop up to 48 hours after thermal injury, with increasing APTT, BCR, and FDPs, with falling plasma fibrinogen and thrombocytopenia (below $100 \times 10^9/l$).

Burns

In the peripheral blood, following burns, the whole-blood haemoglobin concentration varies with the balance of fluid loss, bleeding into the burn, dehydration, treatment with plasma, etc. Schistocytes (fragmented red cells with a diameter of less than 3 μ) appear in the peripheral blood a few hours after a severe burn. Spherocytes may also appear. In severe burns some red cells may be so badly damaged during passage through the burnt area that some D-positive cases temporarily appear to be D-negative on grouping (due to heat lability of the D antigen). Destruction of damaged circulating cells causes an increased plasma haemoglobin, with haemoglobinuria if the plasma haemoglobin exceeds 140 mg/100 ml. Within a few hours of a burn, the reticulocyte count rises to 2–4 per cent, and an increase in the siderocyte count has been reported. In summary, some red cells are destroyed in the burnt area, others survive for a few hours as fragments, others, moderately damaged, circulate as spherocytes with increased saline fragility. Later, erythropoiesis is depressed, remaining so until the burnt area has healed.

The TWBC increases within a few hours of the burn, with a neutrophilia peak at 6–12 hours. With colonization of the burnt area by bacteria later, there is a second neutrophilia. In the early stages, neutrophils frequently contain toxic granules and Döhle bodies may be seen. In some cases there is a leukaemoid reaction with excessively high white-cell counts. Leucocyte antibodies increase rapidly, regardless of thermal agent, patient's age or sex, or methods of resuscitation. Peripheral blood eosinophils increase within a few hours temporarily, with a second increase about 4–6 weeks later (? allergic reaction). Lymphopenia occurs immediately after a burn and tends to persist for a few days. Thrombocytopenia occurs immediately, with subsequent rise to peak counts by 7–10 days.

Plasma fibrinogen increases after a burn, whilst various clotting factors may be temporarily reduced following loss into the burnt area and possibly impaired production by the liver. Plasma fibrinolysin activity increases after a burn.

The serum total protein concentration varies very much with the rate of loss into the burnt area, type and rate of resuscitation, dehydration, etc. but more albumin is lost via the burnt area than are other protein fractions. Similarly, the blood urea varies with the clinical state, tending to rise with dehydration plus catabolism of damaged tissues. With severe shock renal tubular necrosis may develop. With the red-cell destruction, plus muscle damage, the serum bilirubin may be raised during the first few days.

Some patients develop hyperglycaemia: (a) In pre-existing diabetes the insulin requirement is increased. (b) Adrenal medullary hyperglycaemia following release of adrenaline in the first few hours. (c) Adrenal cortical hyperglycaemia developing after a few days. In severe burns the patient tends to develop the 'sick cell syndrome' with loss of intracellular potassium and increasing protein catabolism; this is being treated with intensive glucose plus insulin therapy in some centres.

Peptides from the burnt tissue circulate, resulting in increased plasma amino acids. Blood vitamin C virtually disappears until healing is complete, and serum properdin activity is depressed.

In the urine, amino-acid output is increased, with both free amino acids and peptides. Similarly, derived from damaged muscle, the urine creatine output is increased. The body is in marked negative nitrogen balance. As a further manifestation of the metabolic changes associated with the 'sick cell syndrome' urine sodium output is reduced with increased potassium output. Following red-cell breakdown, plus interference in erythropoiesis, urine protoporphyrin and coproporphyrin may be increased.

Infection of Wounds following Trauma and Burns

Identification of infecting organisms can be determined by microscopy and culture of material from wounds or burnt areas, taken by swabs, preferably moistened with broth if the surface to be sampled is dry. If the raw area is covered by granulation tissue or eschar, viable bacteria may be present beneath this, although the surface may be sterile.

With large areas, separate swabs should be used for different sites.

In extensive burning, the pattern has gradually changed from death in the early stages from severe shock, dehydration, and hypovolaemia, to the present state of survival for the first 2 or 3 weeks following adequate resuscitative measures, rehydration, and correction of electrolyte balance, followed by death from gross infection of the burnt area.

The pattern of organisms isolated from wounds and burns in a hospital can be useful in cross-infection studies, e.g. an increase in the incidence of a particular phage-type of staphylococcus, *Pseudomonas pyocyanea*, *Streptococcus pyogenes*, etc.

Opportunistic Infection

Infection with unusual organisms, or by organisms usually regarded as saprophytes, occurs in patients with compromised immunity, and also in:
1. Intensive Therapy Units.
2. Post-tracheostomy.
3. Patients on ventilators.
4. Central venous lines.
5. Humidifiers.
6. 'Routine prophylactic' administration of antibiotics, especially:
    a. 'Covering' urethral catheterization.
    b. Prolonged antibiotic therapy in respiratory infection.
    c. Acute leukaemia.

Frost-bite

Apart from local damage to frozen parts, haemoglobinuria and raised plasma-haemoglobin levels occur on warming the patient.

Severe Hypothermia

Hypothermia is defined as a body core temperature below 35 °C, and can occur in premature infants in cold rooms, the elderly without food or heating, cases of hypothyroidism, drug overdose, or accidental exposure to cold. Acute pancreatitis may develop, with abnormally raised serum amylase activity. Cold may damage muscle, resulting in abnormally raised serum creatine phosphokinase activity. Varying increases in serum alaninine and aspartate aminotransferases, and alpha-hydroxybutyrate dehydrogenase activities may occur. Renal damage may also be detected.

TESTS OF PROGRESS

During recovery, tissue anoxia may develop during rewarming, with the development of metabolic acidosis and low plasma pH.

Immersion in Water (Near-drowning)

Following inhalation of water, the Pa_{O_2} falls dramatically. Inhalation of more than 22 ml/kg body weight is fatal. Salt water perfuses the alveoli, whereas fresh water removes surfactant and causes alveolar collapse. In most cases there are no significant changes in plasma sodium, potassium, chloride, haematocrit or whole blood haemoglobin concentration.

TESTS OF PROGRESS

Secondary drowning may develop 15 minutes–72 hours after removal from water, and this consists of loss of surfactant activity in the lungs. There is deterioration in pulmonary function with deficient gaseous exchange.

Exercise

ACUTE

Immediately after prolonged severe exercise, blood lactate is increased, with plasma pyruvate concentration rising, especially in untrained subjects. Serum creatine phosphokinase activity is also increased, again to higher levels in the untrained. While plasma fibrinogen and prothrombin time remain unchanged, the total white blood cell count increases, and the APTT and euglobulin lysis time are reduced. Plasma Factor VIIIc and fibrin degradation products (FDPs) are increased. Haemoglobinuria occurs following long periods of running over hard surfaces (e.g. road racing). Proteinuria is very common in normal subjects, even after moderate exercise.

CHRONIC (TRAINED INDIVIDUALS)

There is more effective distribution of blood to muscles and a greater extraction of oxygen occurs. The degree of lactic acidosis is less, and there is evidence that serum HDL levels rise (with ? a fall in serum VLDL).

Post-convulsion

After very severe convulsions, myoglobinuria may rarely occur. Petechial haemorrhages in the skin may be seen, which are said to have occurred because of increased capillary fragility associated with anoxia. Similarly the CSF protein content may be moderately increased.

Crush Injury

Evidence of damage to tissues following crush injury includes increase in plasma-potassium concentration and in serum aspartate aminotransferase and creatine phosphokinase activity, released from damaged muscle. Myoglobin from damaged muscle cells may appear in the urine, with increased urine creatine.

There is a neutrophilia with eosinopenia and a fall in the platelet count soon after the injury, with diminution in plasma fibrinogen. After a few days plasma fibrinogen increases and thrombocytosis is found.

In very severe damage, renal damage follows with azotaemia. The clearance of myoglobin from plasma is so rapid that myoglobin should be looked for in the urine, and not the plasma.

Head Injury

Following head injury or after some intracranial surgery, damage to the hypothalamus may lead to either (1) Hypernatraemia due to dehydration and/or salt retention, or (2) Hyponatraemia due to 'salt wasting', or inappropriate antidiuretic hormone syndrome.

The blood-glucose concentration may fall, or there may be impairment of glucose tolerance with hyperglycaemia and glycosuria.

The CSF may contain excess red cells and increased protein concentration.

Irradiation Injury

Following irradiation, evidence of tissue damage is found which is in proportion to the severity of the damage.

Within a few hours the peripheral blood lymphocytes begin to fall, reaching minimum values by the fourth day, and disappearing altogether if a very large dose of radiation has been received. Peripheral blood neutrophils fall to very low levels by early in the second week, tending to rise again by the tenth to twelfth days and falling a second time with minimal counts by 5–6 weeks. The platelet count falls within a few days of irradiation damage, reaching a minimum by 28–32 days. The red-cell count falls gradually for 26–28 days, when there is a much more rapid fall accompanied by bleeding associated with the low platelet count. At this time, the bleeding time is prolonged in proportion to the depression of the platelet count. There may be nucleated red cells and early myelocytes in the peripheral blood.

Serum aspartate aminotransferase activity may be increased with increased alpha- and gammaglobulins.

Urine creatine output and amino-acid output are increased with increased β-amino-isobutyric acid and taurine.

TESTS OF PROGRESS

With recovery, the peripheral blood recovers in the same order as it deteriorated. Lymphocytes recover first, followed by neutrophils, then platelets, and finally red cells. Progressive and continuous fall in all elements indicates irreversible aplastic anaemia.

Following recovery, subsequent development of either acute or chronic myeloid leukaemia (but never lymphatic leukaemia) may occur. Apart from this, hypoplastic anaemia affecting different elements in the blood may develop (e.g. persistent moderate anemia with neutropenia or thrombocytopenia). Chromosomal studies may reveal a much higher incidence than normal of 'breaks'.

High-voltage Electric Shock

Following muscle damage, serum creatine phosphokinase activity and serum aspartate and alanine aminotransferase activities are increased. Neutrophilia is common for the first 24 hours after damage. In severe cases myoglobinuria may occur.

Post-traumatic Shock

Following traumatic shock, various changes may occur; these changes are not of diagnostic significance, but they will affect results due to other disease processes. The changes which may occur in the haemoglobin and haematocrit vary with the combined effects of haemorrhage and redistribution of the body fluids. There is neutrophilia with lymphocytopenia and eosinopenia, with a temporary increase in the platelet count. Both the blood glucose and lactic acid increase for a short time.

Following damage to tissues with release of intracellular enzymes, serum lactate dehydrogenase and aspartate aminotransferase activities increase. If there has been much muscle damage, then serum creatine phosphokinase activity increases.

Plasma potassium concentrations may be increased as a result of release of intracellular potassium following tissue damage and also reduced urinary flow.

Protein appears in the urine. Later, if there has been bone injury, urinary calcium output increases. The body is in a state of negative nitrogen balance.

Postoperative State

The changes which may occur after operation depend on the duration of the operation, its nature and severity, as well as the condition of the patient.

Immediately after the operation the platelet count falls, rising after the fourth day to reach peak values by the tenth to fourteenth days after operation and falling to normal subsequently. The adhesive platelet count is also at its peak at the tenth to fourteenth days. The plasma fibrinogen increases to peak values about the fifth day, falling to normal by 3 weeks. Similarly, the heparin-retarded clotting time and the plasma-activated partial thromboplastin clotting times reach their lowest values about the fifth day, and return to normal by the end of the second week. At the same time fibrinolytic activity in the blood is increased after operation.

Immediately after operation there is neutrophilia with eosinopenia and lymphopenia, which lasts for the first 2 or 3 days. Serum iron is reduced, the normal diurnal variation is lost, and iron absorption is reduced. C-reactive protein appears in the blood about 12–18 hours after operation, persists for a few days, and then disappears.

Depending on the degree of tissue damage, the activity of serum lactate dehydrogenase, aspartate aminotransferase and creatine phosphokinase may be variably increased.

During the first 48 hours there is water and sodium retention with reduced urine output, with a high specific gravity. Normal rates of excretion return after 2–3 days. There is an increase in the excretion of potassium, which is related to the degree of injury and to the presence of any traumatic shock, and the body is in a state of negative nitrogen balance. Fluid overload, particularly in the elderly, during the first 48 hours after surgical operation, results in hyponatraemia with overhydration. Subsequent treatment with diuretics increases the severity of the hyponatraemia.

Snake-bite

1. Elapidae (cobras, mambas). Very poisonous snakes. Poisons include powerful neurotoxic substances and powerful haemolysins.
2. Colubridae (tree snakes). Not often dangerous to man.
3. Viperidae (vipers). Venoms contain various substances capable of causing rapid thrombosis.
4. Sea snakes. Venom contains a tissue-destroying substance causing lysis of muscle with liberation of myoglobin into the plasma and rapidly into the urine.

Following snake-bite, infection of the wound is very common. There is a non-specific neutrophilia with normal or reduced platelet counts. Coagulation defects may develop with the onset of a disseminated intravascular coagulopathy. With reduced renal function, the blood urea and plasma potassium may rise. The urine output drops, and protein is excreted in the urine, with casts and red cells.

MALIGNANCY

Carcinomatosis

Diagnosis of carcinoma, whether primary or secondary, depends on the demonstration of carcinoma cells in: surgical biopsy material; bone-marrow biopsy material; pleural fluid, ascitic fluid, sputum, gastric washings, CSF, etc. The presence of carcinoma in the body can cause a great variety of changes, with great variation in degree.

A moderate refractory anaemia may develop and there may be neutrophilia. Serum iron falls with reduced TIBC and with marrow stainable iron present. Rarely, an autoimmune haemolytic anaemia may develop.

Serum alphaglobulins, serum hepatoglobins, and serum mucoproteins may be increased.

A. With Secondary Deposits in Bone: Following destruction of bone and local repair processes, serum alkaline phosphatase and non-specific acid phosphatase activities may be increased. If destruction of bone is rapid, then serum calcium levels are increased and the urinary output of calcium is increased. Leucoerythroblastic anaemia may develop, if the marrow is invaded, and carcinoma cells may be found in bone-marrow aspirates.

B. With Secondary Deposits in the Liver: Serum alkaline phosphatase activity is increased, with increases in serum aspartate aminotransferase, lactate dehydrogenase and leucine aminopeptidase activities.

Bilirubin may be detectable in the urine, and some cases become progressively more jaundiced as secondary deposits interfere with the free flow of bile.

C. With Intracranial Deposits: The CSF lactate dehydrogenase activity may be increased with intracerebral or meningeal deposits. Meningeal carcinoma may be associated with a moderate increase in CSF cell count, increased CSF protein concentration, and a very low CSF glucose. Careful cytological examination may reveal carcinoma cells in the CSF.

D. With Deposits invading the Pleural Space: The pleural fluid lactate dehydrogenase activity is increased, and cytological examination of the fluid may reveal carcinoma cells.

E. Malignant Ascites: The ascitic fluid is often bloodstained and its lactate dehydrogenase activity is increased. Cytological examination may reveal the presence of carcinoma cells.

Unusual Manifestations of Malignancy

1. *Ectopic ACTH syndrome*, i.e. ectopic hormone production by malignant cells: Plasma cortisol concentrations are increased, with loss of diurnal variation. Plasma potassium falls. Carbohydrate intolerance is present and there is polyuria with thirst.

2. *Inappropriate ADH syndrome*: Plasma sodium concentration falls, with low plasma osmolality and increased urine osmolality in relation to the plasma.

3. *Hypercalcaemia*: Ectopic secretion of parathormone.

4. *Spontaneous hypoglycaemia*: Pancreatic beta-cell tumour secreting inappropriate insulin.

5. *Thyrotoxicosis*.

6. *Erythrocytosis*:
   - *a.* Erythropoietin-secreting tumour.
   - *b.* Cerebellar haemangioblastoma.
   - *c.* Hepatoma.
   - *d.* Phaeochromocytoma.

7. *Precocious puberty*: Secretion of gonadotrophins.

8. *Gynaecomastia*: Gonadotrophins secreted cause rise in gonadal oestrogen levels.

9. *Multiple hormone system*.

10. *Carcinomatous neuropathy and myopathy*.

11. *Polymyositis, dermatomyositis, scleroderma*.

12. *Acanthosis nigra*.

13. *Arterial and venous thromboses*.

14. *Hypertrophic pulmonary osteoarthropathy*.

15. *Zollinger–Ellison syndrome*.

Metastatic Mucin-secreting Carcinoma and Micro-angiopathic Haemolytic Anaemia

Severe haemolytic anaemia may develop, with marked anisocytosis and poikilocytosis of red cells, and fragmented red cells in the peripheral blood. Fibrin degradation productions may be found in the serum.

Lymphoma

Diagnosis may be confirmed by microscopy of suitable lymph-gland biopsy material. Anaemia is a frequent finding, and this may be leucoerythroblastic.

There may be leucopenia, or occasionally there may be marked lymphocytosis. Lymphoblasts may be found in 'buffy-layer' preparations of the peripheral blood or in bone-marrow aspirates.

Occasionally an autoimmune haemolytic anaemia develops. Rarely there is pancytopenia.

Over 20 per cent of lymphoma cases excrete monoclonal light-chains in the urine. This can be used as a tumour marker for response to treatment.

Lymphosarcoma

Diagnosis may be confirmed by microscopy of surgical biopsy material. Lymphoblasts and lymphosarcoma cells may be found in the peripheral blood, especially in 'buffy-layer' preparations and in bone-marrow aspirates.

Anaemia develops in many cases and may. be leucoerythroblastic. Occasionally an autoimmune haemolytic anaemia develops. Rarely there is pancytopenia.

Over 20 per cent of lymphoma cases excrete monoclonal light-chains in the urine. This can be used as a tumour marker for response to treatment.

Malignant Melanoma

Diagnosis of malignant melanoma is confirmed by histological examination of surgical biopsy material. In some late cases with disseminated disease, the urine contains colourless melanogen, which oxidizes to black melanin on standing.

The presence of oncofetal melanoma antigen in the patient's serum can be a useful tumour marker during treatment.

Neuroblastoma; Ganglioneuroma; Sympathoblastoma

Diagnosis of this condition, characterized by abdominal enlargement with pain, and tumour developing in the adrenal medulla in one-third of cases, retropleural or retroperitoneal in the remaining two-thirds, is confirmed by histological examination of surgical biopsy material.

Diagnosis is supported by the finding of increased excretion of at least one of: 3-methoxy-4-hydroxymandelic acid, dopamine and/or homovanillic acid in the urine.

In young children, the bone marrow may contain tumour cells.

TESTS OF PROGRESS

Follow-up estimations of urinary excretion of VMA can be used to detect recurrence of a tumour after surgical resection.

Sarcoma

Diagnosis may be confirmed by the demonstration of clusters of sarcoma cells in bone-marrow aspirates. Rarely, sarcoma cells have been isolated from the blood. In cases with destruction of bone, urinary calcium output is increased and serum alkaline phosphatase activity may be increased. In reticulum-cell sarcoma with bone-marrow involvement, the abnormal reticulum cells may be found in bone-marrow aspirates.

Rarely, cases of sarcoma, especially reticulum-cell sarcoma, may develop and auto-immune haemolytic anaemia with 'warm' or 'cold' auto-antibodies.

Thymoma

Thymoma has been decribed as being associated with:
- *a*. Cushing's syndrome
- *b*. Myasthenia gravis
- *c*. Various forms of agammaglobulinaemia and dysglobulinaemia
- *d*. Erythroid hyperplasia
- *e*. Rarely, thrombocytopenia, neutropenia, or erythroid hypoplasia

Carcinoid Syndrome

Diagnosis of the presence of carcinoid tumours (90 per cent in the ileocaecal region, but also occurring in lung, pancreas, stomach, duodenum) characterized by attacks of flushing, abdominal discomfort and diarrhoea, skin lesions, cardiac and pulmonary symptoms, is confirmed by the finding of a urinary excretion of 5-HIAA exceeding 150 µmol/24 hours.

TESTS OF PROGRESS

Following successful removal of the tumour, urine 5-HIAA excretion can be used as a tumour marker, excretion increasing with recurrence.

TESTS PROVIDING USEFUL NEGATIVE RESULTS

Rectal carcinoid tumours do not secrete 5-HIAA. Many drugs and foods increase urine 5-HIAA excretion in normal subjects (e.g. bananas, tomatoes, pineapples, walnuts, reserpine, nicotine, and many cough medicines). Phenothiazine drugs depress 5-HIAA excretion.

DERMATOLOGICAL CONDITIONS

Acrodermatitis Enteropathica [AR] [R]

Diagnosis of this rare inherited condition, characterized by erythematous vesicobullous dermatitis of the extremities with acral and orificial skin lesions, alopecia, diarrhoea and vomiting in infants, is confirmed by the finding of serum zinc levels below 6 µmol/l (normal = 10–17 µmol/l). Paronychia, nail dystrophy and ocular symptoms also occur.

TESTS OF PROGRESS

Prolonged feeding with human breast milk may result in a remission. Treatment with zinc supplements causes clinical recovery.

The possibility of severe zinc deficiency, and very low zinc concentration in the mother's breast milk should be excluded.

Angioneurotic Oedema

Eosinophilia is frequently found. In hereditary angioneurotic oedema, abnormally low levels of C1 esterase inhibitors (complement system) are found.

Cutis Laxa [XR] [R]

Diagnosis of this condition, which is complicated by emphysema with frequent pulmonary infections and cor pulmonale, gastrointestinal diverticula and hernia, is aided by the finding of abnormally low serum copper levels. Skin biopsy and tissue-cell culture reveals abnormally reduced lysyl oxidase activity.

Dermatitis Herpetiformis

TESTS ASSOCIATED WITH THE CONDITION

It has been found that about two-thirds of patients suffering from dermatitis herpetiformis have also an enteropathy similar to adult coeliac disease, as revealed by intestinal biopsy samples. Serum IgM is reduced in many cases and IgA deposits occur in the upper dermis below the basal membrane, when skin-biopsy samples are examined by immunofluorescent techniques.

Antibodies are present in the serum against connective tissue (in 17 per cent of patients), against cell nuclei (in 34 per cent of patients), belonging to the IgG or IgM class.

The significance of these findings is not yet clear.

Eczema

Steatorrhoea is often present until the rash has cleared. Eosinophilia may occur during acute exacerbations.

Epidermolysis Bullosa Letatelis [AR] [R]

This condition is fatal in the homozygote. The condition can be detected by means of electron microscopy of amniotic fluid and fetal skin biopsy at 18 weeks' gestation.

Mastocytosis Syndrome

Diagnosis of this condition which includes skin lesions, attacks of flushing, and diarrhoea, due either to disseminated mast-cell tumour or abnormal proliferation of tissue mast cells, is confirmed by the demonstration of increased mast cells in suitable skin biopsies. Patients may develop anaemia, neutropenia with relative lymphocytosis and monocytosis, thrombocytopenia and eosinophilia. Liver damage may develop and steatorrhoea may be found. The excretion of histamine and imidazoacetic acid is increased in the urine. Increased mast cells are seen in bone-marrow aspirate and in splenic imprints.

Pemphigoid

The serum contains antibodies directed against cell basement membrane.

Pemphigus

Immunoglobulin (IgG) antibodies bind to the suprabasilar epidermal cells in the skin. Circulating IgG antibodies are present in the serum, directed against the epidermal cell and against the intercellular cement.

Damaged cells release hydrolytic enzymes from the keratocytes, resulting in autolysis.

Pilonidal Sinus

Determination of the infecting organism, should these sinuses become infected, follows isolation and identification of the organisms from cultures of pus, or granulation tissues scraped from the sinus.

Pseudoxanthoma Elasticum (Grönblad–Strandberg Syndrome)

Diagnosis of this condition can be confirmed by positive skin biopsy, especially after the second decade.

TESTS ASSOCIATED WITH THE CONDITION

Many patients with this disease suffer from gastrointestinal bleeding, leading to iron-deficiency anaemia.

Psoriasis

Steatorrhoea may occur during active rash. The condition has an association with the HLA group CW6.

Red-cell folate activity may also be below normal in the active state, probably reflecting rapid cell turnover.

5 Intoxications

Poisoning (Accidental or Deliberate)

When poisoning is suspected, all food and drink recently taken, any tablets, medicines, domestic cleaning fluids which may have been ingested, should be noted, and remaining items should be kept for analysis (e.g. bacterial or chemical).

Gastric aspirate, vomit, faeces, urine and blood (and CSF samples, if taken) should also be carefully saved for analysis.

During treatment of poisoning by forced diuresis, urine pH should be checked to ensure either alkaline diuresis (in salicylate poisoning), or acid diuresis if this is indicated. Plasma sodium, potassium, bicarbonate, chloride and pH should be checked regularly during such treatment.

Alcohol (Ethanol) Poisoning

ACUTE POISONING

Absorption is rapid, with peak blood concentration at about 1 hour after a single dose, maintained for 2 hours, and then declining with catabolism in the liver and with some urinary excretion.

Serious hypoglycaemia may develop if alcoholic drinks are consumed when fasting, without any carbohydrate intake at the same time. Symptoms of alcoholic intoxication are slight when the blood alcohol reaches 500 mg/l, with gross ataxia at 3000 mg/l, and loss of consciousness and death at 5000–8000 mg/l. Hyperlipaemia may occur during an acute alcoholic debauch.

Urine alcohol concentration tends to be +20 per cent above the corresponding blood alcohol concentration.

CHRONIC ALCOHOLISM

In chronic heavy drinkers, the MCV and gamma-glutamyl transferase activity are increased, with only slight increase in serum alkaline phosphatase activity. Red cell 5'-pyridoxal phosphate is reduced, and thrombocytopenia may occur. In the bone marrow, pronormoblasts and promyelocytes may contain cytoplasmic vacuoles. Megaloblasts may be present, and 'ring' sideroblasts may be found if the subject is well nourished, and not iron-deficient.

Continued moderate intake of alcohol (2 glasses of wine per day) results in a significant increase in serum HDL (with a negative correlation with

85

myocardial infarction). Unfortunately this benefit is lost when the alcohol intake is increased.

TESTS PROVIDING USEFUL NEGATIVE RESULTS

Serum alkaline phosphatase activity tends to be raised more in non-alcoholic liver damage.

Amanita Poisoning ('Mushroom' Poisoning)

Diagnosis of poisoning with *Amanita phalloides* (mistaken for edible fungus) is characterized by violent nausea, colic, vomiting and diarrhoea after an initial 24-hour symptom-free period. Later, renal and hepatic failure develop. Diagnosis of Amanita poisoning is confirmed by the identification of the eaten fungus.

TESTS OF PROGRESS

Increase in serum aspartate and alanine aminotransferase activities with severe hypoglycaemia and evidence of renal damage with oliguria, are grave omens. Treatment (early) with haemodialysis may be attempted.

Arsenic Poisoning

Diagnosis is confirmed by the finding of abnormal amounts of arsenic in the urine (if arsenic is being absorbed by the patient), and arsenic in the nails and hair. Normal output of arsenic in the urine is less than 0·04 mg/day, in arsenic poisoning the arsenic output exceeds 0·1 mg/day, and urine coproporphyrin output is increased.

Normal hair contains less than 0·09 mg/100 g, whereas after prolonged arsenic poisoning, hair contains more than 0·1 mg/100 g. Examination of the hair can give a guide as to when and for how long arsenic has been absorbed, since arsenic is deposited in the growing hair following absorption.

Arsine Gas Poisoning

Diagnosis is confirmed by analysis of the gas to which the patient was exposed, and the finding of variable degrees of haemolytic anaemia and renal damage with oliguria.

Aspirin (Salicylate) Poisoning

Poisoning with aspirin (or salicylate) is characterized by initial vertigo, tinnitus and impairment of hearing. With increasing toxicity, there is nausea, vomiting, sweating, diarrhoea, fever and drowsiness. Later mental aberration develops, with hot dry flushed skin. Initially there is a short period of respiratory alkalosis followed by progressive severe metabolic acidosis. Toxicity is proportional to the dose taken, and when the plasma salicylate exceeds 2·9 mmol/l (40 mg/dl), tinnitus develops.

TESTS OF PROGRESS

Dangerous hypokalaemia and severe dehydration can develop, with a risk of sudden pulmonary oedema, cardiovascular collapse and sudden death. Active forced alkaline diuresis is indicated if plasma salicylate exceeds 3·6 mmol/l (50 mg/dl) or more than 2·2 mmol/l (30 mg/dl) in children.

With increasing toxicity, serum aspartate and alanine aminotransferase activities increase, with slight increase in serum bilirubin. The prothrombin time increases with liver damage (the BCR exceeding 2·0).

Blood gas, pH and electrolyte estimations reveal a combination of respiratory alkalosis (due to stimulation of the respiratory centre), severe metabolic acidosis plus increasing dehydration, unless treatment is instituted. A repeat plasma salicylate estimation 1 hour after the initial estimation is useful as an indicator of further absorption of salicylate from the gut (important now that slow-release salicylate compounds are available).

Barbiturate Poisoning

After barbiturate poisoning, samples of urine and the entire gastric washings should be saved for identification of the barbiturate ingested.

1. *Long-acting* (peak blood concentration 4–8 hours after oral ingestion)—phenobarbitone, barbitone.
2. *Medium duration* (peak blood concentration 1–2 hours after ingestion)—pentobarbitone, amylobarbitone, butobarbitone.
3. *Short-acting* (peak blood concentration 1–2 hours after oral ingestion)—quinalbarbitone, cyclobarbitone.
4. *Ultra-short acting*—? thiopentone sodium.

'Short' and 'medium' duration barbiturates are dangerous because they can cause rapid and profound coma. Alcohol taken with the barbiturate substantially reduces the lethal dose.

TESTS OF PROGRESS

The barbiturate may be identified by chromatographic analysis. The relation between blood levels of barbiturate and clinical state are variable. For example, a dose having little effect on an epileptic treated for many years with phenobarbitone would be potentially lethal to a person unused to barbiturate. Treatment includes ventilation and mechanical respiration, if necessary, with monitoring of blood gases, prevention and treatment of pulmonary oedema, forced diuresis, and haemodialysis of long-acting barbiturate overdose.

Berylliosis

Diagnosis of berylliosis is confirmed by the demonstration of abnormally increased urinary excretion of beryllium. Unfortunately patch skin tests for sensitivity to beryllium are not always positive in affected individuals, and the test itself may sensitize patients and exacerbate symptoms.

Berylliosis may be accompanied by hypercalciuria and increased serum gammaglobulin levels.

Bromide Poisoning

Blood bromide levels exceeding 600 mg/l are found.

Cadmium poisoning

Diagnosis is strongly supported by the finding of increased excretion of cadmium in the urine (normal less than 5 µg/l).

There is an increased frequency of renal stone disease in cadmium workers. In acute poisoning, the urine contains abnormally increased protein, and renal cortical necrosis may occur.

In chronic cadmium poisoning, renal tubular damage is revealed by the increased excretion of low molecular weight proteins in the urine, with glycosuria, amino aciduria, hypercalciuria, increased excretion of urate, and impaired concentration and dilution ability.

Cannabis Usage

Radioimmunoassay of tetrahydrocannabinol-cross-reacting cannabinoids (THC-CRC) is available in some laboratories.

Carbon Monoxide Poisoning

1. ACUTE POISONING

Carboxyhaemoglobin concentrations of 0–20 per cent are not associated with symptoms, 20–40 per cent with headache, nausea, vomiting and loss of manual dexterity, 40–60 per cent with visual and intellectual impairment.

Carbon monoxide forms a stable carboxyhaemoglobin compound in the blood, reducing oxygen carriage by the blood, and shifting the oxygen dissociation to the left so that tissues obtain oxygen from circulating oxyhaemoglobin with greater difficulty. A similar stable compound forms with myoglobin, interfering with muscle function.

Breathing an atmosphere containing 0·1 per cent carbon monoxide results in a carboxyhaemoglobin concentration of 50 per cent in one hour. Breathing an atmosphere containing 1 per cent carbon monoxide is fatal in less than 10 min.

TESTS OF PROGRESS

Room air respiration—half-life of 50 per cent carboxyhaemoglobin is over 200 min. Pure oxygen respiration—half-life of 50 per cent carboxyhaemoglobin is over 40–60 min. Hyperbaric oxygen (2 atmos)—half-life of 50 per cent carboxyhaemoglobin is over 25 min, and the tissues are oxygenated as plasma carries adequate oxygen. Subsequently after recovery, the serum creatine phosphokinase activity reflects tissue damage.

2. SUBACUTE CARBON MONOXIDE POISONING

Patients suffer from dystonic movements, cerebellar ataxia, throbbing headache, vertigo, nausea, vomiting, dyspnoea on exertion. Blood carboxy-haemoglobin levels are found to be 20–30 per cent with consciousness retained, in the home environment often associated with faulty heating equipment.

Discrepancy between the calculated oxygen saturation from the Pao_2 and the actual measured oxygen saturation suggests underlying carboxyhaemo-globin poisoning.

Sodium Chlorate Poisoning

Poisoning following ingestion of this common weedkiller, results in marked methaemoglobinaemia, with detectable cyanosis at 10 per cent and death at 70 per cent methaemoglobin. There is also massive intravascular haemolysis, rising plasma potassium concentration, acute renal tubular necrosis and haematuria.

TESTS OF PROGRESS

Ascorbic acid should be used to treat the methaemoglobinaemia. If intravenous methylene blue is used, chlorate is converted to chlorite, and the patient dies.

Cyanide Poisoning

Normal blood cyanide levels are less than 200 μg/l. Following inhalation of polymer fire fumes (household furnishings), cyanide rapidly combines with cytochrome oxidase in its oxidized form, blocking cell respiration, and causing death.

Cyanide does not combine with haemoglobin in the blood, and therapy is aimed at converting enough haemoglobin to methaemoglobin, to bond with cyanide to form cyanmethaemoglobin, preventing gross inhibition of cellular cytochrome oxidase activity.

Sodium nitrite in solution is injected intravenously over 4 min. This may produce some cyanosis due to methaemoglobin production. Methaemoglobin concentration may reach 15 per cent. Then slow infusion of 12·5 g sodium thiosulphate solution intravenously over 10 min is given, to convert cyanide to thiocyanate, which is excreted in the urine.

In survivors, before treatment, blood thiocyanate levels range from 2 to 125 μmol/l after polymer fume inhalation (normal non-smoker = up to 13 μmol/l).

Digoxin Poisoning

Digoxin poisoning is associated with vomiting, nausea, diarrhoea, headache, confusion, delirium, bradycardia and other disturbances of cardiac rhythm. Metabolic acidosis occurs, with hyperkalaemia. The plasma digoxin level taken at more than 6 hours after ingestion can be used to assess the original intake.

Ethylene Glycol Poisoning (Antifreeze Ingestion)

Following ingestion of ethylene glycol, there is marked reduction in serum calcium with severe metabolic acidosis. Serum oxalate levels are increased, and urine oxalate is also increased, with oxalate crystals visible in freshly voided urine.

Endemic Skeletal Fluorosis

Diagnosis of this condition which occurs in areas in which excessive concentration of fluoride is present in the drinking water is confirmed by the demonstration of increased excretion of fluoride in the urine, and a marked increase in bone fluoride content in bone biopsy material. Serum alkaline phosphatase activity is increased, and serum calcium concentrations are also increased.

TESTS PROVIDING USEFUL NEGATIVE RESULTS

Serum inorganic phosphate and serum magnesium concentrations are normal.

Transfusion Haemosiderosis

Following repeated transfusions without blood loss (e.g. aplastic anaemia, thalassaemia) iron from the transfused blood accumulates. Each unit of blood contributes 200–250 mg of iron. Within two years of regular blood transfusion, serum iron is increased, with 80 per cent saturation of plasma transferrin. There is no simple direct relationship between serum ferritin levels and reticulo-endothelial iron deposition. Liver stainable iron is increased, as is bone-marrow stainable iron in extracellular deposits.

Haemosiderosis also follows excessive iron intake (alcohol, iron cooking pots etc.).

TESTS OF PROGRESS

Iron is removed from the body stores by the chelating agent desferrioxamine. Haemosiderosis not resulting from repeated blood transfusions can also be treated successfully by repeated regular venesections.

USEFUL NEGATIVE RESULTS

There is no prominent deposition of iron in the skin (cf. haemochromatosis).

'Haff' Disease

Following ingestion of unidentified toxic substances found in fish in contaminated rivers in northern Germany myoglobinuria resulted.

Halothane Hepatitis

Following repeat halothane anaesthesia and surgery, after 2–5 days the occasional patient develops fever, anorexia, nausea and vomiting, and occasionally an eosinophilia appears in the peripheral blood with evidence of hepatitis. Mitochondrial antibodies may be detected in the serum.

This syndrome can occur after repeated halothane anaesthesia over a short period, but can follow anaesthesia with other potent inhalational agents also. The initial interval between anaesthesia and symptoms is 8–14 days, but with repeat anaesthesia the interval gets shorter, and the symptoms more severe.

Hypervitaminosis A

Diagnosis of this condition, occurring in infants and young children given excessive amounts of vitamin A (and in adults following the eating of polar bear liver), characterized by nausea, vomiting, drowsiness, diplopia (and papilloedema in infants), is confirmed by the demonstration of abnormally increased serum vitamin A levels. (Plasma retinol concentrations can reach 35 μmol/l (1000 μg/dl) in infants and 700 μmol/l (20 mg/dl) in adults.)

Vitamin D Overdose

Diagnosis is confirmed by the demonstration of high serum vitamin D levels, with abnormally raised serum calcium and inorganic phosphate. Calcinosis affects joints, synovial membranes, kidneys, myocardium, pulmonary alveoli, parathyroid glands, pancreas, skin, arteries, conjunctivae and cornea. Later, demineralization of bones occurs, if the excessive dose continues to be taken.

Hypercalcaemia will be associated with polyuria and nocturia, plus loss of the normal renal ability to concentrate urine.

Heavy-metal Poisoning

Diagnosis is made by estimation of toxic levels of the particular metal in blood, urine, or (at post-mortem) in tissues. These metals cause renal damage; a non-specific clue to possible heavy-metal poisoning in an exposed patient is the finding of proteinuria with amino aciduria.

Acute Iron Toxicity

Diagnosis of this condition affecting infants and young children with access to iron tablets prescribed for adults, and characterized by acute abdominal pain within 30 min of ingestion, a period of 10–14 hours of clinical improvement, followed by profound shock and coma, is confirmed by the finding of serum iron concentrations which may exceed 150 μmol/l (1000 μg/dl), accompanied by severe necrotizing gastritis. The increased serum iron is present mainly in the ferric state, and not bound to transferrin, which is saturated.

TESTS OF PROGRESS
Following gastric lavage, and desferrixoamine therapy, iron is eliminated in a chelated form in the urine.

Lead Poisoning

Diagnosis of lead poisoning is confirmed by the demonstration of serum lead levels exceeding 4·8 μmol/l (100 μg/dl). Excessive exposure to lead is reflected by serum lead levels greater than 1·5 μmol/l (30 μg/dl). Urine lead excretion exceeds 4·8 μmol/day (100 μg/24 hours).

The peripheral blood may show an increased stippled red cell count (punctate basophilia), anaemia and neutrophilia. 'Ring sideroblasts' may be present in bone marrow aspirate. Urine coproporphyrin and delta-amino-laevulinic acid excretion is increased, and prolonged lead poisoning eventually results in amino aciduria, glycosuria and proteinuria.

In acute lead encephalopathy the CSF protein concentration is increased without a corresponding pleocytosis.

TESTS OF PROGRESS

Treatment with calcium disodium edetate results in increased urinary lead excretion and reduction in blood lead levels. Acetyl-D-penicillamine can also be used to sequestrate lead and facilitate its safe excretion in the urine. Screening of potentially exposed people can be by blood lead estimation, or alternatively by initial screening for raised free erythrocyte protoporphyrin with subsequent blood lead estimations on subjects with raised levels.

Lithium Poisoning

Used in long-term prophylaxis of cyclothymic disorder, lithium has a poor therapeutic index, necessitating regular monitoring of blood levels in patients.

Below 0·75 mmol/l treatment with lithium is thought to be ineffective, whereas plasma lithium levels exceeding 1·5 mmol/l can be associated with increasing thirst, nausea and vomiting, progressing to drowsiness, tremor and hyper-reflexia.

TESTS OF PROGRESS

Forced alkaline diuresis is effective in bringing increased blood levels down, if plasma electrolyte balance is maintained. Haemodialysis is not often necessary.

Diuretics which cause increased loss of sodium in the urine may exaggerate lithium toxicity.

Mercury Poisoning

1. ACUTE MERCURY POISONING

There is metabolic disturbance with diarrhoea and anuria. Before complete anuria, the urine contains protein, red blood cells and casts. There may be a peripheral blood neutrophilia.

2. CHRONIC MERCURY POISONING

Urine mercury excretion exceeds 300 μg/l (normal excretion = up to 1 μg/l). Urine mercury of 100 μg/l indicates toxic exposure.

Following chronic poisoning renal tubular damage may result in abnormal excretion of protein, glucose, phosphate and amino acids (Fanconi-type damage).

Acrodynia

Chronic mercury poisoning occurring in infants following ingestion of 'teething powders' containing mercury must no longer occur. Urine mercury excretion reached 100 µg/day.

3. ORGANIC MERCURY POISONING

When workers exposed to organic mercury compounds excrete more than 30 µg/day, they must be considered to be at risk. Organic mercury caused the outbreak of Minamata disease in Japan.

Methanol Poisoning

Following ingestion of methanol, blood methanol levels of more than 50 mg/dl are associated with death or irreversible blindness. Blood formate levels reach 11–26 mmol/l.

TESTS OF PROGRESS

Early haemodialysis results in falling blood methanol levels. Ethanol therapy should be started, to attain a blood ethanol level of 100 mg/dl. This results in competition for the enzyme system producing formic acid and formaldehyde from methanol, and producing acetate and acetaldehyde instead.

Nickel Poisoning

In nickel poisoning plasma nickel can rise to 3 mg/dl. Excess intake has occurred following the use of a nickel-plated water heater in repeated dialysis.

Organophosphorous Insecticide Poisoning (e.g. Malathion)

Poisoning is characterized by bronchospasm, excess bronchial mucus and pulmonary oedema, salivation, diarrhoea, vomiting and sweating, tachycardia, hypotension, convulsions and coma. Serum and red cell cholinesterase levels are markedly reduced.

TESTS OF PROGRESS

Atropinization and pralidoxime therapy with maintenance of ventilation.

Paracetamol poisoning

Following paracetamol overdose, haemorrhage, liver damage, encephalopathy and ultimately death, may follow. Toxicity correlates with blood paracetamol levels. When blood paracetamol exceeds 2 mmol/l (300 mg/100 ml) 4 hours after the overdose, overt liver damage will occur unless the patient receives active treatment.

If a blood concentration of 2 mmol/l at 4 hours and 0·2 mmol/l at 15 hours is plotted on semilog paper, then results falling above the joining line show that a patient is in danger, and requires active treatment with intravenous acetylcysteine (or oral methionine—if the patient can swallow, and is not vomiting). The first 72 hours of such treatment may be associated with hypokalaemia, falling plasma bicarbonate, and sometimes thrombocytopenia.

TESTS OF PROGRESS

Aspartate and alanine aminotransferases rise above normal in proportion to the severity of any liver cell necrosis.

A prothrombin ratio (BCR) exceeding 2·0 indicates a bad prognosis. Disseminated intravascular coagulopathy may develop later.

Paracetamol interferes with some blood glucose methods, giving false high glucose readings, in the presence of a real dangerous hypoglycaemia.

Paraquat Poisoning

Poisoning with the herbicide, paraquat, is followed by burning sore throat, severe abdominal pain, and if enough has been absorbed, by agitation, tremor and convulsions. There is a symptom-free period of 2–5 days, followed by pulmonary, and later, renal and hepatic failure. A simple test using alkaline dithionite is available, and if urine paraquat tests are negative during the first 48 hours after suspected ingestion, insufficient has been absorbed to be dangerous.

TESTS OF PROGRESS

After urgent gastric aspiration, forced diuresis, or if available, haemodialysis, is necessary, with suitable biochemical monitoring.

Blood paraquat estimation is available using gas chromatography.

Serum Reaction

A high titre of antibodies which agglutinate sheep red cells (as in the Paul–Bunnell test) which are absorbed on both guinea pig kidney and ox red cells. Plasma cells may be seen in the peripheral blood, and the marrow plasma cell count increases.

6 Disorders of Metabolism

HEREDITARY DISORDERS

Acatalasaemia [R]

Diagnosis of this rare condition is confirmed by the demonstration in patients subject to infected oral lesions of reduced blood catalase activity.

Albinism

Diagnosis of albinism is clinical. The condition is associated with a mild bleeding tendency. The Hess capillary fragility test is abnormal, and the bleeding time is prolonged. Platelet aggregation response to ADP is variable and the second wave of aggregation is defective. Platelet 5-hydroxytryptamine uptake and retention are defective, and the platelets reveal abnormalities on electron microscopy.

Immune Deficiency Syndrome with Thrombocytopenia and Eczema (Wiskott–Aldrich Syndrome) [AR]

Diagnosis of this sex-linked recessive disorder, characterized by severe infection with thrombocytopenia and an atopic type of eczema, with death in affected boys before 4 years, is supported by the finding of defective platelet function with thrombocytopenia, with normal numbers of megakaryocytes in the marrow, persistent lymphopenia, normal or raised serum IgG, reduced serum IgM, and absence in many cases of iso-agglutinins from the blood. There is no antibody response to typhoid vaccination. Lymph-gland biopsy reveals large follicles with numerous plasma cells, lymphocytes and reticulum cells.

TESTS OF PROGRESS

There is no treatment, and there is a high incidence of malignant lymphoma.

Fibrous Dysplasia of Bone (McCune–Albright Syndrome)

Diagnosis of this condition associated with precocious puberty, cutaneous pigmentation (café-au-lait spots), and tendency to fracture of affected bones, which heal readily with much callus. The affected bones have very thin cortices. While the serum calcium concentration is normal, serum alkaline phosphatase activity and urine hydroxyproline excretion are both increased (indicating high bone turnover).

MUCOPOLYSACCHARIDOSES

Mucopolysaccharidosis Type IH (Hurler's Syndrome) [AR]

Diagnosis of this rare condition, characterized by 'gargoyle' features, hepatosplenomegaly, mental retardation, corneal clouding, and skeletal abnormalities (dysostosis multiplex), is confirmed by the demonstration of reduced activity of alpha-L-iduronohydrolase in leucocytes, cultured fibroblasts, and organ extracts.

The urine contains abnormal amounts of dermatan sulphate and heparan sulphate in the ratio of 3:1.

TESTS OF PROGRESS

During pregnancy amniotic fluid cells, on culture, also show the reduced activity of alpha-L-iduronohydrolase when the fetus is an affected homozygote.

Mucopolysaccharidosis Type IS (Scheie's Syndrome) [AR]

Diagnosis of this rare condition, characterized by signs and symptoms similar to, but less severe than those of mucopolysaccharidosis Type IH (Hurler), with normal intelligence, but with severe corneal clouding, is confirmed by the demonstration of reduced activity of alpha-L-iduronohydrolase in leucocytes, cultured skin fibroblasts and organ extracts.

As in Hurler's syndrome the urine contains dermatan sulphate and heparan sulphate in abnormal amounts in a ratio of 3:1.

Mucopolysaccharidosis Type IH/S [AR]

Diagnosis of this disease, with severity intermediate between Type IH and Type IS (which is thought to be doubly heterozygous for the two mutant genes), again depends on the demonstration of reduced activity of alpha-L-iduronohydrolase in leucocytes, cultured skin fibroblasts, and organ extracts, with abnormal excretion of dermatan sulphate and heparan sulphate.

Mucopolysaccharidosis Type II (Hunter's Syndrome) [XR] [? AR]

CLINICAL VARIANTS

  a. Severe
Rapid mental and neurological degeneration in pre-puberty.
  b. Mild
Normal or moderately impaired intelligence, with mild skeletal abnormalities. These patients often survive into adulthood.

Diagnosis of this rare sex-linked recessive condition is confirmed by the demonstration of deficiency in activity of the enzyme iduronate sulphatase in leucocytes, cultured fibroblasts and organ extracts, with abnormally increased excretion of dermatan sulphate and heparan sulphate in the urine.

Mucopolysaccharidosis Type IIIA (Sanfilippo A Syndrome) [AR]

Diagnosis of this rare condition, characterized by slight dwarfing, moderate skeletal abnormalities, moderate corneal clouding, with hepatosplenomegaly, and severe mental retardation, is confirmed by the demonstration of deficiency of activity of the enzyme heparan-N-sulphatase and also heparan-N-sulphate sulphamidase, in leucocytes and cultured skin fibroblasts. Excessive amounts of heparan sulphate are excreted in the urine.

Mucopolysaccharidosis Type IIIB (Sanfilippo B Syndrome) [AR]

Diagnosis of this rare condition, which is clinically indistinguishable from mucopolysaccharidosis Type IIIA, with severe central nervous system damage and mental retardation, is confirmed by the demonstration of deficiency of activity of the enzyme alpha-N-acetylglucosaminidase in serum and also in cultured skin fibroblasts. There is excessive excretion of heparan sulphate in the urine.

Mucopolysaccharidosis Type IIIC (Sanfilippo C Syndrome) [AR]

Diagnosis of this rare condition, which is clinically indistinguishable from Type IIIA and Type IIIB, is confirmed by the demonstration of deficiency of activity of the enzyme acetyl-CoA:α-glucosaminide N-acetyltransferase in cultured skin fibroblasts. The urine contains excessive amounts of heparan sulphate.

Mucopolysaccharidosis Type IIID (Sanfilippo D Syndrome [AR]

Diagnosis of this rare condition, which is clinically indistinguishable from Types IIIA, IIIB, and Type IIIC, is confirmed by the demonstration of deficiency of activity of the enzyme N-acetylglucosamine-6-sulphate sulphatase in cultured skin fibroblasts. The urine contains excessive amounts of heparan sulphate.

Mucopolysaccharidosis Type IVA (Morquio's A Syndrome) [AR]

Diagnosis of this rare condition, which is characterized bynpronounced bony deformities in the second year (often with atlanto-axial dislocation), dwarfing and frequently deafness, but rare mental retardation or corneal opacity, is confirmed by the demonstration of deficiency of activity of the enzyme N-acetyl hexosamine-6-sulphate sulphatase in cultured skin fibroblasts. The urine contains keratan sulphate in children, but keratan sulphate is not excreted by the adult case.

Mucopolysaccharidosis Type IV B (Morquio's B Syndrome) [AR]

Enzyme deficiency in cultured skin fibroblasts = β-galactosidase deficiency.

Mucopolysaccharidosis Type V

This is now mucopolysaccharidosis Type I, Scheie's syndrome.

Mucopolysaccharidosis Type VI (Marotaux–Lamy Syndrome) [AR]

a. Severe

Diagnosis of this rare condition, characterized by growth retardation from the 2nd–3rd year, dystosis multiplex, and normal intellect, is confirmed by the demonstration of deficiency of activity of the enzyme aryl sulphatase B (N-acetylgalactosamine-4-sulphatase), in cultured skin fibroblasts, liver, kidney or spleen.

The urine contains abnormal amounts of dermatan sulphate. 5–50 per cent of the circulating leucocytes contain Reilly granules (large acid mucosubstance granular inclusions in the cells).

These patients reach adult life, but die of progressive heart disease.

b. Intermediate

Moderately severe clinical manifestations, but laboratory results as in the severe type.

c. Mild

Mild osseous and corneal changes occur, with a normal intellect. Aortic stenosis is present. The laboratory results are as in the severe type.

Mucopolysaccharidosis Type VII [AR]

Diagnosis of this rare condition, characterized by short stature, hepatomegaly, skeletal abnormalities, and possible mental development lagging later, is confirmed by the demonstration of deficiency of activity of the enzyme β-glucuronidase in leucocytes, cultured skin fibroblasts, liver, spleen, kidney or brain. The peripheral blood leucocytes contain granular inclusions, and the urine contains excessive amounts of dermatan sulphate and heparan sulphate.

Mucopolysaccharidosis Type VIII [AR]

Diagnosis of this rare condition, characterized by short stature and mild dysostosis multiplex, is confirmed by demonstration of deficiency of activity of the enzyme glucosamine-6-sulphate sulphatase in leucocytes and cultured fibroblasts. Lymphocytes show ring-shaped metachromasia, and the urine contains increased amounts of keratan sulphate and heparan sulphate.

Gout

Diagnosis of this condition is clinical, with supporting evidence of raised serum uric acid concentration, if uricosuric drugs are not being taken (> 0.36 mmol/l, > 6 mg/100 ml in males, > 0.3 mmol/l, > 5 mg/100 ml in females). During acute attacks of gout, neutrophilia is found with mild increases in plasma fibrinogen, plasma viscosity and erythrocyte sedimentation rate.

Crystals of monosodium urate can be demonstrated in gouty tophi and in fluid aspirated from inflamed joint cavities.

Twenty five per cent of cases produce excessive quantities of uric acid, while 75 per cent excrete uric acid satisfactorily when the plasma uric acid concentration is abnormally raised. On a purine-free diet, the overproducers excrete more than 3·57 mmol uric acid/day in urine (> 600 mg/24 hr) while the undersecretors excrete less than 3·57 mmol/day. A rare form with partial deficiency of hypoxanthine guanine phosphoryl transferase can be detected by demonstration of reduced enzyme activity in cultured fibroblasts, after the finding of urine uric acid/creatinine ratio > 1·13 (mmol/1) (> 0·76 mg/100 ml).

TESTS OF PROGRESS

After an acute attack of gout has been relieved with phenylbutazone, etc. maintenance therapy with probenecid will prevent further attacks in undersecretors, while allopurinol will control oversecretors. Allopurinol should be used if there is a risk of uric acid stone formation, and many centres use it for maintenance therapy in all cases. The serum uric acid can be monitored for satisfactory control.

Adenine Phosphoribosyl Transferase Deficiency [R]

Diagnosis of this very rare condition can only be made by demonstration of deficiency of the specific enzyme, and the estimation is available only in a limited number of laboratories. In homozygotes there are increased concentrations of both adenine and 2-8-dihydroxyadenine (relatively insoluble). The presenting signs and symptoms result from the development of urinary tract calculi.

2,8-Dihydroxyadenine Renal Stones [AR] [R]

Diagnosis of this rare condition, characterized by the development of renal stones in children, is confirmed by the demonstration of deficiency of activity of the enzyme adenine phosphoribosyl transferase in cultured skin fibroblasts. The chemical structure of renal stones can be confirmed, and crystals of 2,8-dihydroxyadenine can be seen in concentrated urine samples, *Variant*: Partial deficiency of the enzyme may be associated with attacks of gout.

Pyrophosphate Arthropathy (Pseudogout)

Diagnosis of this condition of crystal deposition disease, characterized by acute attacks of crystal synovitis occurring in the middle-aged and elderly, is confirmed by the demonstration of crystals of calcium pyrophosphate dihydrate in joint fluid, aspirated during acute attacks of arthritis. Deposition of calcium pyrophosphate dihydrate occurs in hyaline and fibrocartilage, especially in the knee joint menisci. Other joints may also be affected.

TESTS OF PROGRESS

Fifty per cent of cases suffer from haemochromatosis. A few cases have primary hyperparathyroidism.

During acute attacks there is often neutrophilia, with raised ESR and plasma viscosity.

TESTS PROVIDING USEFUL NEGATIVE RESULTS

There is no evidence of suppurative arthritis, and culture of joint fluid is sterile. No uric acid crystals are seen in joint fluid aspirate.

Haemochromatosis

Diagnosis of this condition, characterized by the progressive deposition of iron, hyperpigmentation, diabetes mellitus and later, cirrhosis, is confirmed by the finding of raised serum iron levels (exceeding 30 μmol/l, early), with almost complete saturation of the TIBC (which itself tends to fall), and serum ferritin levels rising to 5–10 × normal. Skin biopsy, liver biopsy and gastric mucosal biopsy, and bone marrow aspirate, all contain much stainable iron. The differential ^{59}Fe desferrioxamine iron excretion test results in a gross excretion of iron in the urine. Progressive iron deposition results in tissue damage. Pancreatic damage results in diabetes mellitus. Liver damage results in cirrhosis, with falling serum albumin and rising serum gammaglobulin levels. Iron-containing renal tubular cells can be found in urine deposits. The peripheral blood contains up to 3–7 per cent siderocytes. Deposition in the joints is associated with arthritis in 20 per cent of cases (predominantly males).

TESTS OF PROGRESS

In suitable cases, weekly phlebotomy of 50 ml blood removes the excess iron, and iron stores are depleted in this way by 6 months to 3 years, the haematocrit stabilizing at about 0·35 (35 per cent). When the serum ferritin concentration has fallen to 10 μg/l, the patient has reached borderline iron deficiency, liver biopsy will not show any stainable iron. Subsequently, phlebotomy can be carried out every 3 months, with the haemoglobin level settling at about 11 g/dl. In cases unable to stand repeated phlebotomies (patients with cardiac disease, anaemia or hypoproteinaemia), chelation therapy can be used to remove the excess iron.

First-degree relatives aged more than 10 years, should be screened by estimation of serum iron, TIBC and ferritin, with liver biopsy for stainable iron if abnormal results are obtained, and followed up.

Serum iron concentration falls with the development of hepatoma in a cirrhotic patient.

Serum ferritin is useful in separating homozygote male patients from male heterozygotes and normal subjects.

USEFUL NEGATIVE RESULTS

In alcoholic liver disease serum ferritin levels can exceed 1000 μg/l, but the level fluctuates, and aminotransferases and gamma-GT activities are also increased.

Hepatolenticular Degeneration (Wilson's Disease) [R] [AR]

Diagnosis of this rare disease, characterized by neurological symptoms (basal ganglion damage) and/or symptoms of liver damage, appearing in childhood, is confirmed by the demonstration of gross reduction in plasma caeruloplasmin (the specific copper-carrying plasma protein–copper oxidase activity), decreased serum copper (less than 13 μmol/l, 80 μg/dl) and abnormally increased urine copper excretion (3·14 μmol, 200 μg per 24 hours). Liver biopsy reveals abnormal ballooning of liver cells with fatty change, and liver copper is increased to more than 25 mg/100 g dry weight.

TESTS OF PROGRESS

Progressive damage to liver cells by deposited copper results eventually in death from liver damage. Renal function is also affected by deposition of copper, with generalized amino aciduria and abnormally low serum uric acid (Fanconi's syndrome).

Penicillamine therapy reduces the rate of cell damage and enables the elimination of copper. Monitoring of the blood is necessary during this lifelong therapy, for the detection of toxic side-effects of penicillamine. Even with this treatment, liver damage slowly progresses. Treatment with triethylene tetramine dihydrochloride can also be used, and should be given to homozygotes detected before symptoms have appeared.

Hypocupraemia with Mental Retardation [R]

Diagnosis of this rare condition was confirmed by the finding of abnormally reduced serum caeruloplasmin, serum copper and markedly reduced urine copper excretion (cf. hepatolenticular degeneration) in a mentally retarded female infant.

Primary Hypomagnesaemia [R]

Diagnosis of this very rare condition presenting in early infancy with convulsions and tetany is made by exclusion of other causes of severe hypomagnesaemia. Plasma magnesium levels as low as 0·084 mmol/l have been reported (normal 0·7–0·93 mmol/l), with plasma inorganic phosphate of 2·78 mmol/l (normal 1·29–1·78 mmol/l), and reduced serum albumin. The condition is due to a defect in the carrier-mediated transport of magnesium from low intraluminal concentrations of magnesium in the gut.

TESTS OF PROGRESS

Oral supplements with magnesium salts maintain normal plasma magnesium levels, but cause diarrhoea.

Hypophosphatasia [AR] [R]

This rare condition is characterized by premature synostosis of the cranial vault bones resulting in raised intracranial pressure and exophthalmos. Presenting later in childhood, it resembles rickets. 'Pseudofractures' develop in middle age.

Diagnosis is confirmed by the demonstration of serum alkaline phosphatase activity markedly reduced for the age of the patient, with raised serum calcium in severe cases plus hypercalciuria, with a very low excretion rate of hydroxyproline in the urine (low bone turnover).

Both plasma and urine contain abnormally increased amounts of phospho-ethanolamine.

TESTS OF PROGRESS

Vitamin D therapy induces or aggravates hypercalcaemia, and must be avoided.

Nephrocalcinosis and renal failure develop later.

Heterozygotes can be detected by the demonstration of serum alkaline phosphatase activity midway between affected homozygotes and normal subjects.

TESTS PROVIDING USEFUL NEGATIVE RESULTS

Fasting plasma inorganic phosphate levels are normal.

Kinky Hair Syndrome [R]

Diagnosis of this sex-linked recessive rare condition, which presents with hypothermia in infancy, feeding difficulties, jaundice in some cases, feeding difficulties at 2–3 months, and short stubby twisted hair developing after normal hair at birth, is confirmed by the finding of markedly reduced serum copper levels, reduced liver copper concentration, with increased copper content of hair, muscle, pancreas, kidney. There is increased uptake of copper into fibroblasts, with reduced egress.

Infants develop increasing drowsiness, seborrhoeic dermatitis and die early in infancy, following mental deterioration.

Marfan's Syndrome [AD]

Diagnosis of this dominant condition is clinical. The condition is characterized by abnormal bodily proportion with disproportionately long extremities and long distal bones (arachnodactyly), most obvious after puberty, with incompetence of the aortic valve and even dissecting aortic aneurysm in some. At post-mortem the great vessels show cystic medial necrosis.

TESTS PROVIDING USEFUL NEGATIVE RESULTS

Tests for homocystinuria are negative. Patients with homocystinuria have a similar body configuration, but some are mentally retarded, and some have lens dislocation.

Congenital Methaemoglobinaemia [R]

Two forms of familial methaemoglobinaemia are known:

1. Deficiency of NADP-dependent methaemoglobin reductase [AR]—characterized by persistent cyanosis and mild polycythaemia, plus mental retardation in some cases.

Oral ascorbic acid or injection of methylene blue will reduce the circulating methaemoglobin level temporarily.

2. Deficiency of NAD-dependent methaemoglobin reductase [AR].

TESTS PROVIDING USEFUL NEGATIVE RESULTS

It is important to diagnose and treat temporary methaemoglobinaemia in otherwise normal cyanosed infants, where abnormal levels of methaemoglobin have resulted from excessive nitrite ingestion.

Several abnormal haemoglobins, referred to as haemoglobins M, are associated with persistent cyanosis due to methaemoglobinaemia, and do not respond to treatment with either ascorbic acid or methylene blue. In HbM with alpha-chain abnormality, cyanosis is present at birth, whereas with beta-chain abnormality, cyanosis appears a few weeks after birth when HbF synthesis is markedly reduced. These abnormal haemoglobins can be detected by haemoglobin electrophoresis.

Primary Hyperoxaluria [R]

TYPE *I*

Diagnosis is confirmed in patients suffering with recurrent calcium oxalate nephrolithiasis, chronic renal failure and oxalosis, by the demonstration of deficiency of activity of 2-ketoglutarate glyoxylate carboligase.

There is markedly increased excretion of oxalate in the urine before renal failure develops, often with increased excretion of glycolate.

TESTS OF PROGRESS

In the infantile type there is rapid deterioration with fits and renal failure. The less rare milder variety is characterized by survival into adult life, and in these cases, oxalate synthesis and excretion may be reduced by a low oxalate intake, with pyridoxine and thiamine supplements.

TYPE *II*

Diagnosis of this rare condition is confirmed by the demonstration of deficiency of the enzyme D-glycerate dehydrogenase, with excessive urinary oxalate and L-glycerate.

Suxamethonium Sensitivity (Scoline Apnoea)

Diagnosis of abnormal sensitivity to the action of the muscle relaxant suxamethonium (scoline), characterized by abnormally prolonged apnoea following its use during anaesthesia, is confirmed either by demonstration of abnormally reduced inhibition of plasma cholinesterase activity in vitro by the spinal anaesthetic dibucaine (hence low 'dibucaine number'), or rarely by the failure to detect plasma cholinesterase activity ('silent gene').

TESTS OF PROGRESS

Heterozygotes carrying the abnormal cholinesterase give intermediate 'dibucaine numbers' between normal subjects and affected homozygotes.

The family of an affected homozygote should be screened and warning cards supplied to affected individuals.

Xanthinuria [R]

Diagnosis of this rare autosomal recessive condition is only likely to be made in random surveys, since the incidence of xanthine stone formation is extremely rare and the condition is otherwise harmless. There is a gross deficiency of xanthine oxidase activity in liver and jejunal biopsy material. Myopathy can develop with crystals of xanthine and hypoxanthine visible in muscle biopsy material. Serum uric acid levels are extremely low (0·1 mmol/l, 0·05–1·6 mg/10 ml) and urine uric acid output is very low (0·01–0·07 mmol/day, 2–12 mg/day). Urine xanthine output is raised to 100–500 mg/day (normal 5–9 mg/day) with hypoxanthine excreted at 0–60 mg/day (normal 6–13 mg/day). Cases of gout treated with allopurinol (xanthine oxidase inhibitor) excrete xanthine and hypoxanthine in increased amounts, but in these latter cases xanthine stone formation has not been reported.

TESTS OF PROGRESS

Following increased fluid intake, with allopurinol to increase hypoxanthine excretion relative to xanthine, the urine excretion pattern is changed and the risk of further stone formation is reduced.

Hereditary Fructose Intolerance [R] [AR]

This rare condition is characterized by the onset of vomiting, poor feeding, failure to thrive, hepatosplenomegaly, spontaneous bleeding, jaundice and convulsions, beginning at the time of weaning with addition of fructose, sorbitol or invert sugar to the infant's diet. Older children become drowsy and vomit after fructose-containing food. Fructose given postoperatively to affected adults can be very dangerous.

Diagnosis is confirmed by the demonstration of abnormally low activity of the enzyme fructose-1-phosphate aldolase in liver or small intestinal mucous membrane biopsy material. Untreated, liver steatosis develops, with hepatocellular necrosis, and portal tract fibrosis leading to cirrhosis. Since there is impaired glycogen breakdown and gluconeogenesis is inhibited, these patients develop severe hypoglycaemia after ingestion of fructose.

TESTS OF PROGRESS

In the acute state, intravenous glucose should be given. After confirmation of the enzyme deficiency (with secondary deficiency of fructose-1,6-diphosphate aldolase), a fructose-free diet with added vitamin C results in clinical recovery.

Urinary 'T' Substance Anomaly

Originally described as a substance related to alloxan, excreted in excess in the urine of some mentally retarded children, it has since been discovered that a fault in an electrolytic desalter produces the substance in any urine. The clinical condition therefore does not exist.

CARBOHYDRATE METABOLIC DISORDERS

Essential Fructosuria

Diagnosis of this harmless condition is confirmed by the finding of large amounts of fructose in the urine, after ingestion of fructose-containing food. Glucose is not excreted in abnormal amounts. The condition is transmitted by an autosomal recessive gene.

Hereditary Fructose-1,6-Diphosphatase Deficiency [AR] [R]

Diagnosis of this rare condition, characterized by severe hypoglycaemia with marked ketosis and lactic acidosis on fasting, and hepatomegaly, lactic acidosis and hypoglycaemia after fructose ingestion, is confirmed by the demonstration of deficiency of fructose-1,6-diphosphatase activity in leucocytes and liver biopsy material. Infections aggravate attacks of hypoglycaemia. Plasma lactate, pyruvate, and aspartate amino transferase activity are increased, with amino aciduria including alanine and glutamine.

TESTS OF PROGRESS

Following intravenous glucose plus bicarbonate in an acute attack, after diagnosis, a fructose-free diet results in clinical improvement.

TESTS PROVIDING USEFUL NEGATIVE RESULTS

Glucagon 1 mg i.v. does not cause any increase in plasma glucose.

Galactosaemia [R] [AR]

Various clinical forms exist:
    1. *Classic*, with severe symptoms in homozygotes, including:
        a. Acute onset with haemorrhagic diathesis and sepsis.
        b. Gastrointestinal symptoms, jaundice and bleeding disorder in the first 2 weeks.
        c. Mild degree of failure to thrive, developing hepatic cirrhosis by 2–6 months.
        d. Mental retardation, cataracts and liver disease.
    2. *Duarte variant.* An apparently partially active enzyme, with activity in homozygote red cells of equivalent activity to that of the heterozygote from the classic variety.
    3. *Negro variant.* The capacity to metabolize galactose increases with age.

Diagnosis of this condition, characterized by anorexia and vomiting appearing towards the end of the first week of life, followed rapidly by jaundice, hepatomegaly and bleeding diathesis, is confirmed by the demonstration of absence or greatly reduced activity of galactose-l-phosphate uridyltransferase in red cells. After galactose-containing feed, blood galactose increases and blood glucose falls to dangerous hypoglycaemia. There is abnormal amino aciduria.

Urine galactose excretion occurs 39–120 min after oral galactose. In the presence of jaundice, bilirubin appears in the urine. Later, tests reveal evidence of liver damage.

TESTS OF PROGRESS

The degree of recovery following galactose-free feeds, depends on the initial liver and brain damage. Death from sepsis occurs in 30 per cent of untreated infants. Screening tests in suspected infants should be carried out on the 3rd–4th day of life (the disease has an incidence of 1 in 30 000–1 in 76 000 live births). Prenatal diagnosis by measurement of the specific enzyme activity in cultured amniotic cells is now possible, for use in known affected families. Carriers of classic galactosaemia have red cell enzyme activity midway between affected homozygotes and normal control subjects.

Congenital Glucose-galactose Malabsorption [R]

Diagnosis of this rare condition, thought to be due to a brush-border translocation defect, characterized by severe gastro-enteritis after each milk feed, occurring in neonates, resulting in severe dehydration, and fatal unless galactose- and glucose-containing foods are withdrawn, is confirmed by the finding of more rapid absorption of fructose than of glucose given at the same time. (Fructose is absorbed passively, while glucose requires active absorption.) The condition improves with age.

USEFUL NEGATIVE RESULTS

Absorption of fructose, xylose, leucine and alanine is normal.

Galactose Kinase Deficiency [R] [AR]

Diagnosis of this rare condition, characterized by the development of cataracts in older patients on an unrestricted diet, and occurring most commonly in people of gypsy extraction, is confirmed by the demonstration of gross reduction in red cell galactose kinase activity in affected homozygotes. After galactose-containing feeds, blood galactose rises, and galactose is excreted in the urine. (Possibly 1 in every 100 patients developing cataracts of unknown origin has this metabolic defect.)

TESTS OF PROGRESS

Patients on a galactose-free diet do not have increased blood galactose levels, and do not excrete galactose. Heterozygotes have specific enzyme activity in their red cells midway between affected homozygotes and normal control subjects.

TESTS PROVIDING USEFUL NEGATIVE RESULTS

Red cell galactose-1-phosphate uridyl transferase activity is normal. There is no jaundice and no failure to thrive. (Mental retardation present in some patients.)

Lactase Deficiency

1. CONGENITAL LACTASE DEFICIENCY

Diagnosis of this condition, characterized by watery, profuse diarrhoea following each milk feed, and fatal unless lactose is eliminated from the infant's diet, is confirmed by the demonstration of the virtual absence of lactase activity in jejunal mucous membrane brush border biopsy material.

Following oral lactose (2 g/kg body weight) the blood glucose rises by less than + 1 mmol/l. The stools have a pH of less than 5·5 and contain lactose. In severe cases there may be amino aciduria.

TESTS OF PROGRESS

Recovery follows elimination of lactose from the diet.

TESTS PROVIDING USEFUL NEGATIVE RESULTS

Glucose absorption is normal when the infant is on a lactose-free diet.

2. ACQUIRED LACTASE DEFICIENCY (ADULT TYPE)

Africans tend to have low intestinal lactase activity, whereas Europeans have high lactase activity. The hypothesis is that high lactase activity is inherited as [AD], and low lactase activity is inherited as [AR]. Possibly 6 per cent of native adult British are unable to hydrolyse lactose adequately in their intestinal brush borders.

Diagnosis of lactose intolerance in adults can be confirmed by the development of symptoms including nausea, bloating, abdominal pain and diarrhoea, following 50 g of oral lactose. The enzyme lactase occurs in the brush border of the villous epithelium of the jejunum in normal infants. Activity drops sharply after weaning in normal Negroes (other than African pastoralists), Asians and South Americans, with consequent malabsorption of lactose, which may lead to lactose intolerance.

Peroral biopsy of the jejunal brush border can be used to demonstrate low lactase activity. Lactose-intolerant infants suffer from watery diarrhoea.

TESTS OF PROGRESS

Removal of milk from the diet results in disappearance of symptoms in lactose intolerance. Following gastric surgery, a subject with lactose malabsorption without symptoms may well develop symptoms of lactose intolerance.

Skimmed milk protein, often used as a dietary protein supplement, may cause diarrhoea when used for this purpose in the Third World.

TESTS PROVIDING USEFUL NEGATIVE RESULTS

Glucose-tolerance tests are normal, with no other evidence of malabsorption, when the infant or adult is taking a lactose-free diet. The rapid disappearance of lactase from the jejunum after weaning is a normal genetic characteristic affecting a large number of people. The enzyme tends to persist in Northern Europeans, African pastoralists and inhabitants of the North-western part of the Indian subcontinent.

FAMILIAL LACTOSE INTOLERANCE

Diagnosis of this condition characterized by severe failure to thrive, liver damage, mental retardation (and hiatus hernia in some cases), thought to be due to increased permeability to lactose and other disaccharides in the gastric mucosa, is confirmed by the demonstration of disacchariduria and amino aciduria from early infancy. Following oral lactose there is no increase in blood galactose.

TESTS OF PROGRESS

Clinical improvement with disappearance of disacchariduria and amino aciduria follows exclusion of lactose from the diet. Tolerance to lactose is recovered between 12 months and 18 months of age.

USEFUL NEGATIVE RESULTS

Small intestinal lactase activity is normal.

Familial Lactic Acidosis [R]

Diagnosis of this rare condition associated with mental retardation is confirmed by the finding of markedly increased plasma lactate levels, with gross reduction of plasma bicarbonate, low blood pH, and low plasma inorganic phosphate levels.

The urine contains abnormally increased amounts of lactic acid (normally present in trace amounts only).

Reactive (Functional) Hypoglycaemia

Diagnosis of this condition, characterized by symptoms associated with hypoglycaemia and relieved by oral glucose, is supported by the finding of normal fasting plasma glucose levels, which rise to a high peak ('lag curve') after oral glucose, falling to hypoglycaemic levels at 3–4 hours.

TESTS PROVIDING USEFUL NEGATIVE RESULTS

Fasting plasma glucose concentration is normal. Prolonged fasting (24–72 hours) does not provoke severe hypoglycaemia (cf. insulinoma). There is no evidence of inappropriate release of insulin into the plasma. There is no evidence of glycogen storage disease.

Idiopathic Neonatal Hypoglycaemia

Diagnosis of this condition, which is probably due to defective gluconeogenesis coupled with increased glucose utilization, is confirmed by the finding of very low blood-glucose concentrations during the first 72 hours after birth. It is particularly liable to occur in premature babies and in babies born to mothers with toxaemia of pregnancy.

Severe hypoglycaemia develops after 3–4 hours of fasting, but this test is dangerous unless the infant is in hospital and intravenous glucose is immediately available.

TESTS OF PROGRESS

Following intravenous glucose therapy (glucose by mouth is often ineffective) and intramuscular cortisone therapy the condition improves.

Ketotic Hypoglycaemia in Infants

Diagnosis of this condition is confirmed by the finding of low blood glucose in infants (usually detected at about 1 year of age) with drowsiness, lethargy, and, in some cases, convulsions in the early morning. The infants often have a history of a small birth weight, hypoglycaemia in the neonatal period, and are thin.

If a high-carbohydrate diet is given for 3 days, followed by a low-carbohydrate, high-fat diet, hypoglycaemia and ketosis develop in many cases within 24 hours (ketogenic provocation).

TESTS OF PROGRESS

Following the giving of carbohydrate supplements at bedtime, the condition improves.

TESTS PROVIDING USEFUL NEGATIVE RESULTS

Fructose tolerance is normal. Leucine tolerance is normal. The response to intravenous tolbutamide is normal.

Leucine-sensitivity Hypoglycaemia

Diagnosis is confirmed in infants with attacks of hypoglycaemia, by demonstrating severe hypoglycaemia developing in an affected infant ½–1 hour after protein or leucine.

TESTS OF PROGRESS

Affected infants recover rapidly when maintained on leucine-poor diets.

Glycogen-storage Disease

A. TYPE I (VON GIERKE'S DISEASE [AR])

Diagnosis of this condition, characterized by hypoglycaemia unless the child is fed every 2–3 hours night and day, is confirmed by the demonstration of reduced glucose-6-phosphatase activity in liver biopsy material, which also shows greatly increased liver glycogen content.

The newborn infant has hepatosplenomegaly with metabolic acidosis plus lactic acidosis. 0·5 mg glucagon i.m. does not cause any increase in blood glucose. Hyperlipidaemia with increased lipolysis in adipose tissue occurs.

Some children may survive the first 4 years of life without serious intellectual defect, but many die during the first 2 years, and are mentally retarded. There is poor excretion of uric acid in the urine, and any child surviving to the age of 10 suffers from attacks of gout.

TESTS OF PROGRESS

Hypoglycaemic attacks can be reduced if the child is fed every 2–3 hours night and day, but becomes obese in the process. Surgical diversion of the portal blood flow has been very successful in a few cases.

Heterozygote carriers in known families can be detected by measuring glucose-6-phosphatase activity in liver or small intestinal mucous membrane biopsy material, enzyme activity falling midway between affected homozygote and normal subject.

VARIANT

A variant has been described with identical clinical features, but with normal glucose-6-phosphatase activity (? a defect in transport of glucose-6-phosphate).

B. TYPE II (POMPE'S DISEASE)

Diagnosis of this condition, characterized by heart failure, gross cardiomegaly and severe hypotonia of all voluntary muscles, including respiratory muscles, appearing after the first 3 months, is confirmed by the demonstration of deficiency of alpha-1:4-glucosidase in leucocytes, cultured skin fibroblasts, liver and muscle biopsy material. Microscopically, it can be seen that there is excess glycogen in both liver and muscle, and a lysosomal membrane can be seen to be surrounding the glycogen accumulation in the liver, using electron microscopy.

TESTS OF PROGRESS

Prenatal diagnosis is possible, as uncultured amniotic cells show the typical accumulation of glycogen and lysosomal membrane on electron microscopy. No satisfactory treatment of affected homozygotes has yet been discovered. The specific enzyme activity in leucocytes and cultured skin fibroblasts lies midway between that of affected homozygotes and normal subjects.

TESTS PROVIDING USEFUL NEGATIVE RESULTS

Blood glucose, lipids and uric acid concentrations are normal. No attacks of hypoglycaemia occur, and there is a normal increase in blood glucose after 0·5 mg glucagon i.m.

VARIANT

A milder adult form also occurs.

C. TYPE III (CORI'S DISEASE; FORBES'S DISEASE; DEBRANCHER DISEASE) [AR]

Diagnosis of this condition, characterized by muscular wasting and weakness in early childhood, with moderate attacks of hypoglycaemia after fasting and mental retardation in the more severe cases, is confirmed by the demonstration of no response to 0·5 mg glucagon i.m. when fasting, but a normal increase in blood glucose 2 hours after a carbohydrate-rich meal when 0·5 mg glucagon i.m. is given (i.e. the outer chains of the glycogen molecules have built up again to normal length).

Limit dextrin can be demonstrated in red and white blood cells, and also in liver and muscle biopsy material. Since the 'debrancher enzyme system' includes at least two distinct enzymes working together, tissue enzyme assays can give different results in different cases (suggesting that this disease is really a collection of related diseases). In some cases an abnormal enzyme rather than enzyme absence is the biochemical defect. The severity of the condition varies from family to family, from manifestation in early childhood to asymptomatic adults.

TESTS OF PROGRESS

Patients suffering from attacks of hypoglycaemia require food by day and night, with some improvement with age. Phenytoin has been used moderately successfully in some cases (? by inhibiting insulin secretion, as there has been no induction of enzyme activity).

D. TYPE IV (ANDERSEN'S DISEASE; BRANCHER DEFICIENCY) [R]

Diagnosis of this rare condition, characterized by progressive cirrhosis beginning in the second or third month with death by the second year, is confirmed by demonstration of amylopectin (lavender colour with iodine) deposited in most tissues, and absent brancher enzyme activity in leucocytes and all tissues. Liver function tests eventually suggest the development of portal cirrhosis.

TESTS WHICH PROVIDE USEFUL NEGATIVE RESULTS

Attacks of hypoglycaemia do not occur, and there is a normal increase in blood glucose following 0·5 glucagon i.m.

E. TYPE V (MCARDLE'S DISEASE) [R]

Diagnosis of this rare condition, characterized by pain and stiffness after moderately strenuous exercise, appearing towards the end of the second decade, and including pain and stiffness in the jaw muscles after vigorous chewing, progressing to 'cramp', is confirmed by the demonstration of the absence of lactic acid production after ischaemic exercise (arm exercises for 1 min with a blood pressure cuff set above systolic blood pressure, and venous blood sampled 1 min after the release of the cuff).

Absence of phosphorylase activity can be demonstrated in muscle biopsy material. After severe exercise, the electromyograph is electrically silent (i.e. there is no active contraction of muscle as would occur in a true 'cramp').

TESTS OF PROGRESS

Glucose or fructose supplements may be taken immediately before expected vigorous exercise.

F. TYPE VI (HERS' DISEASE; HEPATIC PHOSPHORYLASE DEFICIENCY) [AR] [R]

Diagnosis of this rare mild condition, characterized by hepatomegaly and mild or absent hypoglycaemia, is confirmed by the demonstration of deficiency of phosphorylase activity in leucocytes and liver biopsy material. Electron microscopy of liver biopsy material reveals rosette-shaped glycogen particles. A dose of 0·5 mg glucagon i.m. either in the fasting or the postprandial state does not result in any increase in blood glucose.

TESTS OF PROGRESS

Phenytoin reduces liver glycogen content, but does not increase the specific enzyme activity.

G. TYPE VII (MUSCLE PHOSPHOFRUCTOKINASE DEFICIENCY) [AR]/[R]

Diagnosis of this rare condition, characterized by signs and symptoms as in Type V glycogen storage disease, is confirmed by the demonstration of deficient phosphofructokinase activity in red cells and muscle biopsy material, with absence of the immunologically normal enzyme protein; 50 per cent of the phosphofructokinase activity in red cells is of the muscle type, and red cells in this disease have a reduced half-life with a persistent reticulocytosis. As in Type V disease, there is no increase in blood lactic acid after ischaemic muscular exercise.

TESTS OF PROGRESS

Heterozygote carriers in affected families have detectable reduced erythrocyte phosphofructokinase activity.

TESTS WHICH PROVIDE USEFUL NEGATIVE RESULTS

A dose of 0·5 mg glucagon i.m. produces a normal increase in blood glucose.

H. TYPE VIII [R]

Diagnosis of this rare condition, characterized by drowsiness, lethargy, spasticity, decerebration, convulsions and death in infancy, is confirmed by the demonstration of reduced phosphorylase activity in liver biopsy material. Brain histology reveals glycogen deposition and brain phosphorylase activity is abnormally low.

TESTS WHICH PROVIDE USEFUL NEGATIVE RESULTS

Hypoglycaemic attacks do not occur, and after 0·5 mg glucagon i.m. there is a normal increase in blood glucose.

I. TYPE IX (LIVER PHOSPHORYLASE KINASE DEFICIENCY) [R]

Two varieties have been described:

A. TYPE IXa [AR]

There is hepatomegaly, no hypoglycaemic attacks, and a normal blood glucose response to 0·5 mg glucagon i.m.

B. TYPE IXb [*XR*]

There is hepatomegaly, fasting hypoglycaemia and a poor response to 0·5 mg glucagon i.m. There is some retardation of both growth and motor development, but mental development is normal. Girls have only mild symptoms.

Diagnosis of both these conditions is confirmed by the demonstration of deficiency of phosphorylase kinase (but not its absence) in red cells, leucocytes, cultured skin fibrobalsts and in liver biopsy material.

J. TYPE X (LIVER AND MUSCLE GLYCOGENOSIS)

One case has been reported with asymptomatic hepatomegaly. There were no attacks of hypoglycaemia, but also there was no response in blood glucose to 0·5 mg glucagon i.m.

Liver and muscle biopsy material revealed inactive phosphorylase, due to deficient activity of cyclic-AMP-dependent kinase. Both muscle and liver contained excess glycogen.

Uridine Diphosphate Galactose-4-epimerase Deficiency [R]

Some families have been found during screening programmes for glycogen storage disease, with complete absence of activity of the enzyme uridine diphosphate galactose-4-epimerase, in homozygotes. These subjects showed no signs of symptoms of glycogen storage disease and appeared to be clinically normal. This enzyme deficiency is therefore of no clinical significance.

Hypertrophic Steatosis of Debré (Hepatomegalic Gluco-adiposity)[R]

Laboratory findings as in glycogen-storage diseases.

Simple Screening Tests for Glycogen-storage Diseases

Following oral glucose tolerance test dose of glucose:

A. Abnormally increased blood lactate in the fasting state, following fall in blood lactate after glucose load
   ⎰Suggestive of glucose-6-phosphatase deficiency, Type I.⎱
B. Normal fasting blood lactate, with marked rise in blood lactate following glucose load
   Suggestive of:
      1. Debrancher enzyme deficiency, Type III.
      2. Phosphorylase deficiency, Type VI.
   Follow with glucagon tolerance test:
      1. Flat blood-glucose curve = debrancher deficiency.
      2. Normal blood-glucose curve = phosphorylase deficiency.
C. Blood-lactate curve following glucose load at the upper level of normal
   Suggestive of:
      1. No glycogen-storage disorder.
      2. Phosphorylase deficiency.
   Follow with galactose tolerance test:
      1. Normal rise in blood glucose = normal.
      2. Excessive rise in blood lactate = phosphorylase deficiency.

D. Following 0·5 mg glucagon i.m.
   Blood glucose increases normally in Types II, IV, V, VII, VIII, IX and X. Blood glucose rises slightly in fasting patient, but is normal 2 hours after carbohydrate in Type III. Blood glucose fails to rise in Types I and VI.
E. Hypoglycaemic attacks in fasting patients
   These occur in Types I and III, VI (mild or absent), IXb in boys.

Essential Pentosuria

Diagnosis of this harmless recessive condition is confirmed by the finding of increased output of L-xylulose in the urine (a reducing substance) with no abnormal increase in glucose output. The metabolic error is due to a deficiency in the liver of NADP-L-xylulose dehydrogenase activity, and the output of L-xylulose is increased following ingestion of glycuronate-containing substances. Red-cell xylitol dehydrogenase activity is reduced. Heterozygotes can be identified; following oral glucuronlactone, they excrete excessive amounts of L-xylulose in the urine, and serum L-xylulose levels rise abnormally.

TESTS PROVIDING USEFUL NEGATIVE RESULTS

Renal function tests are normal.

Hyperglucaric Aciduria [R]

Diagnosis of this rare condition was confirmed by the finding of excretion of excessive amounts of D-glucaric acid in the urine in a mentally retarded patient.

Sucrase-isomaltase Deficiency [AR] [R]

Diagnosis of this rare condition, presenting in infancy with intolerance to sucrose, with increasing tolerance with age, and characterized by diarrhoea, carbohydrate intolerance, and 'irritable colon', is confirmed by the demonstration of abnormally low activity of sucrase, maltase and isomaltase, in small intestinal biopsy material. There is only a small increase in blood glucose during either sucrose or starch tolerance tests (normally blood glucose should rise by more than 1·2 mmol/l). The stool pH is low.

TESTS OF PROGRESS

The condition improves when sucrose is eliminated from the diet. This enzyme deficiency occurs in up to 10 per cent of Greenland Eskimoes.

TESTS PROVIDING USEFUL NEGATIVE RESULTS

Both glucose and lactose tolerance tests are normal.

Infantile Sucrosuria

Although originally thought to be a congenital anomaly associated with mental defect and hiatus hernia, it has since been shown that sucrosuria occurs normally in new born infants if enough sucrose is added to their feeds.

Trehalase Deficiency [R]

Probably only a few people eat sufficient mushrooms to develop symptoms due to this deficiency. One family has been described, in which inheritance of the enzyme deficiency appeared to be autosomal dominant.

Beta-xylosidase Deficiency [R]

Diagnosis of this very rare condition was made by the demonstration of deficiency of beta-xylosidase activity in lymphocytes in a mentally retarded epileptic patient.

LIPID DISORDERS

SECONDARY HYPERLIPIDAEMIC DISORDERS

USING FREDRICKSON'S CLASSIFICATION

The following conditions may be associated with the electrophoretic patterns of:

Type I (persisting chylomicronaemia)
Dysglobulinaemia
Systemic lupus erythematosus

Type IIa (increased LDL)
Nephrotic syndrome
Hypothyroidism
Dysglobulinaemia
Cushing's syndrome
Acute intermittent porphyria
Hepatoma

Type IIb (increased LDL and VLDL)
Nephrotic syndrome
Hypothyroidism
Dysglobulinaemia
Cushing's syndrome

Type III (increased IDL)
Hypothyroidism
Systemic lupus erythematosus
Long-term maintenance dialysis

Type IV (Increased VLDL)
Diabetes mellitus with severe prolonged insulin deficiency
Glycogen storage disease Type I
Lipodystrophies
Dysglobulinaemia

Uraemia
Hypopituitarism (with secondary hypothyroidism).

Type V (Increased chylomicra, increased VLDL)
Diabetes mellitus with severe prolonged insulin deficiency
Glycogen storage disease Type I.
Lipodystrophies
Dysglobulinaemia
Uraemia
Hypopituitarism (with secondary hypothyroidism)
Nephrotic syndrome

Primary Hyperlipidaemias

Diabetes mellitus
Alcoholism ⎫
Oestrogen therapy ⎬ These conditions may aggravate a primary hyperlipidaemia
Glucocorticoid therapy ⎭ (Types IIb, IV and V).
'Stress'

The primary hyperlipidaemias have been classified, where possible, defining the specific defect causing the abnormality. The Fredrickson classification is also shown in *Table* 1, p. 118.

PRIMARY HYPERLIPIDAEMIC DISORDERS

Familial Lipoprotein Lipase Deficiency

Diagnosis of this rare autosomal recessive condition is made by the finding of a *Type-1 plasma lipoprotein phenotype*—chylomicra circulating in the fasting state. The chilled serum has a creamy layer of chylomicra on top, with clear serum below, due to defective hydrolysis of chylomicron triglyceride. Post-heparin plasma lipolytic activity is below normal. Serum triglyceride levels are grossly increased, with normal or moderately increased serum cholesterol values. Plasma LDL level is low.

TESTS OF PROGRESS

While a high fat intake may result in attacks of severe abdominal pain, a therapeutic trial of dietary fat restriction with added medium-chain triglyceride intake (less than 5 g fat per day for 4–5 days) results in disappearance of circulating chylomicra and the plasma triglyceride level falls to normal (cf. familial hypertriglyceridaemia). For satisfactory maintenance, fat intake should be restricted to 20–30 g per day, with added medium-chain triglycerides. When chylomicronaemia is reduced by diet, the high untreated serum cholesterol can fall to low levels.

Apoprotein-CII Deficiency

Diagnosis of this extremely rare autosomal recessive condition is made by the finding of a *Type-1 plasma lipoprotein phenotype*—chylomicra circulating in the fasting state. The chilled serum has a creamy layer of chylomicra on top, with clear serum below, due to defective hydrolysis of chylomicron trigly-ceride. Apoprotein CII, the essential activator for lipoprotein lipase activity, is absent. Post-heparin plasma lipolytic activity is below normal. Serum triglyceride levels are grossly increased with normal or moderately raised serum cholesterol values.

TESTS OF PROGRESS

Restriction of dietary fat to less than 5 g per day for 4–5 days results in plasma triglycerides falling to normal values, with virtual disappearance of circulating chylomicra (cf. familial hypertriglyceridaemia). For satisfactory maintenance, fat intake should be restricted to 20–30 g per day, with added medium-chain triglycerides.

Plasma transfusion from a normal subject results in a dramatic fall in plasma triglycerides (e.g. from 1000 mg/dl to less than 250 mg/dl in 24 hours, i.e. activation by normal plasma apoprotein CII of lipoprotein lipase).

Familial Hypercholesterolaemia

Diagnosis of this autosomal dominant condition, which is associated with accelerated atherosclerosis and xanthomatosis, is made by the demonstration of a *Type IIa plasma lipoprotein phenotype*—marked increase in serum LDL, with raised serum cholesterol and normal plasma triglycerides. The chilled serum is usually clear. Three defects have been described in this condition. There may be a 50 per cent reduction in LDL receptors on peripheral cell surface in heterozygotes, with almost total absence in homozygotes. There may be defects in 80–90 per cent of LDL receptor sites in homozygotes. Alternatively, there may be receptor mislocation, with a normal number of receptors, but with failure of these sites to aggregate in 'coated pits' of the cell membrane, and hence reduced rate of endocytosis of receptor-LDL com-plexes. Assay of LDL receptor function can be carried out using cultured fibroblasts or blood lymphocytes. The consequence of these defects is defective removal of LDL from the circulation. Failure of uptake into cells fails to inhibit intracellular cholesterol synthesis.

TESTS OF PROGRESS

A fat-modified diet containing about 36 per cent of the total calorie intake as the total fat intake, with reduced saturated fat proportion, partly replaced by polyunsaturated fat, and a total intake of not more than 300 mg cholesterol per day, may result in improvement. If response is incomplete, then 16–28 g of cholestyramine or colestipol may be given per day with meals. If the response is still unsatisfactory, then clofibrate can be added.

In homozygotes an ileal bypass may be necessary. Plasmapheresis has been used in young homozygotes, where diet and medication have been ineffective.

Recently, successful treatment with inhibition of the rate-limiting enzyme 3-hydroxy-3-methylglutaryl coenzyme A reductase, with compactin or mevinolin has been reported.

Table 1. Fredrickson classification of primary hyperlipidaemias

Fredrickson type	Hereditary/ acquired	Atherosclerosis risk	Fasting serum electrophoresis	Fasting chilled serum (12 h)	Serum total triglycerides	Serum total cholesterol	Incidence (%)
Type I	Hereditary acquired	Slight	Chylomicra +++	Creamy supernatant, clear below	Gross increase	Normal	1
Type IIa	Hereditary acquired	Very high	LDL +++	Clear	< 2·29 mmol/l < 200 mg/100 ml	> 6·7 mmol/l > 260 mg/100 ml	20
Type IIb	Hereditary acquired	Very high	LDL and VLDL greatly increased	Clear–turbid	> 2·29 mmol/l > 200 mg/100 ml	> 6·7 mmol/l > 260 mg/100 ml	
Type III	Hereditary acquired	Very high	Broad 'beta' VLDL ++ IDL ++ true LDL low	Clear–turbid	Gross increase	Gross increase	5
Type IV	Hereditary acquired	High	VLDL ++ LDL normal	Turbid– opalescent	> 2·29 mmol/l > 200 mg/100 ml	< 6·7 mmol/l < 260 mg/100 ml	70
Type V	Hereditary acquired	Slight	VLDL +++ Chylomicra ++	Creamy supernatant, turbid below	> 2·29 mmol/l > 200 mg/100 ml	< 6·7 mmol/l < 260 mg/100 ml	5

Polygenic Hypercholesterolaemia

Diagnosis of this polygenic condition, associated with 10 times the 'normal' incidence of ischaemic heart disease in males, and accelerated atherosclerosis, is made by the finding of a *Type IIa serum lipoprotein phenotype*—marked increase in serum LDL with serum cholesterol levels 2–3 times normal and serum triglyceride levels normal or slightly increased. The chilled serum is clear. LDL receptor sites on peripheral cells are normal.

TESTS OF PROGRESS

The total fat intake is restricted to about 36 per cent of the total calorie intake, partly replaced by polyunsaturated fats, and the daily cholesterol intake is restricted to less than 300 mg per day. If dietary restriction does not result in improvement, then clofibrate and cholestyramine may be given.

Familial Combined Hyperlipidaemia

Diagnosis of this autosomal dominant condition, which is associated with accelerated atherosclerosis, is made by the demonstration of *Type IIa, IIb or IV serum lipoprotein phenotype*—raised LDL, raised LDL + VLDL, or excess VLDL, normal LDL and no fasting chylomicra. The chilled serum is turbid, but rarely creamy. The condition probably results from overproduction of VLDL apoprotein-B, which results in increased VLDL secretion, and consequent increased LDL production from VLDL.

One third of cases have hypercholesterolaemia, one third have hypertriglyceridaemia, and one third have hypercholesterolaemia plus hypertriglyceridaemia. Type IV lipoprotein phenotype is found in familial combined hyperlipidaemia with obesity.

TESTS OF PROGRESS

Dietary restriction with low fat intake may result in improvement, but treatment with clofibrate and/or cholestyramine is often necessary. Clofibrate results in a significant fall in the abnormally raised serum triglyceride concentration.

Broad-beta Disease

Diagnosis of this condition with an uncertain form of inheritance, is made by the demonstration of a *Type III serum hyperlipoproteinaemia phenotype*—a broad 'beta-band' with increased VLDL and raised serum triglyceride and cholesterol levels. The 'broad-beta' band consists of IDL, with greatly reduced LDL. There is defective catabolism of chylomicra remnants and of IDL in the liver, with absence of apoprotein EIII and another unknown factor (1 per cent of normolipidaemic subjects lack apoprotein EIII). The condition is associated with accelerated atherosclerosis. Fasting chilled serum is turbid, and often has a small creamy top layer. Serum cholesterol : triglyceride = 3 : 2.

TESTS OF PROGRESS

High carbohydrate intake aggravates the condition. Clofibrate tends to reduce the serum triglyceride levels towards normal.

Familial Hypertriglyceridaemia

Diagnosis of this autosomal dominant condition, which is associated with attacks of abdominal pain, pancreatitis and lipaemia retinalis (occasional), is made by the demonstration of a *Type IV* or *Type V serum hyperlipo-proteinaemia phenotype*—excess VLDL, normal LDL without fasting chylomicra, or increased VLDL with increased chylomicra plus severe hyper-triglyceridaemia. The condition is probably caused by excessive hepatic tri-glyceride synthesis. Rarely the taking of oral contraceptives may result in massive hypertriglyceridaemia complicated by acute pancreatitis.

Chilled fasting serum is usually turbid, and rarely creamy, and fasting serum triglycerides are markedly increased. Serum cholesterol: triglyceride = 1:5.

TESTS OF PROGRESS

Clofibrate results in reduction in serum triglycerides. Therapeutic trial of dietary fat restriction (cf. lipoprotein lipase deficiency) does not cause a marked fall in serum triglycerides.

Familial LCAT Deficiency [R]

Diagnosis of this inherited condition [AR] is confirmed by the finding of grossly reduced plasma LCAT activity. Plasma cholesterol-ester is virtually absent, with an ester-free cholesterol ratio of less than 0·1. Serum HDL is reduced, which is in discoidal nascent form; LDL is present in discoidal form, and there is an accumulation of abnormal cholesterol-rich remanants of chylomicra and catabolized VLDL with abnormally increased levels of *lipoprotein-X*. Impaired triglyceride-rich lipoprotein catabolism with failure of cholesterol esterification in plasma results in plasma total cholesterol and triglyceride levels which may be normal or raised. Serum albumin levels tend to be low, with reduced serum acid phosphatase activity. There is often anaemia with circulating target cells, the result of abnormal red cell membrane. Proteinuria is present, and renal failure is the major cause of death. Accumulation of unesterified cholesterol in the tissues is associated with accelerated atherosclerosis.

There is no specific treatment.

Hyperalphalipoproteinaemia [R]

Diagnosis of this rare condition, associated with reduced risk of atheroscler-otic disease, and with longevity, is confirmed by the finding of serum HDL levels raised significantly above the normal range, and no other abnormality.

HYPOLIPOPROTEINAEMIC DISORDERS

A-Betalipoproteinaemia [R] [AR]

Diagnosis of this rare condition, characterized by steatorrhoea, distorted red cells (possibly with haemolysis), mental retardation (in some cases), plus very low serum cholesterol (1–2 mmol/l, 40–80 mg/dl) and barely detectable plasma triglyceride, is confirmed by the demonstration of the virtual absence of apolipoprotein B. After a fatty meal, there is complete absence of chylomicra, VLDL, IDL or LDL, with increased HDL, in the serum. There is complete inability to assemble VLDL or chylomicra in the intestinal mucosal cells, or liver. Jejunal biopsy may reveal fat accumulation, as globules, in the mucosal cells.

TESTS OF PROGRESS

Partial substitution of dietary fat with medium-chain triglycerides and fat-soluble vitamin supplements, may reduce the steatorrhoea and possibly delay the neurological and retinal changes which develop eventually.

Hypobetalipoproteinaemia [R] [AD]

Diagnosis of this rare condition is confirmed by the finding of low serum cholesterol (1·5–3·5 mmol/l, 60–135 mg/dl), with low serum VLDL and LDL levels (due to reduced synthesis of apolipoprotein B, and hence low rate of synthesis of VLDL, causing low production of LDL). Distorted red cells may be seen in some cases, and fat-engorged intestinal mucosal cells may be seen in biopsy specimens. There appears to be a reduced risk of atherosclerosis in these patients, with a tendency to longevity.

USEFUL NEGATIVE RESULTS

Unlike A-betalipoproteinaemia, chylomicra are formed after a fatty meal, and malabsorption is uncommon.

Familial Alpha-lipoprotein Deficiency [R] [AR]

Diagnosis of this rare condition, associated with corneal opacities, motor and sensory neuropathy, and enlarged tonsils, adenoids, spleen and sometimes liver, due to enhanced catabolism of apoprotein AI and apoprotein AII, is confirmed by the demonstration via serum protein electrophoresis of the virtual absence of alpha-lipoprotein (high-density lipoprotein, HDL). Serum protein electrophoresis also shows a broad band of IDL and VLDL (as seen in Type III hyperlipoproteinaemia). Traces of abnormal HDL may be detected in the serum, with no apoprotein AI present (less than 1 per cent of normal), and apoprotein AII at 5–7 per cent of normal.

Serum cholesterol is reduced (1–3 mmol/l, 40–120 mg/dl) with normal-to-raised serum triglycerides (1·8–2·8 mmol/l, 150–256 mg/dl), and these two findings also suggest the possibility of this diagnosis. Plasma LCAT activity is normal, or moderately reduced *in vivo*. Hepatic secretion of nascent discoidal HDL is normal, reverse cholesterol transfer is normal, and HDL ester cholesterol turnover is also normal. Cholesteryl esters and remnants of chylomicron catabolism accumulate in the tonsils, adenoids, spleen and liver, and can be seen as visible deposits phagocytosed by the reticulo-endothelial system.

There is no specific treatment.

LIPID STORAGE DISEASES

Amaurotic Familial Idiocy (GM$_2$ Gangliosidosis Types 1 and 3; Infantile Type 1 and Juvenile Type 3 Tay–Sachs' Disease) [R]

Diagnosis of this recessive neurodegenerative disorder, with progressive distension of neurons with GM$_2$ ganglioside, is confirmed by the demonstration of deficiency of activity of beta-N-acetylhexosaminidase-isoenzyme A, in leucocytes, urine, cultured fibroblasts, muscle, spleen, liver, kidney and brain. After demonstration of the specific enzyme deficiency in leucocytes, the deficiency should be confirmed in cultured skin fibroblasts. Varieties of this disease, reflecting time of onset and severity of signs and symptoms (Norman–Wood disease, Tay–Sachs' disease, Batten's disease and Kuf's disease), occur.

In Type 1 disease, the deficiency of hexosaminidase A is almost complete.

In Type 3 disease, the deficiency of hexosaminidase A is less, but still severe. Many of the circulating neutrophils and monocytes contain abnormal cytoplasmic granular inclusions. Serum aspartate aminotransferase and lactate dehydrogenase activities may be increased. CSF aspartate aminotransferase and lactate dehydrogenase activities may be increased.

TESTS OF PROGRESS

Prenatal amniotic fluid monitoring enables fibroblast culture to be undertaken, with subsequent detection of affected fetuses in utero, in members of known affected families when they become pregnant.

Sandhoff's Disease (GM$_2$ Gangliosidosis Type 2; Globoside Storage Disease) [R]

Diagnosis of this rare recessive neurodegenerative disorder, clinically indistinguishable from infantile Tay–Sachs' (Type 1) disease, is confirmed by the demonstration of deficiency of both iso-enzymes A and B of beta-N-acetylhexosaminidase. The deficiency of activity is detectable in leucocytes, urine, cultured fibroblasts, liver, spleen, kidney, muscle and brain. After demonstration of the specific enzyme deficiency in leucocytes, the deficiency should be confirmed in cultured fibroblasts.

Cephalin Lipidosis [R]

Diagnosis of this rare condition was made by the finding of reduced serum phospholipids with virtual absence of lecithin, with excessive storage of a cephalin in the spleen, liver, brain, and spinal cord.

Cholesterol Ester Storage Disease [R] [AR]

Diagnosis of this rare condition, characterized by hepatomegaly followed later by splenomegaly, is confirmed by the demonstration of the virtual absence of lysosomal cholesterol esterase in liver biopsy material. Affected infants may initially be asymptomatic, but the condition is associated with premature atherosclerosis.

There is a moderate increase in serum cholesterol, with increases in serum VLDL and LDL, and low HDL levels.

Farber's Lipogranulomatosis (Ceramidase Deficiency) [R]

Diagnosis of this rare recessive condition, associated with arthropathy, subcutaneous, periarticular and visceral nodules and mild macular degeneration, is confirmed by the demonstration of deficiency of acid ceramidase activity in leucocytes, cultured fibroblasts, kidney and cerebellum. After initial finding of deficiency of the enzyme activity in leucocytes, the result should be confirmed using cultured skin fibroblasts.

The CSF protein is increased. Affected homozygote patients survive for two years.

TESTS OF PROGRESS

Culture of amniotic fluid cells in members of known affected families, during pregnancy, enables the detection of normal, heterozygote and homozygote affected fetuses. There is no treatment for affected cases.

Fabry's Disease (Angiokeratoma Corporis Diffuse) [R]

Diagnosis of this rare sex-linked dominant recessive condition, which produces severe symptoms in hemizygous males including painful neuropathy plus cataracts and corneal dystrophy and only slight symptoms in heterozygous females, is made by the demonstration of deficiency of activity of heat-labile alpha-D-galactosidase in cultured skin fibroblasts. Infiltration with ceramide occurs in skin, causing a papular rash on the trunk and buttocks, in the lungs causing impaired ventilation, in the kidneys causing tubular and glomerular impairment, uraemia and high blood pressure, cardiovascular damage, and accumulation in muscle, enables histological diagnosis to be made. The galactosyl-galactosyl-glucosyl ceramide stains metachromatically with toluidine blue. 'Foamy' macrophages may be seen in bone marrow aspirate. The specific heat-labile enzyme is deficient in liver, kidney, spleen, intestinal mucosa, lymph nodes, heart, white blood cells, cultured skin fibroblasts, serum and urine.

CSF protein may be increased without any increase in cells.

TESTS OF PROGRESS

Screening of possible cases and carriers can be carried out by examination of filter-paper through which 24-hour collection of urine has been filtered, for excess ceramide. Fibroblast tissue cultures should be carried out on positive screen results.

Fucosidosis [R]

Diagnosis of this rare recessive condition is confirmed by the demonstration of the virtual absence of the lysosomal enzyme alpha-L-fucosidase in cultures of skin fibroblasts. Clinically, the disease resembles Hurler's syndrome (muco-polysaccharidosis Type IH), with progressive neurological degeneration, mental subnormality, muscle hypotonia and spasticity, with death in 5–6 years. Very low activity of alpha-L-fucosidase is found in liver, brain, lung, kidney, pancreas, fibroblasts, white blood cells, serum and urine. There is hepatomegaly, cardiomegaly, thickened skin with infiltration with storage polysaccharide, with lung infiltration (causing respiratory infections), which can be detected histologically.

Screening of suspected cases can be carried out by examination of enzyme activity in white blood cells, followed by tissue fibroblast culture examination if low enzyme levels are found.

GM₁ Gangliosidosis [R]

TYPE I

Diagnosis of this rare neurodegenerative disorder of infancy, which is accompanied by hepatosplenomegaly and skeletal abnormalities resembling Hurler Type I mycopolysaccharidosis is confirmed by the demonstration of deficiency of beta-D-galactoside-galactohydrolase (galactosidase) which occurs in brain, liver, spleen, kidney, leucocytes, cultured fibroblasts and urine. There are a number of iso-enzyme forms of the enzyme, and deficiency
of liver iso-enzymes A, B and C galactosidase is found.

Peripheral blood lymphocytes contain vacuoles, and the urine deposit contains foamy mononuclear cells.

USEFUL NEGATIVE RESULTS

The urine mucopolysaccharide content is normal or slightly increased (i.e. distinguishing this disease from Type I mucopolysaccharidosis H).

TYPE II

Diagnosis of this rare clinically milder juvenile form of the disease is confirmed by the demonstration of severe deficiency of galactosidase deficiency in brain, liver, spleen, kidney, leucocytes, cultured fibroblasts and urine. It is reported that there is a deficiency of liver iso-enzymes B and C galactosidase (cf. Type I). The peripheral blood lymphocytes contain vacuoles in some cases, and foamy mononuclear cells are present in the bone marrow.

USEFUL NEGATIVE RESULTS

The urine mucopolysaccharide content is normal or slightly increased (i.e. distinguishing this disease from Type I mucopolysaccharidosis H).

Rare Gangliosidoses [R]

Cases have been reported with various different patterns of abnormal accumulation of gangliosides, e.g.

GM₃ and GM₄ without GM₂ and with small amounts of GM₁.

GM_3 sphingolipodystrophy, with accumulation of GM_3 in brain and liver. GM_1, GM_3, GM_4, accumulation in the brain.

Gaucher's Disease (Kerasinosis) [AR]

Diagnosis of this recessive condition is confirmed by the demonstration of gross reduction in activity of the enzyme beta-D-glucosidase, in leucocytes, cultured fibroblasts, urine, spleen, liver and brain. After demonstration of the specific enzyme deficiency in leucocytes, the result should be confirmed on cultured skin fibroblasts.

Three clinical types occur:
1. Adult chronic non-neuropathic form.
2. Acute neuropathic type.
3. Subacute juvenile neuropathic form.

Typical infiltration with Gaucher cells filled with glucocerebroside occurs in the bone-marrow, spleen, liver and lymph glands, and suitable histochemical stains of biopsy material can be used to demonstrate this.

Serum acid phosphatase activity is increased above normal if phenyl phosphate is used as substrate for the estimation, but not if glycerophosphate is used as substrate. Serum alkaline phosphatase activity is also increased if there is much bone resorption with consecutive repair. A moderate normochromic, normocytic anaemia is commonly found, although leuco-erythroblastic anaemia may occur. Neutropenia with relative lymphocytosis and also thrombocytopenia is found, due to hypersplenism.

Aspartate aminotransferase activity is increased both in serum and CSF. On tissue culture of skin fibroblasts, giant cells full of metachromic material are grown in non-cerebral forms and in carriers of the non-cerebral type of the disease.

TESTS OF PROGRESS

Following splenectomy, serum acid phosphatase activity is reduced and hypersplenism is relieved.

Although it should be possible to detect the enzyme deficiency in tissue cultures from amniotic fluid aspiration, this has not yet been reported.

It is possible to screen both potential cases and carriers by examination of a filter-paper through which a 24-hour collection of urine has been filtered, for abnormal amounts of glycosphingolipid. The filter-paper can be sent through the post after it has been dried.

Krabbe's Leucodystrophy (Globoid Leucodystrophy) [R]

Diagnosis of this rare neurodegenerative disease of infancy, associated with deafness, blindness, cerebral degeneration and death within 2 years, is confirmed by the demonstration of a gross deficiency of galactoceramide beta-D-galactosidase activity in brain, kidney, liver, spleen, leucocytes, cultured fibroblasts and serum. Abnormal globoid cells of mesodermal origin are present in the white matter in brain biopsy material.

Heterozygotes, clinically normal, have enzyme activity levels between the normal and affected homozygote values. When amniocentesis is carried out to detect affected homozygote fetuses in utero, in affected families, the amniotic fluid activity in an affected homozygote fetus has a galactosidase activity of less than 20 per cent of normal.

Green Acyl Dehydrogenase Deficiency [R]

Diagnosis of this very rare condition is confirmed by the finding of urine which smells of 'sweaty feet' and which contains butyric and hexanoic acids.

Mucoliposis Type II (I-Cell Disease) [R]

Diagnosis of this very rare neurodegenerative disease is confirmed by the demonstration of reduction in activity of alpha-L-iduronidase and iduronate sulphatase in brain biopsy material and cultured fibroblasts. The finding of low iduronidase activity in peripheral blood leucocytes should be confirmed by enzyme assays using cultured fibroblasts. Very large numbers of inclusion bodies develop in cultured fibroblasts.

Urine contains increased amounts of dermatan sulphate.

Lecithin-cholesterol Acyl Transferase Deficiency (Norum's Disease) [R]

Diagnosis of this rare condition, associated with anaemia, proteinuria, corneal opacities and premature atherosclerosis, and compatible with adult life, is confirmed by the demonstration of deficiency of lecithin-cholesterol acyl transferase activity in liver, plasma and lymph.

Total serum cholesterol and total serum lecithin levels are often increased, with very low levels of serum ester cholesterol, and HDL (high-density lipoprotein, alpha-lipoprotein) and VLDL (very low-density lipoproteins, pre-beta-lipoproteins) below normal. All the plasma lipoproteins may show qualitative changes with abnormal electrophoretic mobilities. Serum triglyceride and uric acid concentrations are increased above normal.

Foam macrophages are found in bone marrow aspirate, and in glomeruli in renal biopsy material. Anaemia with target cells and proteinuria may be found. The detection of lipoprotein-X (an abnormal low-density lipoprotein) can be used as a screening test before specific enzyme estimation in suspected cases.

USEFUL NEGATIVE RESULTS

Liver function tests are normal.

Mannosidosis [R]

Diagnosis of this rare disease, fatal within a few years of onset, which clinically resembles mucopolysaccharidosis Type IH (Hurler), with hepatomegaly, splenomegaly, muscular hypotonia, bone abnormalities and lens opacities, is confirmed by the demonstration of deficiency in activity of alpha-D-mannose mannohydrolase in liver, brain, leucocytes, plasma and cultured fibroblasts.

There is abnormal storage of lipid in the brain.

Metachromatic Leucodystrophy (Metachromatic Leucoencephalopathy)

Diagnosis of this neurodegenerative disease, associated with hypotonia, and progressive paralysis, is confirmed by the demonstration of deficiency of aryl sulphatase iso-enzyme A in brain, liver, spleen, kidney, leucocytes, cultured skin fibroblasts. When the enzyme deficiency has been demonstrated in peripheral blood leucocytes, the deficiency should then be demonstrated using cultured skin fibroblasts.

The condition becomes clinically apparent usually by 2 years of age, and is fatal after a few years. Peripheral nerve (rectal or mesenteric plexus biopsy material) can be examined by electron microscopy for typical abnormalities.

Amniocentesis can be used to detect affected homozygote fetuses. Urine from possible carriers can be screened by examination for excess sulphatide, but confirmation of results should be carried out by leucocyte enzyme estimation.

Niemann–Pick Disease (Sphingomyelin Lipidoses) [AR]

This rare recessive condition presents in various clinical forms:

1. *Infantile* (85 per cent of cases)—characterized by mental retardation, blindness, progressive neurological deterioration, hepatosplenomegaly, enlargement of the lymph glands, cherry red macula spot, and death in infancy.
2. *Childhood*—death by 3 years.
3. *Juvenile*—onset of disease at 3–4 years.
4. *Adult form*—without neurological damage.

Diagnosis of this condition is confirmed by the demonstration of reduced sphingomyelinase activity in cultured skin fibroblasts, peripheral blood leucocytes (also liver, spleen and kidney). Sphingomyelin progressively accumulates in the tissues. Many of the peripheral blood lymphocytes and monocytes are vacuolated. A leuco-erythroblastic anaemia with thrombocytopenia develops later in the disease. Using phenyl phosphate as substrate, the serum acid phosphatase activity is increased.

In the bone marrow, vacuolated and 'foamy' histiocytes are found. 'Foam cells' containing the storage lipid are present in skin, liver, spleen, rectal ganglia and lymph gland biopsy material.

TESTS OF PROGRESS

Sphingomyelinase deficiency can be demonstrated in cell cultures from amniotic fluid. The condition can therefore be detected antenatally in known affected families.

Refsum's Disease [R] [AR]

Diagnosis of this rare condition, associated with chronic neurological degeneration leading to cerebellar ataxia, peripheral neuropathy and retinitis pigmentosa, is confirmed by the demonstration of the abnormal accumulation of phytanic acid in serum, and deficiency of activity of phytanic acid alpha-hydroxylase in cultured skin fibroblasts. Affected peripheral nerves conduct impulses more slowly than normal, and show a typical appearance on biopsy.

Serum creatine phosphokinase activity is increased. In the CSF, protein concentration, lactate dehydrogenase activity and aspartate aminotransferase activity are all increased abnormally, without corresponding increase in serum lactate dehydrogenase or aspartate aminotransferase activities.

A partial alpha-hydroxylase activity defect can be detected in cultured skin fibroblasts of heterozygotes.

TESTS OF PROGRESS

This condition is treatable. Following diagnosis, the patient is placed on a strict phytol-free diet (i.e. no chlorophyll-containing foods). Over a year of such treatment, serum phytanic acid levels fall and peripheral nerve conduction slowly improves, with clinical improvement in the patient.

Lactosyl Ceramidosis (GM₃ Gangliosidosis) [R]

Lactosyl Ceramidosis (GM$_3$ Gangliosidosis) [R]

Diagnosis of this rare neurodegenerative disease of juveniles, associated with hepatosplenomegaly, is confirmed by the demonstration of deficiency of beta-D-galactoside galactohydrolase in brain, kidney, liver, spleen, leucocytes, cultured skin fibroblasts and serum.

Unlike Krabbe's leucodystrophy, lactosyl ceramide accumulates in erythrocytes, plasma, bone marrow, liver cells, and can be found in urine deposits. Early cases were confused with Niemann–Pick disease.

Wolman's Disease (Acyl Lipase Deficiency) [R]

Diagnosis of this rare disease of infancy, characterized by excessive storage of neutral lipids (triglycerides and cholesteryl esters), causing hepatosplenomegaly, is confirmed by the demonstration of deficiency of triglycerylglycerol lipase in liver, spleen and leucocytes.

Liver biopsy material reveals portal fibrosis with early cirrhosis, bile duct proliferation and many vacuolated histiocytes. Lymph gland biopsy reveals lipid deposits. Skin biopsies contain droplets of sudanophilic liquid and cholesterol in, and between, the connective tissue cells. Bone marrow aspirates contain numbers of foamy cells extensively replacing normal marrow cells.

The fasting serum is turbid, with increased VLDL lipoproteins (pre-beta-lipoprotein) and chylomicra (i.e. increased triglycerides).

Total Lipodystrophy

Diagnosis of this rare condition in infants and young children is suggested by the clinical appearance, with no obvious subcutaneous fat, hepatomegaly, splenomegaly, cardiomegaly and pigmentation of the skin, and confirmed by skin biopsy which shows normal skin with fibrous tissue replacing all subcutaneous fat.

There is a hyperlipaemia, with raised fasting blood glucose, but otherwise a normal response to a glucose load with normal blood-glucose rise and normal serum-insulin levels.

Cerebrotendinous Xanthomatosis [R]

Diagnosis of this rare condition of progressive cerebellar ataxia, dementia, with cataract formation and tendon xanthomas, is confirmed by the finding of deposition of cholesterol, cholesterol esters and cholestanol in the brain, central nervous system and other tissues. The plasma cholestanol concentration is increased by more than ten times the normal value, whilst the plasma cholesterol level is below normal.

PROTEIN METABOLIC DISORDERS

Analbuminaemia [R]

One family has been described in which there was no demonstrable serum albumin, and in which there was a compensatory increase in alpha-2, beta-, and gammaglobulins. Serum cholesterol and phospholipid concentrations were also increased.

TESTS OF PROGRESS

Following infusion of albumin, the increased plasma gammaglobulin, fibrinogen and transferrin levels, previously elevated, temporarily return to normal.

Bisalbuminaemia [R]

One family has been described in which two separate serum-albumin fractions were separated on paper electrophoresis. The affected members of the family presented with acrocyanosis and hyperkeratosis over the interphalangeal joints and nailfolds.

Familial Idiopathic Hypercatabolic Hypoproteinaemia [R]

Diagnosis of this very rare condition was confirmed by the finding of marked reduction in serum albumin and IgG immunoglobulin, with normal or slightly increased IgM and IgA immunoglobulins. The total body pool of IgG and albumin was reduced, with an increased turnover rate for these two groups of proteins.

TESTS PROVIDING USEFUL NEGATIVE RESULTS

There was no gastrointestinal or renal loss of protein, and thyroid, liver and kidney functions were normal.

IMMUNOGLOBULIN DISORDERS

Marked reduction in IgG, IgM and IgA represents 'agammaglobulinaemia'. When not all the three main immunoglobulin fractions are reduced, the condition may be described as 'dysgammaglobulinaemia', and this latter condition has been classified as:

Type I	IgA ↓	IgM ↓	IgG N
Type II	IgA ↓	IgM ↑	IgG ↓
Type III	IgA N	IgM N	IgG ↓
Type IV	IgA ↓	IgM N	IgG N
Type V	IgA N	IgM ↓	IgG N
Type VI	IgA N	IgM N	IgG N (probably ineffective protein)
Type VII	IgA ↑	IgM ↓	IgG ↓

(Types IV and V are found far more frequently than the other types.)

The clinical separation of the various disorders is based on:

Clinical signs and symptoms, plus family history including repeated persisting infections

The number of circulating lymphocytes

The number of plasma cells

Immunoglobulin deficiency

Humoral antibody response

Cellular immunity response

State of the thymus

Peripheral lymphoid tissues appearance

Associated disorders

Infantile Sex-linked Agammaglobulinaemia (Bruton's Disease) [R]

Diagnosis of this uncommon condition, characterized by infections caused by pyogenic cocci, from 9–12 months of age onwards, with increased later incidence of 'autoimmune disease', leukaemia and lymphoma, is confirmed by the demonstration of absence of fully developed B lymphocytes and plasma cells from blood and blood-forming tissues. Serum immunoglobulins IgA, IgM, IgD and IgE are absent, and IgG is absent or in low concentration. The lymph glands show absence of germinal centres, with no plasma cells in the nodes.

Antibody response to pyogenic cocci is nil, but delayed hypersensitivity reaction is normal. Cell-mediated immunity is normal, with normal resistance to tuberculosis, histoplasmosis, fungus and virus infections (other than to infective hepatitis, which can be devastating).

TESTS OF PROGRESS

Death follows repeated severe infections in the untreated case. Regular injections of gammaglobulins and treatment with relevant antibiotics during infection prolong life.

Transient Hypogammaglobulinaemia in Infants

Diagnosis of this condition of delayed synthesis of immunoglobulins in the otherwise normal infant, is confirmed by demonstration of transient hypogammaglobulinaemia (IgG, IgA, and IgM depressed), increasing towards normal by the end of the first year.

Hypogammaglobulinaemia with Thymoma (Good's Syndrome)

Diagnosis of this condition, characterized by frequent infections, anaemia and a higher than normal incidence of autoimmune disease, is confirmed by the demonstration of reduced serum immunoglobulins (IgA, IgG and IgM) with reduced numbers of plasma cells in lymph glands and bone marrow aspirate, in the presence of an enlarged thymus.

Acquired Congenital Non-sex-linked Agammaglobulinaemia

(Non-sex-linked primary deficiency with variable onset and expression)

Diagnosis of this rare condition is confirmed by the finding of normal numbers of circulating lymphocytes and reduced numbers of plasma cells in lymph glands and bone-marrow aspirate. In the lymph glands, germinal centres are usually absent and the paracortex is often deficient. Serum immunoglobulins are invariably reduced, but the class involved and the degree of reduction vary.

There is a high frequency of autoimmune disorders, lymphoreticular malignancy and, rarely, amyloidosis.

TESTS OF PROGRESS

This condition responds to antibiotic therapy (antibacterial antibody production is poor) and to treatment with gammaglobulin concentrates. Viral antibodies are formed normally, and vaccination 'takes'.

Autosomal Recessive Alymphocytic Agammaglobulinaemia

Diagnosis of this rare recessive condition is confirmed by the demonstration of the absence of plasma cells and lymphocytes from both lymph glands and bone-marrow aspirate. Scanty circulating lymphocytes are found. All the serum immunoglobulins are markedly reduced. These patients do not survive beyond infancy. The thymus is hypoplastic.

Severe Combined Immunodeficiency, Swiss Type [R] [XR]

Diagnosis of this rare sex-linked condition, characterized by early death from repeated infections (including bacterial, viral, fungal), is confirmed by the demonstration of deficiency of both T and B lymphocytes, with atrophy of all lymphoid tissue. Peripheral blood lymphocyte counts are less than $1 \times 10^9/1$. All immunoglobulins are grossly reduced in concentration. There is no delayed hypersensitivity reaction.

TESTS OF PROGRESS

Marrow transplant may be successful in matched siblings.

Autosomal Recessive Lymphopenia (Nezelof's Syndrome)

Diagnosis of this rare recessive condition is confirmed by the finding of normal serum immunoglobulins with marked reduction both in the number of circulating lymphocytes and the number of lymphocytes in lymph glands. Plasma cells are present in normal numbers in lymph glands and in bone-marrow aspirate. The thymus is hypoplastic.

Di George's Syndrome (Thymic Aplasia) [R]

Diagnosis of this rare condition, characterized by repeated respiratory tract infections, plus hypocalcaemia and tetany if the parathyroid glands are absent, is confirmed by demonstration of absence of T lymphocytes. The condition results from failure of the third and fourth pharyngeal pouches to develop, with consequent absence of thymus and often absence of parathyroid glands. The infections include virus, fungus and pneumocystic pneumonia.

TESTS OF PROGRESS

Transplantation of thymus from allogenic embryos has apparently been successful, but in some cases host-versus-graft reaction occurs.

USEFUL NEGATIVE RESULTS

Plasma cells and B lymphocytes are present in lymph glands and marrow. The serum immunoglobulins are normal.

Isolated Deficiency of IgA

Diagnosis of this condition, which may be asymptomatic, or characterized by severe atopy, a greater incidence of autoimmune disease, respiratory disease, and/or gastrointestinal disease, is confirmed by the demonstration of an abnormally low serum IgA concentration. It is thought to be a defect of IgA release rather than a synthesis defect (explaining some asymptomatic cases). It is thought to occur in up to 1:700 of the population.

Gluten sensitivity and pernicious anaemia are common associations. *Giardia lamblia* infestation is often found.

USEFUL NEGATIVE RESULTS

The number of circulating B lymphocytes is normal and the structure of lymph glands is normal also.

Ataxia Telangiectasia (Louis–Bar Syndrome; Progressive Cerebellar Ataxia) [AR]

Diagnosis of this rare condition, characterized by presentation with progressive cerebellar ataxia and other neurological damage and cutaneous venous telangiectases during the first 3 years of life, with death usually before 20 years, is strongly supported by biopsy appearance of telangiectatic lesions, with very low serum IgA concentration (due to a very high rate of catabolism), undetectable or low serum IgG_2 and undetectable serum IgG_4. Both serum IgG_1 and IgG_3 concentrations are increased, so that the total serum IgG level is normal.

Antibody response to specific viral and bacterial antigens is often deficient, and there is both humoral and cellular immunodeficiency, with thymic hypoplasia and atrophy, and recurrent sinopulmonary infections. There is also an extreme resistance to insulin with glucose intolerance in many cases, due to defects in the affinity of receptors for insulin. Also there is a high incidence of terminal lymphoreticular and epithelial malignancy. Gonadal agenesis also occurs.

Primary Cryoglobulinaemia

Diagnosis of this rare condition is confirmed by the finding of a cryoglobulin which precipitates out of plasma at room temperature or lower and which redissolves on warming. The ESR is low at room temperature with cryoglobulin precipitated, and increases if the rate is measured at 37 °C. Serum gammaglobulin is increased.

The one-stage prothrombin clotting time may be prolonged as cryoglobulin may act as an anticoagulant.

Adenosine Deaminase Deficiency [R]

Diagnosis of this rare condition, characterized by severe combined immuno-deficiency disease, is confirmed by the demonstration of deficiency of adenosine deaminase activity in red cells.

T-cell function is depressed, and there is a lymphopenia. Serum uric acid levels are very low.

Purine Nucleoside-phosphorylase Deficiency [R]

Diagnosis of this rare condition is supported by the finding of isolated defect in T-cell function, with gross excessive excretion of purines in the urine, and a very low serum uric acid level.

Ecto-purine-5'-nucleotidase Deficiency [R]

Diagnosis is confirmed by the demonstration of abnormally low ecto-purine-5'-nucleotidase activity in B cells, either with adult-onset agammaglobulinaemia or with X-linked agammaglobulinaemia.

Myeloma (Multiple Myelomatosis)

Diagnosis of this tumour of B lymphocytes, a condition characterized by onset most frequently after 40 years of age, with a variety of signs and symptoms including bone pain, but also the effects of anaemia, renal failure, pathological fracture, carpal tunnel syndrome, compression paraplegia, etc. is confirmed by the finding of plasmacytosis in tissue biopsy, more than 30 per cent of plasma cells in bone marrow aspirate, monoclonal gammopathy on serum electrophoresis exceeding 35 g/l for IgG, or 20 g/l for IgA, or light chain (Bence Jones protein) excretion in the urine exceeding 1 g/day without other proteinuria. The light chain κ/λ ratio (normal 1:1–3:1) is abnormal and monoclonal (i.e. predominantly κ or λ). Suppression of normal immunoglobulin in serum may also be found (IgM < 0·5 g/l, < IgA < 1 g/l, or IgG < 6 g/l).

IgG is the commonest variety, with IgA next most frequent. IgD and IgE myeloma are rare, and since normal serum IgD and IgE levels are very low, special tests for these abnormal gammopathies are needed for their detection. IgM myeloma is very rare. Light chain myeloma (10–20 per cent of all cases) is also described, with massive excretion of light chains in the urine, bone lysis, but no accompanying monoclonal heavy chain type.

With progressive bone destruction (lytic lesions visible on X-ray) urine calcium output is increased, and with renal damage, serum calcium may rise abnormally. Amyloid may also be deposited in the kidneys increasing renal failure. The associated anaemia is non-specific, with raised ESR and plasma viscosity if there is gross increase in abnormal immunoglobulin.

TESTS OF PROGRESS

Following treatment with melphalan (or methotrexate) with prednisolone, with monitoring of blood counts and plasma urea, induction therapy followed by regression of the tumour can be monitored by measurement of (a) tritiated thymidine index of marrow plasma cells, (b) light chain excretion rate in the urine, (c) β_2-microglobulin in urine.

Following induction therapy and maintenance therapy with regression of the tumour, there is a later phase of release which is difficult to treat.

Patients with a very high plasma viscosity plus anaemia respond badly to blood transfusion, since the increased haematocrit is associated with a very great increase in whole blood viscosity. Plasmaphoresis can be used to reduce the circulating abnormal immunoglobulin temporarily.

Macroglobulinaemia of Waldenström

Diagnosis of this condition, predominantly affecting elderly patients, and characterized by vague ill-health, infections, bleeding gums and hyperviscosity syndrome, including headache, vertigo, deafness, fits, etc. is confirmed by the demonstration of serum monoclonal IgM gammopathy (10–12 g/l) with abnormal κ/λ ratio. The bone marrow is infiltrated with lymphocytes with an increased number of plasma cells. Excess light chains (Bence Jones protein) are excreted in the urine in 30 per cent of cases.

There is moderate non-specific anaemia with marked increase in ESR and plasma viscosity. The prothrombin time may be slightly prolonged, and the bleeding time is often increased (paraprotein coating platelets).

TESTS OF PROGRESS

Blood transfusion can be dangerous since the whole blood viscosity increases markedly because of the hyperviscosity of the plasma. Plasmapheresis is very useful for relieving the hyperviscosity syndrome.

Treatment with chlorambucil results in a fall in serum IgM in responsive cases.

Heavy Chain Disease [R]

1. γ-HEAVY CHAIN DISEASE (Franklin's Disease)

This rare disease presents as a primary lymphoma in the middle-aged. The bone marrow contains increased lymphocytes and plasma cells. Serum paraprotein γ-heavy chain fragments (2–4 g/100 ml) occur with hypogammaglobulinaemia, and proteinuria (4–15 g/day).

2. α-HEAVY CHAIN DISEASE

This rare disease presents in the second and third decades, especially in non-Ashkenazi Jews and Palestinian Arabs ('Mediterranean-type abdominal lymphoma'), with a malabsorption syndrome. The peripheral blood and bone marrow are not directly invaded. Small intestinal biopsy reveals the lamina propria to be infiltrated with lymphocytes and plasma cells. Alpha-chain fragments are found in the serum but not in the urine. Diagnosis depends on serum immunopheresis into a gel containing a specially developed anti-Fab-antiserum, as the defect in the IgA molecule is a deletion of the variable and first constant region of the α-heavy chains.

Prompt treatment with antibiotics prevents the development of an immunotumour of B-cell origin.

3. μ-HEAVY CHAIN DISEASE

Only a very few cases have been described, presenting as a chronic lymphatic leukaemia, with anaemia and lymphadenopathy, one case excreting excess light chains in the urine.

The abnormal μ-chain appears in the serum.

Light Chain Disease

Light chain disease comprises 10–20 per cent of all myelomas. Excessive amounts of homogeneous light chains are excreted in the urine. The serum does not contain any abnormal heavy chain gammopathy (i.e. no evidence of IgG, IgA, IgM, IgD, or IgE myeloma).

The condition is characterized by anaemia, osteolysis, hypercalcaemia, azotaemia, low serum albumin and the bone-marrow findings of myeloma.

Familial Amyloidosis [R]

Various types of heredofamilial disorders have been described:
1. Neuropathic disorder.
2. Nephropathic disorder.
3. Cardiomyopathic disorder.
4. Miscellaneous.

Diagnosis is confirmed by staining for amyloid with Congo Red or Sirius Red, and/or examination by electron microscopy of affected tissue biopsy. Rectal biopsy may also be useful in diagnosis.

Secondary Amyloidosis

Amyloidosis develops secondarily to chronic disease. Again, diagnosis is confirmed by demonstration of the presence of amyloid in affected tissues using Congo Red or Sirius Red stains, or electron microscopy.

Benign Monoclonal Gammopathy (Benign Paraproteinaemia)

Diagnosis of this condition, in which an abnormal serum paraprotein (less than 10 g/l) is discovered in a patient with no increase in paraprotein concentration over a period of years, is confirmed by negative results of tests.

USEFUL NEGATIVE RESULTS

There is no light chain (Bence Jones protein) excretion in the urine. There is no increase in serum paraprotein over many years. There are no clinical symptoms related to myeloma or macroglobulinaemia, no hepatosplenomegaly, and no enlarged lymph glands. X-rays of bones do not show lesions and bone marrow aspirates appear normal.

TESTS OF PROGRESS

There is no evidence of malignancy during follow-up over at least 5 years.

Deficiencies of Components of Complement

A. Hereditary Angioneurotic Oedema [R]
   Type I—Absence of C_1 inhibitor protein.
   Type II—Presence of C_1 inhibitor protein (demonstrated by immunological techniques) which is biologically ineffective.
B. Deficiency of $C3_b$ Inactivator [R]
C. Deficiency of C2 [R]
Immune adherence is abnormally reduced, and bacteriocidal activity is abnormally reduced.
D. Deficiency of C3 [R]
Both bacteriocidal and chemotactic activity are abnormally reduced.
E. Deficiency of Fifth of Complement (C5) [R]
Cases suffer from repeated local and systemic infections. Both chemotaxis and enhancement of phagocytosis of organisms are abnormally reduced.

METABOLIC DISORDERS

Influence of Diet on the Normal Subject

Diet has a marked effect on many biochemical results. Therefore the effects of starvation, high-carbohydrate intake, high-fat intake, high-protein intake, and some other diets are considered here.

The urinary output of sodium, potassium, chloride, calcium, sulphate and urea is equal to the intake from the diet. After a mixed meal, the total lipids rise within 2 hours to a peak at about 3 hours and reach the prandial level by 10 hours after the meal. Depending on the amount of protein eaten, the average output of urea in the urine per day varies about 20–25 g on a normal mixed diet.

The urine calcium output rarely exceeds 300 mg/day in the normal subject on a normal mixed diet. There is a slight temporary increase in serum calcium following a meal, with a coincident fall in plasma inorganic phosphate, inversely proportional to the rise in blood glucose.

It is because of the variations occurring following ingestion of food that fasting blood samples are best for most tests.

STARVATION

After a day or two of complete starvation with adequate fluid intake, body fat and protein are mobilized. Serum neutral fats increase and ketones appear in increasing amounts in the blood, with a fall in blood pH, standard bicarbonate and P_{CO_2}. The BMR falls and the subject is increasingly sensitive to insulin (since liver glycogen has been used up). The results of serum cholesterol estimations are variable. Serum protein-bound iodine falls.

The urine contains increased ketone bodies and increased ammonium salts, and urine titratable acid is increased. Increased amounts of β-aminobutyric acid appear in the urine. Following cell breakdown, urine potassium output increases, and urine creatine output increases as muscle cells are catabolized. The urine urea output falls, but not as greatly as when a small carbohydrate supplement is given. Urine 17-oxosteroid output falls, but urine 17-hydroxy-corticosteroid output remains normal, and the response to ACTH is normal.

HIGH-CARBOHYDRATE–LOW-PROTEIN DIET

Serum total cholesterol tends to fall, with blood-urea concentration at the lower limit of normal, and extremely low output of urea in the urine (e.g. 5 g/day). The blood glucose may rise unexpectedly in some people, with plasma inorganic phosphate falling at the same time. If the diet is very strictly vegetarian, with absolutely no animal products at all, eventually the serum vitamin-B_{12} level falls below normal, and megaloblastic anaemia may develop.

The urine titratable acid and ammonium output are reduced, and both urine creatine and uric acid outputs are reduced.

HIGH-FAT DIET

The serum triglyceride (chylomicra) is increased with peak values 2–3 hours after meals, and the serum cholesterol concentration tends to rise, especially after animal fats. If the diet does not contain enough carbohydrate, then ketone bodies appear in the blood and are excreted in the urine in increasing amounts. The urine titratable acid is increased and urine ammonium output is increased.

HIGH-PROTEIN DIET (HIGH-MEAT DIET)

The blood urea rises to the upper limit of normal, and plasma amino acids rise after meals, falling to preprandial levels after 4 hours. Serum creatine levels and urinary creatine output are increased if much meat is eaten raw. On the other hand, if well-roasted or grilled meats are eaten, since the outer layers contain creatinine, both plasma creatinine levels and urinary creatinine output are increased.

Urine urea output increases to about 35 g/day, and both urine titratable acid and ammonium output are increased. The output of both uric acid and sulphate are also increased in the urine. Increased urine histidine and methylhistidine are excreted, and may interfere with the interpretation of urine amino-acid chromatography.

The faecal coproporphyrin output appears to be directly related to the meat content of the diet.

SPECIAL DIETS

1. *Carbohydrate and Fat only, Protein-free*
   With adequate water intake and with a minimum of 100 g glucose or its equivalent daily, the breakdown of the body protein with equivalent excretion of potassium and urea is reduced to a minimum.
2. *High Phytate Content of Diet* (e.g. Oats)
   There may be interference with calcium absorption, if there is also a high phosphate content in the diet.
3. *Low-calcium Content*
   Secondary osteomalacia develops.
4. *Low-salt Diet and/or Salt-removing Resins Orally*
   The urine output of sodium and chloride falls, and eventually plasma sodium and chloride levels fall also.
5. *High-iron with Low-phosphate Content*
   Serum iron and TIBC increase, with eventually haemosiderosis.
6. *Glucose after Starvation*
   There is an excessive rise in blood glucose, often with glycosuria.
7. *After eating Large Amounts of Fruit, especially Stone Fruit*
   Some subjects excrete abnormally increased amounts of pentose in the urine and D-arabinosuria.
8. *Fructosuria*
   May follow eating of grapes and honey.
9. *Large Amounts of Tomato Purée or Bananas*
   Result in increased excretion of 5-HIAA in the urine.
10. *Various Dyes are excreted in the Urine*
    Beetroot
    Eosin
    Phenindione

Normal Geriatrics

In old age, some haematological and biochemical results differ from the normal adult findings:

Haemoglobin levels remain within the normal range, unless there is underlying disease.

The blood urea rises slowly in old age, reflecting the loss of functioning nephrons.

Plasma sodium, potassium and chloride results fall within a wider range of values.

Serum cholesterol falls after 50–60 years.

Serum total protein and serum albumin results tend to fall, but this may reflect the tendency to malnutrition in the aged. In the presence of a low plasma albumin, the ESR may increase (albumin normally protects against rouleaux formation) with a normal plasma viscosity (since neither globulin nor fibrinogen is increased).

Some raised serum uric acid values and some raised blood glucose results are found.

Serum calcium and plasma inorganic phosphate results tend to be lower than the normal adult values.

Serum T3 and T4 levels tend to be lower than in normal younger age groups, with normal serum TSH levels.

Urine 17-oxosteroid output falls by 50 per cent after 50 years of age, as does the serum testosterone in males.

An increasing proportion of otherwise normal old people develop histamine-fast achlorhydria with increasing age, 15 per cent between 40 and 60 years, 25 per cent between 60 and 70 years, and 30 per cent over 70 years.

Metabolic Acidosis (Non-respiratory)

The plasma standard bicarbonate concentration tends to fall, with reduced plasma P_{CO_2}, and with blood pH at the lower limit of the normal range, until decompensation is present. The urine titratable acidity and ammonium excretion rates are increased, with increased output of phosphate and potassium, unless there is also renal impairment.

Respiratory Acidosis

Plasma standard bicarbonate and P_{CO_2} concentrations are increased, with whole-blood pH at the lower limit of normal, until decompensation occurs. Plasma chloride tends to be reduced.

The urine pH falls, and urine titratable acid, chloride and ammonium excretion rates are increased. There is also increase in urinary output of both citrate and phosphate.

Metabolic Alkalosis (Non-respiratory)

Plasma standard bicarbonate and P_{CO_2} increase, with blood pH at the upper limit of normal until decompensation occurs. In severe cases, ketone bodies appear in the blood and are minimally excreted in the urine. The urine output of sodium and potassium in the urine is increased, and urine titratable acid and ammonium output are reduced.

Respiratory Alkalosis

With overbreathing, the plasma standard bicarbonate and P_{CO_2} fall, and the blood pH tends to rise to the upper limit of normal until decompensation occurs. Plasma chloride concentration increases (and intracellular sodium tends to increase with decrease in intracellular potassium).

Urine output of sodium is increased, with increased bicarbonate excretion. Chloride and ammonium output is reduced in the urine. Ketone bodies may appear in very severe cases.

Diarrhoea

Diarrhoea, if severe or prolonged, results in marked changes from normal in many biochemical results.

The stools are bulky, with a high water content, with a high content of sodium, chloride, potassium, and nitrogen. Steatorrhoea occurs in severe diarrhoea.

In the blood evidence is found of developing metabolic acidosis, with reduced plasma bicarbonate, Pco_2, and eventually reduced plasma potassium concentration. The blood pH tends to fall to the lower limit of normal in severe cases.

In very severe prolonged diarrhoea, plasma sodium falls with severe dehydration and the plasma volume falls.

Prolonged diarrhoea eventually leads to some form of malabsorption.

Idiopathic Infantile Hypercalcaemia [R]

Diagnosis of this condition which has become rarer since the toxicity of excessive doses of vitamin D was appreciated is confirmed by the finding of raised serum calcium, with evidence in severe cases of renal damage. Progressive renal damage results in increased blood urea, serum inorganic phosphate, and loss of ability to concentrate urine and proteinuria. The initial increase in urine-calcium output following increased absorption of calcium from the gut is followed by decrease in calcium output.

Serum total cholesterol is increased, and serum alkaline phosphatase activity is lower than expected for the infant's age.

TESTS OF PROGRESS

Urgent reduction of hypercalcaemia is essential. The earlier a low-calcium diet plus carefully judged doses of cortisone to reduce calcium absorption from the gut are instituted, the more likely is it that permanent brain damage may be avoided.

Familial Hypocalciuric Hypercalcaemia [AD] [R]

Diagnosis of this rare condition, with a mild clinical course, is confirmed by the finding of hypercalcaemia (but less than 3·2 mmol/l) with normal but inappropriate parathyroid hormone levels for the serum calcium concentration. Fasting plasma inorganic phosphate concentration is at the lower end of the normal range. Urinary calcium output is less than 5 mmol/day (less than 200 mg/24 hours). The calcium clearance/creatinine clearance and calcium excretion expressed as mmol of the GFR are both reduced (cf. primary hyperparathyroidism). Fifty per cent of cases have hypermagnesaemia.

TESTS OF PROGRESS

Surgery is not indicated, and subtotal parathyroidectomy does not cure the hypercalcaemia. Phosphate or cellulose phosphate added to the diet is not helpful. The patient should not take drugs which reduce calcium excretion as a side-effect.

TESTS WHICH PROVIDE USEFUL NEGATIVE RESULTS

There is no evidence of primary hyperparathyroidism, and there is no fall in serum calcium levels following cortisone suppression test.

Tests for vitamin D excess are negative, and serum 1,25-dihydro-cholecalciferol is normal. Tests for renal insufficiency are negative.

Familial Dysautonomia (Riley–Day Syndrome) [R]

Clinical diagnosis of this rare condition is supported by the finding of reduced urinary output of vanillyl mandelic acid (VMA) and increased output of homovanillic acid (HVA).

Lesch–Nyhan Syndrome [R]

Diagnosis of this rare sex-linked recessive condition is confirmed by the demonstration of almost complete deficiency of HGPR (hypoxanthine guanine phosphoryl) transferase in fibroblasts grown in skin-tissue culture. After a normal birth, affected male patients develop slowly with hypotonia and vomiting starting at 3 months, with athetosis following from 8 months onwards. The patients are mentally retarded, aggressive and suffer self-mutilation. The urine contains a grossly increased deposit of orange-pink pigmented urates, insoluble on standing. Urine uric acid output is 150–850 µmol/kg/day (25–143 mg/kg/day) (normal < 110 µmol/kg/day, < 18 mg/kg/day) with urine uric acid : creatinine ratio > 1·4 (SI) (> 2·0 (mg)). The serum uric acid levels are increased above 0·4 mmol/l (7 mg/100 ml). Cerebrospinal fluid xanthine and hypoxanthine levels are 4 × normal with normal uric acid levels. Heterozygote female carriers can be detected by estimation of red-cell HGPR transferase activity, reduced to levels intermediate between those of patients and normal controls.

TESTS OF PROGRESS

Treatment with allopurinol reduces the urine uric acid output and reduces serum uric acid concentration.

Milk-alkali Syndrome

Diagnosis of this condition, usually a complication of excessive intake of milk with calcium carbonate for relief of peptic ulcer pain, is supported by the finding of hypercalcaemia, with moderate alkalosis and raised plasma urea. There is polyuria with protein and casts in the urine, and a low urinary excretion of calcium. The condition is worse if there is pre-existing renal disease.

TESTS OF PROGRESS

Reduction of intake of milk and alkali results in return to normal, unless there is permanent renal damage. The serum calcium returns to normal.

TESTS PROVIDING USEFUL NEGATIVE RESULTS

Serum alkaline phosphatase activity is normal or only slightly increased.

Idiopathic Hypercalcuria

Diagnosis of this condition is supported by elimination of other known causes of increased urine-calcium output. Following provocative deprivation of dietary phosphate plus administration of chorothiazide diuretic, some cases develop hypercalcaemia and are subsequently found to have a parathyroid adenoma or hyperparathyroidism.

Cases of idiopathic hypercalciuria do not suffer from hyperparathyroidism, but appear to absorb more calcium from the diet than normal and excrete more calcium in the urine, even on low calcium intake. They are liable to renal stone formation.

Congenital Chloridorrhoea [R]

Diagnosis of this rare condition, characterized by severe watery diarrhoea, and hypokalaemic metabolic alkalosis, is confirmed by the demonstration of a stool chloride concentration of about 150 mmol/l, which always exceeds the sum of the faecal potassium plus sodium concentration. There is hypochloraemic, hypokalaemic metabolic alkalosis.

TESTS OF PROGRESS

Sodium chloride, potassium chloride and water supplements reduce the plasma abnormalities with clinical improvement. So far, of the 44 cases described, 22 have been diagnosed in North-east Finland.

Familial Pseudohyperkalaemia [R]

Diagnosis of this rare condition is confirmed by the finding of spuriously raised plasma potassium concentrations in plasma separated from red cells after some delay. No such increase is found in plasma potassium levels when plasma is separated from red cells as soon as blood has been collected from the patient. The condition has no clinical significance, if it is detected and identified.

Primary Hypomagnesaemia [R]

Diagnosis of this rare condition, characterized by a normal infant at birth who develops convulsions at 3–5 weeks, preceded by eye rolling and/or latent tetany and hypotonia, is confirmed by severe hypomagnesaemia (plasma magnesium down to 0·2 mmol/l), hypoproteinaemia, secondary hypocalcaemia, steatorrhoea, with an excessive excretion of magnesium in the urine.

TESTS OF PROGRESS

Following magnesium sulphate 0·4–0·5 mmol/kg/day i.m. there is both clinical and biochemical improvement. Oral replacement is possible, if the dose is adjusted to avoid diarrhoea.

Menkes' Steely Hair Syndrome (X-linked Copper Malabsorption) [R] [XR]

Diagnosis of this rare inherited condition, characterized by neurodegeneration, failure to thrive, seizures and peculiar hair, with mental retardation, is confirmed by the finding of abnormally low plasma copper and caeruloplasmin levels, reduced liver copper concentration, with abnormally increased urinary (and also amniotic fluid) copper content. Microscopy of the hair reveals pili torti and trichorrhexis nodosa (which also occurs in argininosuccinuria).

No treatment has yet been discovered.

PORPHYRIA

Symptomatic Porphyria

Diagnosis of this condition, which may be caused by ingestion of hexachlorbenzene or of hepatotoxic substances in adulterated drinks, is supported by the finding of excessive excretion in the urine of uroporphyrin and coproporphyrin, and occasionally porphobilinogen and δ-amino laevulinic acid. The serum iron is increased. Photosensitive skin changes occur in this condition.

TESTS PROVIDING USEFUL NEGATIVE RESULTS

It is important to distinguish this acquired condition from hereditary porphyrias. In this acquired condition, there is no increase in faecal porphyrin excretion, unlike acute intermittent porphyria, congenital porphyria, or porphyria cutanea tarda.

Congenital Porphyria ('Erythropoietic Type') [AR]

Diagnosis of this autosomal recessive condition associated with excessive production of porphyrins in the bone marrow is confirmed by the demonstration of deficiency of the enzyme uroporphyrinogen III co-synthase (porphobilinogen isomerase) in erythrocytes or fibroblasts after culture. During an acute attack severe haemolysis of the red cells occurs, and there is a greatly increased output in the urine of uroporphyrin and coproporphyrin (mainly Type I isomer), with increased faecal coproporphyrin (Type I) and protoporphyrin. Red-cell protoporphyrin and coproporphyrin concentrations are also increased.

TESTS OF PROGRESS

In remission urine findings are normal. In this rare autosomal recessive condition, symptoms develop from early infancy onwards, unlike cutaneous hepatic porphyria (porphyria cutanea tarda).

TESTS PROVIDING USEFUL NEGATIVE RESULTS

The plasma and urine do not contain porphobilinogen in the acute attack.

Erythropoietic Protoporphyria [AD]

Diagnosis of this autosomal dominant condition is confirmed by the demonstration of deficiency of the enzyme haem synthase (ferrochetolase). In an acute attack red-cell protoporphyrin, plasma protoporphyrin concentrations are markedly increased, with great increase in faecal coproporphyrin and protoporphyrin.

TESTS OF PROGRESS

In remission red-cell protoporphyrin remains abnormally increased, with increased faecal excretion of protoporphyrin and coproporphyrin. In this rare condition photosensitivity begins in childhood.

TESTS PROVIDING USEFUL NEGATIVE RESULTS

There is no excessive excretion of porphobilinogen, δ-aminolaevulinic acid, uroporphyrin, or coproporphyrin in the urine.

Cutaneous Hepatic Porphyria (Porphyria Cutanea Tarda) [AD]

Diagnosis of this autosomal dominant condition is confirmed by the demonstration of deficiency of the enzyme uroporphyrinogen decarboxylase in erythrocytes or in liver biopsy material. In an acute attack there is a gross increase in urine uroporphyrin excretion (70 per cent uroporphyrin I), with a corresponding increase in plasma uroporphyrin, and photosensitivity of the skin.

TESTS OF PROGRESS

In remission there is a moderate increase in urinary and faecal excretion of coproporphyrin and protoporphyrin. Evidence of liver damage associated with acute attacks of the disease is shown by increased serum bilirubin, alkaline phosphatase, aminotransferase activities, serum iron and serum transferrin levels.

Plasmapheresis or phlebotomy may relieve acute attacks.

Cutaneous hepatic porphyria is the commonest form of porphyria in Europe, and includes:
1. Familial porphyria cutanea tarda [AD].
2. Genetically disposed — drug provoked;
                              — alcohol provoked;
                              — cirrhosis associated.
3. Acquired — hexachlorobenzene induced.

TESTS PROVIDING USEFUL NEGATIVE RESULTS

The bone-marrow aspirate does not fluoresce, unlike erythropoietic congenital porphyria.

Acute Intermittent Porphyria (Swedish Type) [AD]

Diagnosis of this autosomal dominant condition is confirmed by the demonstration of deficiency of the enzyme uroporphyrinogen I synthase (porphobilinogen deaminase) in erythrocyte, cultured skin fibroblasts, amniotic cells, or liver biopsy material. There is a 50 per cent decrease in enzyme activity in patients. In acute attacks, in which neuropsychiatric disorders may develop, there is a gross excretion of porphobilinogen and δ-aminolaevulinic acid in the urine, with a moderate increase in urine uroporphyrin output.

TESTS OF PROGRESS

The acute attacks are precipitated by barbiturates, hormones, late pregnancy, infection and/or starvation. When the precipitating agent is eliminated, the abnormal excretion of δ-aminolaevulinic acid and of porphobilinogen fall to low levels, but persist.

TESTS PROVIDING USEFUL NEGATIVE RESULTS

These patients do not suffer from photosensitivity. During acute attacks neither the bone marrow nor the plasma fluoresce. Also during acute attacks severe abdominal pain may develop, but neutrophilia and abdominal rigidity do not occur unless other disease processes are also present.

Erythrocyte uroporphyrinogen synthetase ↓ in carrier (but overlap of values with normal).

Variegate Porphyria (South African Genetic Porphyria)[AD]

Diagnosis of this autosomal dominant condition, common in both South Africa and Finland, is confirmed by the demonstration of deficiency of the enzyme protoporphyrinogen oxidase in affected patients, with associated photosensitivity. In acute attacks there is gross increase in urinary excretion of δ-aminolaevulinic acid and porphobilinogen (5–50 × upper limit of normal), with markedly increased faecal excretion of protoporphyrin and faecal X-porphyrin and moderate increase in faecal coproporphyrin III excretion. Up to 25 per cent of patients are delirious and may be psychotic in an acute attack.

TESTS OF PROGRESS

In remission there is no increase in urinary δ-aminolaevulinic acid or porphobilinogen (cf. acute intermittent porphyria). Some cases excrete increased amounts of coproporphyrin in the urine. Faecal X-porphyrin estimation does not assist in the diagnosis.

TESTS PROVIDING USEFUL NEGATIVE RESULTS

In remission, urine δ-aminolaevulinic acid and porphobilinogen are normal, unlike patients with acute intermittent porphyria, even though they suffer from photosensitivity (again, unlike acute intermittent porphyria).

Hereditary Coproporphyria [AD]

Diagnosis of this autosomal dominant condition is confirmed by the finding of deficiency of the enzyme coproporphyrinogen oxidase in cultured fibroblasts and liver biopsy material (decarboxylase plus dehydrogenase) in affected patients. In acute attacks there is a gross increase in excretion of coproporphyrin in the urine, with moderate increases in δ-aminolaevulinic acid and porphobilinogen excretion. Red-cell coproporphyrin levels may be increased in some cases.

TESTS OF PROGRESS

In remission urine coproporphyrin output varies between normal and moderately increased. Faecal coproporphyrin output is also moderately increased. Photosensitivity is apparent in 30 per cent of cases in the acute attack.

TESTS PROVIDING USEFUL NEGATIVE RESULTS

Faecal protoporphyrin excretion normal.

HEREDITARY AMINO ACIDURIA

(Many of these conditions are very rare.)

Inherited Amino Acid Disorders of the Krebs–Henseleit Urea Cycle [R]

Inherited deficiency of individual enzymes of the Krebs–Henseleit urea cycle are associated with degeneration and atrophy of the cerebrum, cerebellum and basal ganglia, fatty liver, irritability, lethargy, poor feeding, convulsions, coma and eventual death in infancy. Hyperammonaemia with convulsions occur after protein intake. Children with less severe enzyme deficiency survive into childhood, but are mentally retarded and suffer from seizures. The only treatment available at the moment consists of limiting the daily protein intake, and giving small frequent feeds, in an attempt to limit the degree of hyperammonaemia, since the defective Krebs–Henseleit cycle is not very effective in rapidly producing urea from minute amounts of ammonia (as occurs in the normal subject). (Arginine supplements to infants with argininosuccinate synthetase deficiency and argininosuccinase deficiency, and sodium benzoate supplements to carbamyl phosphate synthetase deficiency, ornithine transcarbamylase deficiency and argininosuccinate synthetase deficiency, show promise in therapy. They allow citrulline, argininosuccinate and hippuric acid to act as waste nitrogenous products, and reduce the incidence and severity of attacks of hyperammonaemia.) The specific deficiences include:

1. *Carbamyl phosphate synthetase deficiency [AR].* The enzyme deficiency can be demonstrated in liver biopsy material.

2. *Citrullinuria [AR].* Argininosuccinic acid synthetase deficiency can be demonstrated in cultured skin fibroblasts and in liver biopsy material.

3. *Ornithine transcarbamylase deficiency [XR].* The enzyme deficiency can be demonstrated in liver biopsy material. Some female carriers develop:

   a. Hyperammonaemia after protein feeds.
   b. Hyperorotic aciduria after protein feeds.
   c. Both hyperammonaemia and hyperorotic aciduria after protein feeds.

4. *Argininosuccinic aciduria [AR].* Gross deficiency of argininosuccinate lyase can be demonstrated in cultured skin fibroblasts and in liver biopsy material.

5. *Argininuria [AR]*. Gross deficiency of arginase activity can be demonstrated in red blood cells.

Hereditary Disorders of Tyrosine Metabolism [R]

Transient tyrosinaemia occurs in neonates, especially in low birthweight infants. They rapidly improve following treatment with vitamin C.

HEREDITARY HYPERTYROSINAEMIAS

1. *Hereditary Tyrosinaemia [AR]*
   a. Acute

Vomiting, diarrhoea, failure to thrive, oedema, ascites, hepatosplenomegaly and bleeding develop within 1–6 months of birth. One-third of babies develop jaundice, and there is rapid deterioration with liver failure. One-third die in the first year.

   b. Subacute or Chronic

Symptoms appear after the first year, with failure to thrive, cirrhosis and rickets developing. Death occurs within 10 years.

Diagnosis is confirmed by the demonstration of deficiency of the enzyme *p*-hydroxyphenylpyruvic acid oxidase in liver biopsy material. There is a general amino aciduria with *p*-hydroxyphenyllactic acid, and especially tyrosine, proline, threonine and phenylalanine. The urine also contains δ-aminolaevulinic acid, glucose, protein and increased phosphate. With developing liver damage, liver function tests become positive. Attacks of hypoglycaemia occur.

TESTS OF PROGRESS

A diet low in both tyrosine and phenylalanine (and, in some cases, methionine) reduces the rate of development of cirrhosis and renal failure.

2. *Richner–Hanhart Syndrome of Tyrosinaemia [AR]*

These infants have palmar and plantar punctate hyperkeratosis, herpetiform corneal ulceration, mental retardation, and tyrosinaemia and tyrosinuria, without liver damage. A diet with reduced tyrosine content results in clinical improvement.

3. *Deficiency of Tyrosine Aminotransferase*

One child has been described, with deficiency of tyrosine aminotransferase in liver biopsy material. The urine contained excessive amounts of *p*-hydroxyphenylpyruvic acid; blood tyrosine was greatly increased, and the child was mentally retarded.

4. *Alcaptonuria [AR]*

Diagnosis of this condition, characterized by passage of urine which becomes black on standing, beginning in infancy (or first noted in first or second decade), is confirmed by demonstration of the presence of a reducing substance in the urine, deficiency of the enzyme homogentisic acid oxidase. The reducing substance in the urine is homogentisic acid. Cartilages become pigmented and eventually undergo premature degeneration.

TESTS WHICH PROVIDE USEFUL NEGATIVE RESULTS

Homogentisic acid does not react with glucose oxidase, and the dark urine of phenol poisoning and urine from a patient with a melanotic tumour do not have reducing properties.

Inherited Disorders of Lysine Metabolism and Associated Substances

1.   LYSINE PROTEIN INTOLERANCE

Diagnosis of this condition, characterized by hyperammonaemia after protein feeds, hepatosplenomegaly, osteoporosis, diarrhoea and vomiting, is supported by the finding of hyperammonaemia after protein feeds, and increased urinary excretion of lysine and arginine, with increased plasma lysine levels. The condition is due to defective transport of arginine and ornithine from the gastrointestinal tract. Some cases are mentally retarded. Twenty cases have been reported in Finland.

TESTS OF PROGRESS

Hyperammonaemia after protein intake is relieved by supplement of arginine or ornithine.

2.   LYSINAEMIA [R]

Persistent lysinaemia with increased lysinuria has been described in patients ranging from those clinically normal apart from being of short stature to mentally retarded cases with muscle weakness.
Diagnosis is confirmed by the demonstration of deficiency of activity of the enzyme lysine ketoglutarate reductase in cultured skin fibroblasts.

TESTS PROVIDING USEFUL NEGATIVE RESULTS

Attacks of hyperammonaemia do not follow protein feeds.

3.   HYDROXYLYSINURIA

Eight patients with hydroxylysinuria and a variety of symptoms have been described.

4.   CONGENITAL LYSINE INTOLERANCE [R]

Two patients with hyperammonaemia after feeds have been described, with deficiency of activity of the enzyme lysine dehydrogenase in liver biopsy material. It is thought that the increased plasma lysine levels inhibited arginase activity in the Krebs–Henseleit urea cycle.

5.   SACCHAROPINURIA [R]

A condition, characterized by failure to thrive and mental retardation, has

been described, with increased lysine, citrulline, homocitrulline and saccharo-pine increased in both plasma and urine.
Diagnosis is confirmed by the demonstration of deficiency of activity of the enzyme saccharopine dehydrogenase in cultured skin fibroblasts.

6. PIPECOLATAEMIA [R]

One infant has been described with degenerative disease of the central nervous system, hepatomegaly and increased plasma pipecolic acid.

7. ALPHA-AMINO ADIPIC ACIDAEMIA [R]

Two siblings with alpha-amino adipic acidaemia have been discovered on screening.

8. GLUTARIC ACIDAEMIA [R]

Type I

Diagnosis of this rare condition, characterized by hyperkinaesia, dysarthria, and possibly mental retardation, was confirmed by the demonstration of deficiency of activity of the enzyme glutaryl-CoA-dehydrogenase in leuco-cytes and cultured skin fibroblasts. The urine contained excessive amounts of glutaric acid (approximately 40 mmol/g creatinine—normally absent from the urine), and also abnormal amounts of 3-hydroxyglutaric and glutaconic acids.

Type II

Diagnosis of this rare condition is confirmed by the demonstration of deficiency of activity of the enzyme acyl-CoA-dehydrogenase in cultured skin fibroblasts. The urine contains excessive amounts of glutaric and lactic acids.

9. ALPHA-KETO ADIPIC ACIDURIA [R]

Diagnosis of this rare condition, characterized by psychomotor retardation and failure to thrive, was confirmed by the demonstration of deficiency of activity of the enzyme converting alpha-keto adipic acid to glutaric acid in cultured skin fibroblasts. The urine contained excess of alpha-adipic acid and related substances in the urine.

Inherited Disorders of Tryptophan Metabolism and Related Substances

1. HARTNUP DISEASE [AR]

Mental retardation described in the first family diagnosed, is an incidental finding in this metabolic disorder, which is characterized by cutaneous photosensitivity resulting in a pellagroid rash and cerebellar ataxia (both of which may develop during febrile illness).

Diagnosis is confirmed by the demonstration of gross amino aciduria, with excessive excretion of asparagine, but no proline, excessive amounts of indican derived from indole, and indoylacetic acid and indoylacetyl glutamine derived from tryptamine, in the urine. Plasma tryptophan levels are very low, with increased free tryptophan in the stools (normally present in very small amounts). Urine excretion of N-methylnicotinamide is also very low.

TESTS OF PROGRESS

There is no severe nutritional defect in these patients, even though there is a specific amino acid transport defect, as the 'affected' amino acids are absorbed normally when in the form of dipeptides. Following supplements of nicotinamide (25–50 mg/day) there is clinical improvement and N-methyl-nicotinamide is excreted in the urine as long as the supplements are given.

2. TRYPTOPHANAEMIA [R]

Two patients, dwarfs with cerebellar ataxia, pellagroid rash and mental retardation, have been described, with tryptophanaemia and tryptophanuria.

3. KYNURENINURIA

Four generations of one family have been described, with excessive amounts of tryptophan metabolites in the urine both before and after tryptophan. A partial deficiency of activity of the enzyme kynurenine hydroxylase which did not respond to pyridoxine has been demonstrated.

4. KYNURENINASE DEFECTS

a. Hydroxykynureninuria [R]
A rare condition with nicotinic acid deficiency has been described, in which kynurenine, 3-hydroxykynurenine and xanthurenic acid are excreted in the urine. One patient was mentally retarded.
b. Pyridoxine-responsive xanthurenic aciduria [R]
In this rare condition, hydroxykynurenine, kynurenine and xanthurenic acid are excreted in the urine. The enzyme xanthurenic oxidase is defective, and requires supplements of pyridoxal phosphate.

5. INDICANURIA ('BLUE DIAPER')

This rare condition is characterized by indicanuria and accompanied by hypercalcaemia and nephrocalcinosis.

6. HYDROXYINDICANURIA [R]

One mentally retarded child has been described with persistent metabolic acidosis, and with excessive excretion of hydroxyindican in the urine.

7. INDOYLACROYLGLYCINURIA [R]

One family has been described, in which affected patients excreted excess indoylacroylglycinuria, this abnormal excretion being temporarily reduced by neomycin therapy (presumably reducing gut flora).

Inherited Metabolic Disorders of Histidine and Related Substances

1. HISTIDINAEMIA [AR]

Diagnosis of this condition, characterized by impaired growth in some, impaired speech in some, and mental retardation in others, is confirmed by the demonstration of deficiency of the enzyme histidase in skin fibroblasts, and in liver biopsy material (in liver only, in some cases). The plasma histidine level is increased, and the urine contains excess of imidazolepyruvic acid (which gives a positive test result with ferric chloride solution).

2. HISTIDINURIA [R]

An isolated renal tubule defect with excess excretion of histidine in the urine has been described in three children.

3. IMIDAZOLE ACIDURIA [R]

Diagnosis of this rare condition, which clinically resembles juvenile Tay–Sachs' disease, is confirmed by the excessive excretion of carnosine, anserine, histidine, 1-methyl histidine and, occasionally, homocarnosine.

4. CARNOSINAEMIA [R] [AR]

Two children have been described, suffering from severe mental retardation. The diagnosis was confirmed by the demonstration of deficiency of carnosinase in the plasma. The plasma carnosine was abnormally raised, while they were on a carnosine-free diet, and the CSF contained homocarnosine.

5. HOMOCARNOSINOSIS [R]

Three siblings have been described, suffering from spastic paraplegia, mental retardation and retinal pigmentation. The cerebrospinal concentration of homocarnosine was 20 × the upper limit of normal.

6. UROCANIC ACIDURIA [R]

Diagnosis of this very rare condition was made in a mentally retarded male patient by the demonstration of abnormal elevation of plasma histidine levels after oral histidine, with excessive amounts of urocanic acid excreted in the urine.

NEGATIVE FINDINGS

Skin fibroblast histidinase activity normal (unlike congenital histidinaemia).

Inherited Disorders of Methionine Metabolism and Related Substances

1. MALABSORPTION OF METHIONE [AR]

One case with diarrhoea, convulsions, tachypnoea and mental retardation, plus an unusual body odour, has been described. Failure of absorption of methionine from the diet resulted in its fermentation in the gut by bacteria, and subsequent urinary excretion of these absorbed metabolites, alpha-hydroxybutyric acid, alpha-ketobutyric acid and alpha-aminobutyric acid.

2. HOMOCYSTINAEMIA

a. Type I

Diagnosis of this variety of homocystinaemia, characterized by a Marfan-like appearance, ectopia lentis, malar flush and osteoporosis, with mental retardation in 50 per cent, is confirmed by the demonstration of deficiency of cystathionine synthetase. Blood methionine is increased, as is the urinary excretion of homocystine. There is a markedly increased tendency to thromboembolic disease, as the platelets aggregate and adhere much more readily than normal when blood homocystine concentrations increase. The brain is devoid of cystathionine.

TESTS OF PROGRESS

Some cases with a defective form of cystathionine synthetase respond to continued large doses of vitamin B_6. Other cases with total deficiency of the enzyme do not respond to vitamin B_6. Both forms should also be treated with a methionine-restricted diet.

b. Type II

Diagnosis of this variety of homocystinuria is confirmed by the demonstration of deficiency of activity of the enzyme N^5-methyl tetrahydrofolate methyl-transferase in cultured skin fibroblasts, liver biopsy material, brain, or kidney. The enzyme is present in an abnormal form and responds to vitamin B_6.

TESTS OF PROGRESS

A methionine-restricted diet should be given with continued vitamin B_6 supplements, otherwise there is a risk of progressive dementia.

c. Type III

Diagnosis of this condition, characterized by neurological damage and possibly mental retardation (described in two children), is confirmed by demonstration of deficiency of activity of the enzyme $N^{5,10}$-methylene tetrahydrofolate reductase in cultured fibroblasts.

TESTS OF PROGRESS

Methionine restriction is harmful in this variety. Folate supplements plus vitamin B_{12} should be given daily from the time of diagnosis.

3. CYSTATHIONINAEMIA [AR]

Diagnosis of this condition, characterized by various defects, and with mental retardation in less than 50 per cent of cases, is confirmed by the demonstration of reduced activity of the enzyme cystathioninase.

TESTS OF PROGRESS

Continued vitamin B_6 supplements result in a fall in blood and urine cystathionine in some cases (i.e. those with an abnormal form of the enzyme, with defective enzyme-binding sites).

Variant
Latent cystathioninuria with mental retardation in 2 cases. Two homozygote cystathioninaemia cases have been described, who are clinically normal.

Disorders of Cystine Metabolism

1. CYSTINE-LYSINURIA

Diagnosis of this condition, characterized by the eventual presentation of large renal calculi, which are usually branched, is confirmed by the demonstration of excessive excretion of cystine, lysine, arginine and ornithine in the urine, with normal plasma amino acid pattern.

In one form of the disorder, heterozygotes do not have an abnormal amino aciduria, whereas in the second form, heterozygotes excrete cystine and lysine in the urine. There are three distinct closely related recessive conditions with excess cystinuria and various patterns of excretion of arginine, lysine and ornithine.

TESTS OF PROGRESS

Patients should be given adequate oral fluids, and the urine should be kept alkaline with a pH exceeding 7·5. Penicillamine forms penicillamine-cysteine-disulphide, which is excreted in the urine, and which reduces the excretion of cystine, and hence the tendency to form large cystine stones. Pyridoxine supplements should also be given, since D-penicillamine inhibits pyridoxal-5-phosphate. Acetyl cysteine can be used instead of penicillamine (? giving glutamine supplements).

2. CYSTINOSIS (DE TONI–FANCONI SYNDROME; CYSTINE RICKETS) [AR]

Diagnosis of this condition, characterized by failure to thrive, vitamin D-resistant rickets, phosphaturia, glycosuria and amino aciduria with high cystine content, progressive renal failure and metabolic acidosis, is confirmed by the demonstration of excessive deposition of cystine in the reticulo-endothelial system, peripheral blood leucocytes, cultured skin fibroblasts, bone-marrow aspirate, lymph-gland biopsy and parenchymatous organs.

There is metabolic acidosis with low plasma bicarbonate and P_{CO_2}, hypokalaemia and hypophosphataemia. The urine contains glucose, phosphate and amino acids, including cystine.

TESTS OF PROGRESS

There is progressive renal failure. Following high doses of vitamin D, serum inorganic phosphate levels rise and rickets tends to heal. At the same time, the amino aciduria is reduced. The outlook is poor, but added supplements of alkalis and potassium salts give temporary improvement.

Heterozygotes can be detected, as both peripheral blood leucocytes and cultured skin fibroblasts contain increased intracellular free cystine crystals. Also leucocytes can be exposed to cystine dimethyl ester.

3. TAURINURIA [AD]

Seventeen cases of taurinuria in 4 families, with camptodactyly and excess urinary taurine have been described.

4. BETA-MERCAPTOLACTATE-CYSTEINE DISULPHIDURIA

Two normal children and 2 mentally retarded children (1 with dislocated lenses) have been described, with excessive excretion of beta-mercapto-lactate-cysteine disulphide in the urine.

5. SULPHITE OXIDASE DEFICIENCY [AR]

Five cases of this condition, characterized by mental retardation and metabolic disorder, with early death, have been described.

Diagnosis is confirmed by the demonstration of deficiency of sulphite oxidase in cultured skin fibroblasts. The urine contains excess of sulphite, thiosulphate and S-sulpho-L-cysteine.

Inherited Disorders of Metabolism of Glycine and Related Substances

1. GLYCINAEMIA WITHOUT KETOSIS [R]

Diagnosis of this rare condition, characterized by failure to thrive, listlessness, seizures and progressive mental retardation from birth onwards, is confirmed by the demonstration of deficiency of activity of glycine-cleaving enzyme, plus hyperammonaemia. The CSF glycine concentration is 15–20 × normal, and glycine cleavage is not detectable in the brain. Profound coma follows ingestion of valine.

2. SARCOSINAEMIA [AR]

Sarcosinaemia has been demonstrated in 2 siblings, one of whom was mentally retarded, and in 2 other apparently normal siblings. The biochemical defect appears to be deficiency of activity of sarcosine dehydrogenase.

3. D-GLYCERIC ACIDAEMIA [R]

One mentally retarded child has been described excreting excessive amounts of D-glycerate in the urine. The defect was assumed to be deficiency of activity of the enzyme D-glycerate kinase.

4. TRIMETHYLAMINURIA [R]

Children who are asymptomatic apart from having a foul body odour, have been described, who excrete excessive amounts of trimethylamine in their urine. It has been found that liver trimethylamine oxidase activity is abnormally low in liver biopsy material.

Inherited Disorders of Proline Metabolism and Related Substances

1. PROLINAEMIA

a. Type I

Diagnosis of this rare condition, characterized by mild mental retardation, renal abnormalities, nerve deafness and photogenic epilepsy, is confirmed by the demonstration of deficiency of the enzyme proline oxidase in liver biopsy material.

b. Type II

Diagnosis of this rare condition, characterized by mild mental retardation in one child, was confirmed by the demonstration of deficiency of the enzyme delta-pyrroline-5-carboxylic acid dehydrogenase in liver biopsy material. Many asymptomatic cases of hyperprolinaemia have since been discovered.

2. HYDROXYPROLINURIA [AR] [R]

Diagnosis of hydroxyprolinuria is confirmed by demonstration of its excessive excretion in the urine, and deficiency of the enzyme hydroxyproline oxidase. It is possible that its association with mental retardation was fortuitous.

3. PROLINURIA [AR]

A renal tubular defect has been described in which proline, hydroxyproline and glycine are excreted excessively in the urine (a common transport mechanism defect). Its association with mental retardation may be fortuitous.

Inherited Disorders Involving Branched-chain Amino Acids [R]

1. MAPLE-SYRUP URINE DISEASE [AR]

a. Classic

Postnatal failure to thrive occurs, with vomiting, convulsions and progressive mental retardation. Feeding difficulties occur. The urine has a characteristic our. Hypoglycaemia and metabolic acidosis develop.

Diagnosis is confirmed by demonstration of deficiency of branched-chain amino acid decarboxylase in white blood cells (activity 0–2 per cent). The urine contains excess amounts of keto acids of leucine, isoleucine and valine, plus the abnormal substance allo-isoleucine.

Treatment has been attempted with a diet with a low branched-chain amino acid content.

b. Intermittent Branched-chain Ketonuria [AR]

This condition is less severe than the classic form, and children suddenly become very ill when infected. Leucocyte branched-chain amino acid decarboxylase activity is about 8–16 per cent of normal. The urine does not have a 'maple-syrup' odour.

c. Mild Variant

Patients are moderately mentally retarded, the urine may or may not have the 'maple-syrup' odour, and leucocyte branched-chain amino acid decarboxylase activity falls between (a) and (b).

d. Vitamin B₁-responsive Form

Clinically the condition is mild; odour is present in the urine; leucine, isoleucine and valine are present in the blood, and their keto acids are present in the urine. When 10 mg thiamine is given daily, these infants improve. It appears that if the condition is diagnosed early enough and vitamin B_1 supplements given early, then mental retardation can be avoided.

2. HYPERVALINAEMIA [AR]

One case has been described, with failure to thrive, mental retardation, hypervalinaemia and excessive excretion of valine in the urine.

3. HYPERLYSINAEMIA [AR]

Deficiency of branched-chain amino acid aminotransferase has been described, affecting leucine-isoleucine, with 50 per cent of normal activity. Two siblings had CNS damage and mental retardation.

4. ALPHA-METHYLACETO-ACETIC ACIDURIA

Three cases have been described, presenting with attacks of intermittent acidosis, vomiting associated with infection. Isoleucine caused deterioration. Dietary protein reduction resulted in clinical improvement. Deficiency of oxidation of isoleucine was demonstrated in cultured skin fibroblasts.

5. ISOVALERIC ACIDAEMIA

Isovaleric acidaemia has been described in 2 siblings, presenting with episodes of vomiting, hypotonia, ketosis and mental retardation. Attacks of keto acidosis followed infections. The body odour of 'sweaty feet' was due to free isovaleric acid. The specific enzyme deficiency (isovaleryl-CoA dehydrogenase) was demonstrated in leucocytes and in cultured skin fibroblasts.

6. BETA-METHYLCROTONYL GLYCINURIA

A leucine catabolite, which was associated with the smell of 'tomcat's urine'. Prenatal diagnosis using amniocentesis plus tissue culture with demonstration of carboxylase deficiency is possible in known affected families.

Prenatal biotin supplements and continued supplements after birth improve the outlook for this condition.

7. BETA-METHYLGLUTACONIC ACIDURIA

One case has been described.

8. PROPIONIC ACIDAEMIA [R]

Diagnosis of this rare condition, presenting in the first year of life with episodes of vomiting, lethargy, and hypotonia, and keto acidosis with raised blood ammonia levels during infection or after a high protein intake, is confirmed by the demonstration of deficiency of propionyl-CoA-carboxylase in leucocytes and cultured fibroblasts.

Blood concentrations of glycine and propionate are both increased.

TESTS OF PROGRESS

L-Carnitine supplements to the diet reduce the incidence and severity of hyperammonaemia.

Jamaican Vomiting Sickness

Diagnosis of this condition caused by the eating of unripe ackee fruit, is supported by the finding the urinary excretion pattern very similar to that of isovaleric acidaemia (*see above*). The toxins in the unripe fruit inhibit short-chain acyl-CoA dehydrogenase.

Inherited Disorders of Phenylalanine Metabolism and Associated Substances

1. PHENYLKETONURIA [AR]

Diagnosis of this commonest of the amino acid metabolic disorders, characterized by progressive mental retardation, seizures, eczema, psychotic behaviour, pigment dilution, and 'mousy' odour, in the absence of treatment, is supported by the finding of plasma phenylalanine concentrations exceeding 20 mg/100 ml at the third to sixth day after birth. The diagnosis is confirmed by the demonstration of gross phenylalanine intolerance in response to oral phenylalanine.

TESTS OF PROGRESS

On a carefully controlled special diet containing limited amounts of phenylalanine, blood phenylalanine should be maintained between 4 and 12 mg/100 ml, starting as soon after detection as possible, and certainly at least before 60 days after birth (to avoid brain damage).

Adult female homozygotes who become pregnant must immediately go onto this diet with carefully controlled phenylalanine for the entire pregnancy, otherwise the infant will be born severely damaged.

2. MILD PHENYLKETONURIA

In this intermediate variant without mental handicap, blood phenylalanine levels remain below 1·2 mmol/l (less than 20 mg/100 ml), without specific treatment.

3. TRANSIENT PHENYLALANINAEMIA

4. BENIGN PERSISTENT PHENYLALANINAEMIA

5. 'LETHAL' PHENYLKETONURIA

a. Dihydropteridine Reductase Deficiency

The clinical appearance and behaviour are the same as in classic phenylketonuria. The specific enzyme deficiency can be demonstrated in cultured skin fibroblasts and also in amniotic cells (enabling detection in the affected fetus). There is no response to the controlled diet and death occurs in infancy.

b. Dihydropteridine Reductase Normal, with Reduced Cellular Tetrahydropteridine in Liver Biopsy Material [R]

Clinically as classic phenylketonuria, with no response to specific controlled diet, and with death in infancy.

6. METHYLMANDELIC ACIDURIA [R]

Two siblings have been described, with ataxia, convulsions, mental retardation and methylmandelic acid excretion in the urine, varying directly with protein intake.

7. PARAHYDROXYPHENYLACETIC ACIDURIA [R]

One case has been described with cardiomegaly, hepatomegaly, hypotonia and anaemia.

α-Aminobutyric Aciduria (Oculo-otocerebrorenal Syndrome) [R]

Diagnosis of this very rare condition was confirmed by the finding of increased plasma α-aminobutyric acid, increased CSF α-aminobutyric acid and increased output of α-aminobutyric acid in the urine.

Aspartylglycosaminuria [R]

Diagnosis of this rare condition, associated with mental retardation, is confirmed by the demonstration of excretion of aspartylglucosamine in the urine in excessive amounts. Deficiency of activity of the specific lysosomal enzyme has been demonstrated in seminal fluid from affected male patients. Many of the circulating lymphocytes in the blood contain cytoplasmic vacuoles.

Beta-alaninaemia [R]

Diagnosis of this rare condition, characterized by physical and mental retardation, is confirmed by the finding of raised plasma beta-alanine concentration, with excretion of beta-alanine and beta-aminoisobutyric acid in the urine.

Beta-aminoisobutyric Aciduria

There is a genetic variant in some normal subjects, and 10 × the normal rate of excretion of beta-aminoisobutyric acid is found in the urine.

Beta-ketothiolase Deficiency [R]

Diagnosis of this rare condition, presenting with attacks of metabolic acidosis and vomiting soon after birth, is confirmed by the demonstration of a deficiency of beta-ketothiolase in leucocytes and fibroblasts.

The urine contains a gross excess of N-trihydroxyglycine.

Gamma-glutamyl Transpeptidase Deficiency [R]

Diagnosis of this very rare condition was made in a mentally retarded male patient by the demonstration of deficiency in serum gamma-glutamyl transpeptidase activity, with increased plasma glutathione and excessive excretion of glutathione in the urine.

Hydroxylysinuria

Diagnosis of this rare condition is confirmed by the demonstration of abnormally increased hydroxylysine excretion in the urine, in the form of peptides (the traces of hydroxylysine in the urine of normal subjects is in the free form).

2-Hydroxyglutaric Aciduria [R]

Diagnosis of this extremely rare condition (2 cases reported) was made by the demonstration of abnormally increased excretion of 2-hydroxyglutaric acid in urine (more than 5 mmol/l).

3-Hydroxy-3-methylglutaryl-CoA Lyase Deficiency [R]

Diagnosis of this rare condition, presenting with severe metabolic acidosis, hypoglycaemia and failure to thrive, is confirmed by the demonstration of HMG-CoA-lyase deficiency in leucocytes and cultured fibroblasts. The infant suffers from attacks of severe hypoglycaemia and a number of organic acids are excreted in excess in the urine.

Hyperalaninuria [R]

Diagnosis of this very rare condition was confirmed by the finding, with microcephalic dwarfism and clinical diabetes mellitus, of markedly increased blood concentrations of alanine and lactate, with gross output of alanine in the urine.

Hyperornithinaemia, Hyperammonaemia, and Homocitrullinuria [R]

Diagnosis of this very rare condition was made by the demonstration of hyperornithinaemia, hyperammonaemia, and excessive excretion of homo-citrulline in the urine of a mentally retarded boy, suffering from irritability and intermittent ataxia.

Hyperpyruvic Acidaemia, Hyperalaninaemia, and Hyperalaninuria [R]

Diagnosis of this very rare condition was made by the demonstration of the presence of abnormally increased amounts of pyruvic acid and alanine in the plasma, with an excessive excretion of alanine in the urine. A further case, also mentally retarded, with microcephaly, dwarfism and diabetes mellitus, was found to excrete abnormally increased amounts of alanine in the urine.

3-Methylcrotonyl-CoA-carboxylase Deficiency [R]

Diagnosis of this rare condition, presenting as a 'floppy infant' with metabolic acidosis, is supported by the finding of increased urine excretion of 3-methylcrotonylglycine and 3-hydroxyisovaleric acid. The specific enzyme deficiency can be demonstrated in leucocytes and in cultured fibroblasts.

TESTS OF PROGRESS

Biotin-responsive patients can be identified during the specific enzyme assay.

Methylmalonic Acidaemia [R]

Excluding methylmalonic acidaemia due to vitamin B_{12} deficiency, at least 9 rare congenital methylmalonic acidaemia syndromes have been described. Symptoms range from failure to thrive and very severe metabolic acidosis to asymptomatic infants (found during screening programmes).

Definition is important, since some are responsive to continued large doses of vitamin B_{12}.

Oast-house Syndrome (Alpha-hydroxybutyric Aciduria) [R]

Diagnosis of this very rare condition was suspected by the finding that the urine passed by the infant smelt of 'dry celery' or 'burnt sugar', and the diagnosis was confirmed by the finding of excessive excretion of alpha-hydroxybutyric acid, with an excesss of phenylacetic acid, phenylalanine, tyrosine and methionine.

TESTS OF PROGRESS

Some clinical improvement followed the giving of a methionine-poor protein-restricted diet.

Oculocerebrorenal Syndrome (Lowe's Syndrome) [R]

Diagnosis of this rare condition, characterized by mental retardation, ataxia, cataracts, glaucoma, renal disease, metabolic acidosis, proteinuria with generalized hyperamino aciduria and organic aciduria, is confirmed by the demonstration of multiple amino aciduria, renal casts plus protein, and an inability to excrete excess hydrogen ions (e.g. after ammonium chloride the urine does not become acid).

Death from progressive renal failure occurs in late childhood–adolescence.

Orotic Aciduria [R] [AR]

Diagnosis of this rare condition, characterized by physical and mental retardation, with megaloblastic anaemia resistant to treatment with vitamin B_{12}, folic acid and vitamin C, is confirmed by the demonstration of excretion of up to 1·5 g orotic acid in the urine each day. Deficient activities of the enzymes orotidylic acid pyrophosphorylase and orotidylic acid decarboxylase can be demonstrated in liver, leucocytes, red blood cells and fibroblasts on culture.

TESTS OF PROGRESS

Clinical improvement with conversion of the megaloblastic anaemia to normal follows treatment with pyrimidine compounds distal to the metabolic block. Heterozygotes have activity of the specific enzyme midway between the affected homozygotes and normal.

Orotic acid is also excreted in excess in the urine in patients with a primary genetic fault in the urea cycle.

TESTS PROVIDING USEFUL NEGATIVE RESULTS

Patients with gout, being treated with allopurinol, excrete excess orotic acid in their urine, but also excrete xanthine and hypoxanthine with only traces of uric acid.

Propionyl-CoA-carboxylase Deficiency [R]

One child, with severe metabolic ketosis, protein intolerance, developmental retardation, and episodic neutropenia and thrombocytopenia, was found to have increased plasma glycine and deficiency of propionyl-CoA-carboxylase activity.

Pyroglutamic Aciduria [R]

Diagnosis of this rare condition is confirmed by the finding of abnormally increased excretion of 5-oxoproline in the urine (L configuration), with plasma 5-oxoproline levels reaching 2–5 mmol/l.

Deficiency of either 5-oxoprolinase or glutathione synthetase has been demonstrated in the red cells.

Pyruvate Decarboxylase Deficiency [R]

Diagnosis of this very rare condition was made in a boy who suffered from choreoathetosis following fever or excitement. Excessive amounts of pyruvic acid and alanine were present in blood, CSF and urine.

Reye's Syndrome [R]

Diagnosis of this frequently fatal condition of infancy and early childhood, of cerebral oedema and fatty liver, is supported by the finding of marked increase in serum aminotransferase activity and lactate dehydrogenase activity, raised blood ammonia and hypoglycaemia. Serum bilirubin levels are increased, with increased prothrombin times. There is usually marked peripheral blood neutrophilia.

The CSF glucose is also low, but otherwise unremarkable.

Urocanic Aciduria [R]

Diagnosis of this very rare condition was made in a mentally retarded male patient by the demonstration of abnormal elevation of plasma histidine levels after oral histidine, with excessive amounts of urocanic acid excreted in the urine.

NEGATIVE FINDINGS

Skin fibroblast histidinase activity normal (unlike congenital histidinaemia).

Rare Causes of Lactic Acidaemia [R]

Include:
1. Pyruvate decarboxylase deficiency.
2. Dihydrolipoyl acetyl transferase deficiency.
3. Dihydrolysoyl dehydrogenase deficiency.
4. Pyruvate dehydrogenase phosphatase deficiency.

Rare Organic Acidurias [R]

Single cases have been reported of:
1. D-Lactic aciduria.
2. Succinyl-CoA:3-ketoacid CoA transferase deficiency.
3. Acetoacetyl-CoA-thiolase deficiency.
4. Dicarboxylase aciduria.
5. Carnitine deficiency.
6. Ethylmalonic/dicarboxylic aciduria.

DISEASES OF UNKNOWN AETIOLOGY

Sarcoidosis (Boeck's Sarcoid)

Diagnosis of this condition, which can present with respiratory or cutaneous lesions, enlarged lymph nodes, splenomegaly, uveitis and/or enlargement of salivary and lacrimal glands, lesions of bone, joints, muscles (including heart) or nervous system, is confirmed by histological examination of biopsy material. The intradermal Kveim test (injection of suspension of proven lymph node or spleen material) is positive (but may also be positive in some cases of Crohn's regional enteritis, or less commonly ulcerative colitis).

A mild normochromic anaemia may be found, with increased ESR and plasma viscosity, increased serum gammaglobulin and plasma fibrinogen. Splenomegaly may be accompanied by thrombocytopenia, neutropenia and, rarely, haemolytic anaemia.

Patients are hypersensitive to vitamin D, and 25 per cent have hypercalcaemia with hypercalciuria.

TESTS OF PROGRESS

In untreated cases, nephrocalcinosis may progress to uraemia. Serum alkaline phosphatase activity increases with hepatic granuloma formation.

Steroid therapy causes the serum calcium to return to normal (cf. primary hyperparathyroidism), haemoglobin levels to rise towards normal, and serum gammaglobulin levels to fall towards normal.

TESTS PROVIDING USEFUL NEGATIVE RESULTS

Tests for syphilis, tuberculosis, histoplasmosis, coccidioidomycosis and beryllium poisoning are negative.

Behçet's Syndrome

Diagnosis of this chronic relapsing condition, with many different manifestations, including oral ulceration, genital ulceration, skin lesions, uveitis and, less commonly, thrombophlebitis, pericarditis, ulcerative colitis, central nervous system degeneration or arthropathy, occurring especially in Greece, Turkey, Cyprus and the Middle East and Japan, is confirmed by demonstration of vasculitis with C3 and C9 deposited in the vessel walls and C9 deposited in the basement membrane. Tests for circulating immune complexes are positive. The condition tends to be associated with HLA-B5 in Japan, HLA-B12 with uveitis and HLA-27 with arthritis.

During acute exacerbations the ESR and plasma viscosity are increased, with increased globulin and cryoglobulins, and positive C-reactive protein tests. Mild anaemia also occurs.

TESTS OF PROGRESS

The condition is treated with steroids and azathioprine.

7 Deficiency Diseases

Vitamin A Deficiency

Diagnosis of vitamin A deficiency, characterized by a dry scaly skin, impairment of dark adaptation and night blindness and, in severe cases, xerosis conjunctivae and xerosis corneae, progressing to keratomalacia, is supported by the clinical findings and confirmed by the demonstration of low plasma vitamin A concentration (which falls much more slowly than the serum carotene concentration, which fluctuates within hours with the diet). Vitamin A deficiency is rare in healthy children on varied diets, and plasma retinol levels of less than 0.35 μmol/l (10 μg/dl) are associated with night blindness.

TESTS OF PROGRESS

Daily supplements with 5000 iu vitamin A repair the deficiency, unless there is also an impairment of fat absorption.

TESTS PROVIDING USEFUL NEGATIVE RESULTS

A plasma retinol level exceeding 0.7 μmol/l (20 μg/dl) excludes a diagnosis of vitamin A deficiency.

Vitamin B_1 Deficiency (Thiamine Deficiency; Beriberi)

Diagnosis of vitamin B_1 deficiency is confirmed by a daily urine thiamine excretion of less than 50 μg/24 hours, red cell ketolase activity with and without added thiamine pyrophosphate difference exceeding 25 per cent, and excretion of less than 50 μg thiamine in the urine in 4 hours, after oral thiamine (0.35 mg/m^2).

Blood pyruvate estimation is not a useful test for the detection of vitamin B_1 deficiency.

TESTS OF PROGRESS

Rapid clinical improvement follows treatment with thiamine supplements.

TESTS PROVIDING USEFUL NEGATIVE RESULTS

Since thiamine is a non-threshold substance, the detection of vitamin B_1 in the urine in the absence of therapeutic supplements, excludes vitamin B_1 deficiency.

Wernicke's Encephalopathy

This is regarded as a cerebral form of beriberi. Evidence of vitamin B_1

deficiency is found in the blood. The CSF protein is increased without increased cell count.

Pellagra (Niacin Deficiency)

Diagnosis of this deficiency state, characterized by loss of appetite, weakness, dermatitis (which is photosensitive), glossitis, diarrhoea and eventually mental symptoms, is confirmed by clinical examination and the demonstration that urine N-methylnicotinamide is undetectable. Fasting plasma tryptophan concentrations are also low.

TESTS OF PROGRESS

Rapid recovery follows treatment with nicotinamide supplements.

Pyridoxine Deficiency

Pyridoxine deficiency has been produced when artificial diets, grossly deficient in pyridoxine, were fed to infants, some of whom developed convulsions until pyridoxine was restored to the diet. With natural foods, pyridoxine deficiency is very rare, unless the metabolism of pyridoxine is blocked (e.g. isoniazid treatment of tuberculosis).

Diagnosis of pyridoxine deficiency can be demonstrated by giving oral tryptophan (2 g for adults, as larger doses cause tryptophan-induced pyridoxal deficiency—possibly explaining many contradictory reports), following which patients with pyridoxine deficiency excrete increased amounts of xanthurenic acid in the urine.

Alternatively, estimation of the patient's serum alanine and aspartate aminotransferase activities before and after adding pyridoxal phosphate to the estimation may reveal pyridoxine deficiency, since these reactions require pyridoxine.

(For related conditions, *see* Pyridoxine Dependency and Pyridoxine Responsive Sideroblastic Anaemia, p. 238.)

Scurvy (Vitamin C Deficiency)

Diagnosis of this deficiency state, characterized by failure to thrive, with subperiosteal haemorrhages of the long bones in infants, bleeding gums in relation to teeth, purpura, hyperkeratosis, and even sudden death in adults, is confirmed by the demonstration of leucocyte vitamin C concentrations below 85 µg per 18^8 white cells.

Plasma ascorbic acid levels are very variable in the normal population, and vitamin C saturation tests are now obsolete.

TESTS OF PROGRESS

Vitamin C supplements result in clinical recovery. Very high dosage with vitamin C increases the risk of formation of urinary tract oxalate stones.

Hypovitaminosis D (Dietary Rickets; Osteomalacia)

Diagnosis of vitamin-D-deficient rickets is confirmed by the finding of normal or reduced serum calcium, reduced serum inorganic phosphate, and the product of serum calcium in mg per cent and serum inorganic phosphate in mg per cent below 40. Urine-calcium output is reduced, with less absorption of dietary calcium and increased faecal calcium. Serum alkaline phosphatase activity rises with increasing severity and duration of the vitamin deficiency. Plasma 25-hydroxycholecalciferol levels are abnormally low.

TESTS OF PROGRESS

Following treatment with vitamin D, serum calcium and inorganic phosphate return to normal, and the serum alkaline phosphatase activity returns to the normal level for the age of the subject (serum alkaline phosphatase activity is normally higher in growing children than in adults).

TESTS PROVIDING USEFUL NEGATIVE RESULTS

Only small amounts of amino acids appear intermittently in the urine. There is no glycosuria.

Hypovitaminosis K (Haemorrhagic Disease of the Newborn)

Diagnosis of haemorrhagic disease of the newborn due to hypovitaminosis K, characterized by bleeding occurring 24–72 hours after birth, from the umbilical stump, gastrointestinal tract, renal tract, and the site of any birth injury, is confirmed by demonstration of a prolonged prothrombin time and activated partial thromboplastin time (both corrected in vitro by normal plasma 1:10), which are restored to normal following treatment with vitamin K. The normal newborn has lower plasma clotting factor concentrations than the adult, and if the mother is vitamin K-deficient during pregnancy, the infant is born with even lower plasma clotting factor levels. Normally within a few days, normal intestinal bacteria colonize the infant's gastrointestinal tract and synthesize vitamin K, which is absorbed. Premature and low birth weight infants have lower plasma clotting factor levels than normal, and therefore are more susceptible to deficiency of vitamin K.

TESTS OF PROGRESS

Following not more than 1 mg vitamin K_1 i.m., the baby's clotting Factors II, VII, IX and X, prothrombin time and APTT return to normal. Larger doses of vitamin K_1 are unnecessary and can cause haemolytic anaemia.

Copper Deficiency in Infants [R]

Copper deficiency has been produced in experimental animals but it has never been proved to occur in man. It has been reported that some infants with severe hypochromic anaemia only responded to iron therapy when traces of copper were added.

One case of infantile hypocupraemia has been reported, in which there was associated liver damage and brain damage. It appeared that there was a gross deficiency in the mechanism of copper absorption from the diet.

Protein-energy Malnutrition (PEM)

Diagnosis of malnutrition, including marasmus and kwashiorkor, is made clinically.

Liver biopsy material reveals extensive fatty infiltration. There is a moderate normochromic, normocytic anaemia with very low serum iron, TIBC and ferritin levels. Serum albumin is low, and may fall below 20 g/l, often with abnormally raised serum globulin concentrations. The ratio of non-essential to essential amino acids in the serum is increased (> 2·0). With the decrease in muscle mass, urine creatinine falls. There is fasting hypoglycaemia with glucose intolerance, and frequently hypokalaemia. In severe cases, there may also be hyponatraemia. Plasma urea and non-protein nitrogen are low, and the urine contains both protein and amino acids.

TESTS OF PROGRESS

Plasma transferrin, thyroxine-binding prealbumin and retinol-binding protein are all reduced in PEM, and are useful in early diagnosis, and to measure response to careful refeeding.

TESTS PROVIDING USEFUL NEGATIVE RESULTS

A normal serum albumin concentration is against this diagnosis.

8 *Alimentary Tract Diseases*

Food Poisoning

Includes:

1. Food 'allergy', e.g. to shellfish, etc.
2. Unsuitable food, e.g. excess of unripe or over-ripe fruit.
3. Food contaminated with toxic substances.
4. Food contaminated with organisms, or toxins produced by organisms.
   a. Viruses causing 'gastroenteritis'.
   b. Bacteria:
      i. Causing infection, e.g. salmonella species, campylobacter, etc.
      ii. Enterotoxin producers, e.g. *Staphylococcus pyogenes*, clostridia, botulism, etc.
      iii. Travellers' diarrhoea, e.g. viruses, enterogenic *Escherichia coli* (excluding *Giardia intestinalis*, *Entamoeba histolytica* and other diseases acquired 'abroad').

A. SALMONELLOSIS

1. Acute infective food poisoning—over one hundred different strains of faecal pathogens are known. Incubation period 12–24 hours, followed by a biphasic illness, with headache, malaise, nausea, vomiting and diarrhoea. The organism can be isolated on stool culture.

2. Toxic salmonella enteritis—after excessive growth of the organism in food, it is killed by cooking, but heat-stable enterotoxin persists. The onset of diarrhoea and vomiting is 2–6 hours after eating the food. Detection of the cause is difficult, unless samples of the contaminated food before cooking is available.

B. CLOSTRIDIAL ENTERITIS

1. *Cl. welchii*—heat-resistant spores persist, and the organisms later multiply in warmed-up precooked food.

2. *Cl. perfringens*—type A and type F occur in home-preserved meats.

C. STAPHYLOCOCCAL FOOD POISONING

1. *Staph. pyogenes* multiplies in processed meats (e.g. cold ham contaminated by infected food handlers).

2. *Staph. pyogenes* multiplies in food before cooking, but is killed during cooking, with enterotoxin persisting.

D. ESCH. COLI

1. Enterotoxic *Esch. coli* in infancy.

2. Enterotoxic *Esch. coli*—'new organism' acquired on holiday, producing 'travellers' diarrhoea'.

E. CAMPYLOBACTER SPECIES

Organisms acquired from animals, contaminating food, resulting in colicky abdominal pain and foul-smelling watery diarrhoea. The organism can be isolated from stool culture. Serum antibodies rise later.

F. VIBRIO PARAHAEMOLYTICUS

Organisms causing common gastroenteritis associated with the eating of sea-food in the USA and Japan.

G. BACILLUS CEREUS FOOD POISONING

Occurs when rice is cooked in bulk, stored and reheated as required over a period of days (e.g. restaurant).

Staphylococcal Diarrhoea (Staphylococcal Enterocolitis)

Diagnosis of this condition is confirmed by microscopy and culture of faeces. There is sudden collapse of the patient, with the onset of profuse watery diarrhoea, and the incidence is higher after gastrointestinal surgery and treatment with broad-spectrum antibiotics. Stained films of faeces, especially of mucopus, reveal a predominance of gram-positive cocci (and this is strongly suggestive of the diagnosis). Cultures yield *Staphylococcus pyogenes*, and phage typing of the staphylococcus is useful in epidemiological studies.

There is a very rapid and serious loss of body water, sodium and potassium in this condition.

Enteropathogenic Esch. Coli Gastroenteritis

Diagnosis of gastroenteritis, with watery diarrhoea, vomiting, and eventually metabolic disturbances due to enteropathogenic *Esch. coli*, is confirmed by demonstration of the specific *Esch. coli* in stools, using fluorescent-labelled specific antisera. Blood cultures are rarely positive.

TESTS OF PROGRESS

Severity of metabolic disturbance, rapidity of recovery and course depend on the age and state of health of the patient.

TESTS PROVIDING USEFUL NEGATIVE RESULTS

Tests for shigella and salmonella are negative.

Botulism [R]

Diagnosis of poisoning following ingestion of toxins produced by *Clostridium botulinum* growing under strictly anaerobic conditions in stored food, characterized by vomiting, hoarseness of the voice after a few hours, neurological symptoms with paralysis without loss of sensation or conscious-ness, with death from respiratory failure (in the absence of artificial ventilation) about the third day, is supported by the isolation of the organism and toxin from the stools.

Infantile botulism is characterized by constipation at 3–20 weeks, with neurological damage, including weakness, slow feeding and choking, but with intact mental alertness.

Vomiting

Persistent and prolonged vomiting results in metabolic alkalosis with starvation and dehydration, since gastric juice contains water, sodium, potassium, chloride and hydrogen ions.

Constipation

Both urine urobilinogen and indican may be increased above normal.

Peritonitis

There is neutrophilia with increased numbers of 'stab' cells and some myelocytes, with progressive deterioration and toxaemia. The organisms isolated on culture of peritoneal exudate depend on the cause of the peritonitis and its duration.

Salivary-gland Disease

There may be increased serum amylase and urine amylase in conditions such as mumps, suppurative parotitis, or salivary-gland obstruction. Any pyogenic infection affecting salivary glands will also produce its effects.

Hiatus Hernia

Tests for occult blood on stools may be positive in up to one-third of patients, and many patients suffer from moderate iron-deficiency anaemia.

Gastritis

Aspirated gastric secretions contain some blood and much mucus, with hypochlorhydria or achlorhydria. Acid secretion after maximal stimulation with histamine or after insulin-induced hypoglycaemia is often reduced below normal.

TESTS PROVIDING USEFUL NEGATIVE RESULTS

Absence of megaloblastic anaemia with low serum vitamin-B_{12} levels, and absence of visible carcinoma of the stomach by fibrescope examination and barium-meal X-ray studies.

Gastric Ulcer

Gastric aspirates may contain blood, and gastric acid production after maximal stimulation with histamine is increased above normal. The site of the ulcer crater can be demonstrated by barium-meal and X-ray studies, and the ulcer can be viewed and biopsied by means of a fibrescope.

Occult blood may be present in the stools if the ulcer is bleeding, and this may be associated with iron-deficiency anaemia.

TESTS OF PROGRESS

In cases with a benign gastric ulcer, it has been found that the increased volume of maximal acid secretion in the stomach does not indicate the clinical course, nor does it necessarily indicate surgical treatment.

Postvagotomy

Following successful surgical vagotomy, no free hydrochloric acid is obtained in samples of gastric aspirate during insulin-induced hypoglycaemia. The test is not valid unless hypoglycaemia is produced. 'Medical vagotomy' can be tried before surgical division of branches of the vagus nerve to see whether the patient is likely to benefit by the operation.

Secretion of free acid after stimulation of the stomach is reduced, but the total chloride secretion is unchanged, sodium ions replacing hydrogen ions in the gastric juice.

Following vagotomy, after oral glucose the blood glucose rises unusually rapidly to a higher peak than normal, falling rapidly to below the fasting level, frequently with symptoms of hypoglycaemia.

Perforated Peptic Ulcer

Associated with severe shock, the haematocrit and haemoglobin levels rise in the blood. There are also neutrophilia and thrombocytosis. Serum amylase and lipase rise, but not to the same high levels found in acute pancreatitis. Following the increase in serum amylase, the urine amylase output increases.

Gastric Carcinoma

Diagnosis of gastric carcinoma may be confirmed by demonstration of the growth by barium meal, and by finding carcinoma cells in gastric washings (not many laboratories are prepared to carry out this investigation). Gastric aspirates contain blood, excess mucus and no free hydrochloric acid (these findings depend on the size, position and nature of the carcinoma). Occult blood tests on stool samples are frequently positive.

It is very rare for carcinoma of the stomach to be extensive enough to impair vitamin-B_{12} absorption for sufficient time for megaloblastic anaemia to develop, although gastric carcinoma can develop in a patient already suffering from pernicious anaemia.

Pyloric Stenosis

Diagnosis is supported when gastric aspiration reveals a large fasting volume, with evidence of previous meals, e.g. tomato skins. Markers, such as starch (tested for with iodine) or charcoal biscuits, remain in the stomach for an abnormally long time, and no bile pigments appear in any aspirate.

With the progressive loss of gastric contents following vomiting plus lack of food and fluids because of failure of gastric contents to pass into the small intestine, metabolic alkalosis develops. Plasma sodium and potassium tend to fall, with marked fall in plasma chloride and compensatory rise in plasma bicarbonate. The blood P_{CO_2} rises, and the blood pH tends to rise with decompensation. The blood urea and NPN rise progressively.

Urine output is decreased and urinary sodium output is reduced. Although metabolic alkalosis develops, there is a paradoxical fall in the urinary pH, since the urine pH is controlled by the intracellular pH which is falling following loss of intracellular potassium and gain of intracellular hydrogen ion and sodium.

The absence of food entering the small intestine results in starvation ketosis, with ketones in both the blood and urine. The stool bulk is small.

TESTS OF PROGRESS

Adequate water and salt repair the body deficit if adequate potassium salts are given at the same time to repair the intracellular deficit.

Congenital Hypertrophic Pyloric Stenosis

Diagnosis of this condition, characterized by the onset of vomiting in the latter half of the neonatal period, with projectile vomiting after each feed, with consequent severe malnutrition, is clinical, and the treatment is surgical.

TESTS PROVIDING USEFUL NEGATIVE RESULTS

Congenital hiatus hernia is associated with regurgitation of feeds from birth onwards; vomiting may occur between feeds, and the vomitus contains blood and mucus.

Infections, especially urinary tract infections, may be associated with vomiting. Vomiting developing by the second week of life, with low plasma sodium, hyperkalaemia and metabolic acidosis, occurs in congenital adrenal hyperplasia of the salt-losing variety.

Postgastrectomy

Surgical operations on the stomach result in variable biochemical and haematological changes, caused by alteration in both the rate and efficiency of absorption of foodstuffs from the alimentary tract.

TOTAL GASTRECTOMY

Steatorrhoea is common. The 'dumping syndrome', with rapid rise in blood glucose after meals followed soon by hypoglycaemia, hypokalaemia, and fall in plasma volume due to transfer of glucose, potassium, phosphate and water into cells, is also common. The serum vitamin B_{12} (and body stores of vitamin B_{12}) falls, as no intrinsic factor is available for absorption of the vitamin. Megaloblastic anaemia eventually develops. Obviously there is achlorhydria, resistant to histamine.

PARTIAL GASTRECTOMY

Steatorrhoea is common and is more severe after a Polya-type than after a Billroth-type gastrectomy. Acute attacks of abdominal pain, with very high levels of serum amylase activity, may occur with any afferent loop obstruction. The 'dumping syndrome' may also occur after meals, with hypoglycaemia, hypokalaemia and reduced plasma volume following a rapid and excessive rise in blood glucose.

Depending on the extent and site of the partial gastrectomy, there may be either achlorhydria resistant to histamine or reduced acid response to histamine. If all the intrinsic factor-producing area is removed, then megaloblastic anaemia develops after depletion in vitamin B_{12} stores in the body and a fall in the serum vitamin B_{12} level.

Afferent Loop Syndrome

Diagnosis, following a previous history of gastric surgery, is strongly supported by the finding of very high serum amylase levels (e.g. > 1000 i.u./l). Probably the only other condition associated with such high serum amylase levels is early acute pancreatitis.

Zollinger–Ellison Syndrome

Diagnosis of the presence of an active gastrin-secreting gastrinoma, occurring predominantly in pancreas (occasionally in duodenum and rarely in the gastric antrum), which is always malignant, is confirmed by the demonstration of increased gastrin in serum (10 × upper limit of normal) both in the basal state after feeds or injection of secretin, glucagon or calcium.

The resting gastric juice secretion rate is equal to the normal maximum rate and the pH of the juice in the duodenum is 1·5–2·0. The rate of flow does not increase following pentagastrin. The overnight basal gastric secretion exceeds 1000 ml and exceeds 100 mmol hydrogen ion.

Diarrhoea is common, and steatorrhoea may be present. Metabolic alkalosis with hypokalaemia may develop, following continuous faecal potassium loss. Peptic ulceration results in positive occult blood tests in the faeces.

Duodenal Ulcer

Diagnosis is clinical and radiographic. Augmented histamine test-meal results reveal that gastric secretion of acid is above normal, and occult blood tests on stool samples may be positive, indicating bleeding in the gastrointestinal tract.

TESTS PROVIDING USEFUL NEGATIVE RESULTS

Persistent achlorhydria following adequate gastric stimulation virtually excludes a diagnosis of duodenal ulcer.

Mesenteric Adenitis

As this condition may simulate an acute abdominal condition microscopy and culture of lymph glands removed at operation should be performed.

Infection with *Pasteurella pseudotuberculosis* and *Mycobacterium tuberculosis* should be tested for.

Appendicitis

Diagnosis of this condition is essentially a clinical one. The results from blood counts may be misleading, as the white-cell count varies greatly with the rate of development of the condition and the degree of local inflammation.

TESTS OF PROGRESS

Perforation or abscess formation may be accompanied by increased neutrophilia, but again it is unwise to use laboratory data as indicators of the onset of complications.

Crohn's Disease (Regional Ileitis; Regional Enteritis)

Diagnosis of this condition, which can present with chronic abdominal pain, diarrhoea, ill-health, weight loss and fever, is essentially made clinically with radiological examination.

Laboratory results reflect a variable combination of blood loss from intestinal lesions, inflammatory response, and malabsorption: hypoproteinaemia; anaemia due to blood loss, toxic depression of the marrow, iron, folate and vitamin B_{12} deficiency; steatorrhoea.

TESTS OF PROGRESS

Tests reflect the development of intestinal perforation, peritonitis or obstruction, arthritis, varying levels of anaemia and malabsorption.

The full blood count, ESR, plasma viscosity, plasma fibrinogen, C-reactive protein (CRP) and orosomucoid are all useful indicators of disease activity.

Whipple's Disease [R]

Diagnosis of this rare condition, characterized by weight loss, fever, skin pigmentation, abdominal pain, lymphadenopathy and migrating polyarthritis, is confirmed by the demonstration, in intestinal biopsy material, of swollen foamy macrophages in distended villi with distended lymphatic spaces. The foamy cells stain positively with periodic acid Schiff reagent, and the epithelial layer is normal. Electron microscopy reveals an ultrastructure, ? bacteria, and long-term antibiotic treatment results in their disappearance. Intestinal biopsies also reveal a paucity of lymphocytes and plasma cells. Lymphocytes from the peripheral blood do not 'transform' normally.

TESTS OF PROGRESS

Malabsorption occurs, with developing hypochromic anaemia, reduced serum albumin (and maybe reduced serum calcium concentration), with low fasting blood glucose concentrations.

Treatment with streptomycin and lincomycin, followed by 12-months of treatment with tetracycline, results in recovery.

TESTS PROVIDING USEFUL NEGATIVE RESULTS

Serum immunoglobulins are normal, and tests for serum RA factor are negative.

Diverticulitis (Colon)

Chronic diverticulitis is a condition which is difficult to diagnose. It is a cause of *pyrexia of unknown origin*, with vague malaise, neutrophilia, raised ESR and plasma viscosity. The site of inflamed diverticula determines the signs and symptoms. Anaemia develops, with hypochromia, and occult blood tests on stools may be positive.

Enterostomy

Unless an adequate check is kept of fluid intake and loss and vitamin supplements are given by injection, various vitamin deficiency states, dehydration or sodium or potassium deficit may develop.

Protein-losing Enteropathy

Diagnosis is supported by the finding of steatorrhoea, with increased faecal nitrogen due to protein loss. Serum protein levels, particularly serum albumin, are reduced. The diagnosis can be confirmed by injecting polyvinyl pyrrolidone ^{131}I 15–25 µc intravenously, and collecting the stools for the subsequent 4–5 days. Normally less than 2 per cent of the radioactivity appears in the stools. In protein-losing enteropathy more than 2 per cent radioactivity appears in the stools.

External Bile Fistula

If an external bile fistula persists for a long time, deficiency of vitamin K and also steatorrhoea may develop.

Gastrocolic Fistula

Undigested food and partially digested food is found in the faeces, and if a suitable marker is given (e.g. charcoal biscuits) at a particular meal, the time between ingestion and excretion of the marker can be noted. Faecal nitrogen is grossly increased, with failure to absorb protein.

Intestinal Resection

PROXIMAL RESECTION

Resection of jejunum does not cause such a severe degree of malabsorption as resection of a similar length of ileum. After jejunal resection, moderate steatorrhoea may occur, and absorption of both iron and folic acid may be impaired. Obviously the greater the resection, the more severe is the defect produced.

DISTAL RESECTION

Resection of ileum interferes with the absorption of vitamin B_{12}. Steatorrhoea may occur. Again, it is obvious that the greater the resection, the more severe is the defect produced.

Prolonged Steatorrhoea

Prolonged steatorrhoea is associated with malabsorption of many substances resulting in changes in the body:

Faecal loss of fat is associated with abnormal loss in the faeces of calcium, phosphate, fat-soluble vitamins (A, D, E and K), carbohydrate, protein breakdown products before absorption, increasing faecal nitrogen and failure to absorb iron.

There is frequently an iron-deficient anaemia, with low serum iron, a macrocytic anaemia, or less commonly a megaloblastic anaemia. Plasma Factors II, VII, IX and X may be reduced, as they are vitamin K dependent, and the prothrombin time is prolonged.

The oral glucose-tolerance test may show a flattened curve with poor absorption, with a low fasting blood glucose, but with normal response to intravenous glucose. With poor protein absorption, serum albumin falls, xylose-tolerance tests shows impairment, in relation to small intestinal hurry and malfunction.

With poor absorption of calcium from the diet, the serum calcium may be below normal, and osteomalacia may develop with increasing alkaline phosphatase activity.

If the stool bulk is very large and much water is lost in the faeces, faecal potassium output may be increased with resulting depletion of body potassium, which may be associated with a low plasma potassium.

The findings will depend on the effects of the primary condition causing the severe steatorrhoea.

Tropical Sprue

Diagnosis is supported by the finding of steatorrhoea with bulky stools, with iron deficiency and hypochromic anaemia in many cases, which may progress to macrocytic megaloblastic anaemia in some cases. There is malabsorption, with moderately flattened glucose-tolerance curve, poor xylose absorption (and hence excretion in the urine). Serum albumin is reduced, and depression of vitamin-K-dependent plasma clotting factors (II, VII, X) results in moderate increase in the prothrombin clotting time.

Serum folate activity is frequently low, and red-cell folate activity may be reduced.

TESTS OF PROGRESS

Treatment with folate supplements or crude liver injections results in recovery of about one-third of cases. Removal from the tropics results in recovery of most cases.

Peroral jejunal biopsy material rarely shows total villous atrophy, unlike adult coeliac disease (or adult non-tropical sprue). Only a small proportion of cases show any improvement on a gluten-free diet, unlike adult coeliac disease.

Coeliac Disease (Gluten-induced Enteropathy)

Diagnosis of this disease, presenting with generalized malabsorption, is confirmed by the demonstration of abnormal small intestinal biopsy histology, with clinical improvement on a gluten-free diet and return to normal of the intestinal biopsy appearance.

Serum IgA concentration correlates directly with gluten intake, falling to normal on a gluten-free diet.

Serum gluten antibodies are present in 20 per cent of normal subjects, in 90 per cent of coeliac patients ingesting gluten in their diet (becoming negative after 6 months of gluten-free food). Gluten skin test gives a positive Arthus reaction.

In adults, serum IgG and IgM may be abnormally low, rising to normal on a gluten-free diet.

After oral xylose, urinary xylose excretion is defective while gluten is in the diet, returning to normal after some weeks on a gluten-free diet. In severe cases, in the absence of proper dietary control, malabsorption may result in hypocalcaemia, marked hypoproteinaemia, and anaemia with both folate and vitamin B_{12} deficiency.

TESTS OF PROGRESS

In the presence of gut neoplasia, serum IgA levels remain abnormally raised in spite of gluten-free diet.

Cow's Milk Protein Intolerance

Diagnosis of this uncommon condition is supported by the finding after oral xylose ($14 \cdot 5$ g/m^2 in 10 per cent solution) that the blood xylose concentration taken 1 hour after oral xylose is lower when the test is repeated 24 hours after cow's milk has been added to the infant's diet.

Eosinophilia is common, and occult or overt blood may be present in the stools. Small intestinal biopsy histologically resembles that of coeliac disease.

Skin tests to milk protein may be positive, and there is a raised serum titre of antibodies to cow's milk protein, with increased serum IgE.

Anorexia Nervosa

Diagnosis of this condition of devastating anorexia and weight loss is supported by the exclusion of other known illness to explain the patient's state. Serum LH, FSH and oestradiol levels are low. Serum TSH and T4 concentrations are normal, with low serum T3 levels. Serum cortisol and HGH concentrations are normal or raised, with normal serum prolactin concentration. Serum vasopressin levels may be low.

Primary Intestinal Lymphangiectasia [R]

Diagnosis of this rare condition, characterized by intermittent diarrhoea, steatorrhoea with excessive loss of protein into the gut, is confirmed by examination of small intestinal biopsy material. Dilated lymph vessels in the submucosa with chyle leaking into the intestinal lumen is diagnostic.

TESTS OF PROGRESS

Reduction of dietary fat to diminish chyle flow, and the addition of medium-chain triglycerides which are transported by the portal vessels rather than via lymphatic chyle, results in clinical improvement and reduction of steatorrhoea.

Schwachman's Syndrome [R] [AR]

Diagnosis of this rare condition, characterized by malabsorption, diarrhoea, failure to thrive and feeding problems, first apparent at 4–6 months, with repeated infections (pneumonia, meningitis, sepsis), is supported by the finding of steatorrhoea. Serum amylase activity is reduced, and the diagnosis is confirmed by the demonstration of absence of serum pancreatic isoamylase, with neutropenia, often intermittent, thrombocytopenia, with platelets less than $100 \times 10^9/1$ in 60–70 per cent. Anaemia is less frequent.

TESTS OF PROGRESS

Clinical improvement with reduction in steatorrhoea follows continuous pancreatic replacement therapy.

TESTS PROVIDING USEFUL NEGATIVE RESULTS

Sweat sodium chloride concentrations during a sweat test are normal.

Paralytic Ileus, Intestinal Obstruction

The laboratory results obtained vary greatly with the degree of developing toxicity, dehydration and electrolyte imbalance. The TWBC is increased, with neutrophilia and thrombocytosis. Blood urea levels tend to increase, with tissue breakdown and dehydration. Haematocrit readings, plasma sodium, potassium, chloride, standard bicarbonate and urea estimations are useful during the treatment of a patient, but are not helpful diagnostically.

Ulcerative Colitis

Diagnosis of ulcerative colitis is clinical, following colonoscopy. Clinical activity of the condition is associated with the passage of fresh blood and mucus in frequent stools. Hypochromic anaemia results from blood loss. There is a neutrophilia with thrombocytosis, and the ESR and plasma viscosity are increased, with falling serum albumin and increasing serum globulin and plasma fibrinogen. There is no simple relationship between the results of these tests and disease activity.

TESTS OF PROGRESS

Following recovery from an acute attack, serum albumin increases towards normal, with increase in haemoglobin concentration towards normal.

In longstanding ulcerative colitis, acute fatty liver, sclerosing cholangitis, gallstones following ileal resection, or bile-duct carcinoma may develop.

TESTS PROVIDING USEFUL NEGATIVE RESULTS

Stool culture for bacterial pathogens, including *Cl. difficile*, campylobacter species, are negative. Microscopy of stools does not reveal the presence of *Ent. histolytica*.

Large-bowel Villous Tumours

Diagnosis is supported by the demonstration of a greatly increased faecal potassium excretion with excessive amounts of mucus. This continuous loss of potassium may be reflected by a low plasma-potassium concentration.

Peritonitis

Commonly secondary to bowel soiling of the peritoneal cavity, microscopy and culture of fluid or pus from the peritoneal cavity can be used for the identification of infecting organisms and an assessment of suitable antibiotics for their elimination.

Uncommonly, nowadays, the condition may be a primary tuberculous infection.

Laboratory tests (plasma electrolytes and full blood count) reflect changes associated with infection, water, and electrolyte imbalance. The TWBC is increased with neutrophilia and thrombocytosis.

Pelvic Abscess

Identification of the infecting organism or organisms can be made by microscopy and culture of pus obtained at operation. Pelvic abscess is usually secondary to intra-abdominal lesions, such as salpingitis, diverticulitis, ruptured appendix in acute appendicitis, etc.

Neutrophilia, raised ESR and plasma viscosity occur with a pelvic abscess.

Subphrenic Abscess

Identification of the organism or organisms can be made by microscopy and culture of pus obtained either at operation or by aspiration. Subphrenic abscess is most commonly related to intra-abdominal lesions, but can be in association with a pulmonary disease (in which case sputum should also be cultured).

A marked neutrophilia, with increased ESR and plasma viscosity, and progressive anaemia, occurs with untreated subphrenic abscess.

Irritable Bowel Syndrome

Diagnosis of this condition, which can present either with abdominal pain, constipation, diarrhoea or alternating periods of both, or with intermittent or continuous painless diarrhoea, consists of excluding major organic conditions, including:

Infections with bacteria, parasites.
Organic lesions of gastrointestinal tract.

Investigations with normal results, include:
Full blood count plus ESR or plasma viscosity.
Microscopy and culture of stools.
Tests for occult blood in stools.

Acute Ischaemia of the Small Bowel

Diagnosis of this condition is clinical, with confirmation at operation. Laboratory findings include rising haematocrit, neutrophilia, moderate increase in serum amylase activity, and persistent base deficit.

TESTS OF PROGRESS

Regular estimations of plasma sodium, potassium chloride, bicarbonate and urea are necessary for correction of fluid imbalance, with base deficit.

9 *Diseases of the Liver, Gallbladder, and Pancreas*

DISEASES OF THE LIVER

Hepatic Encephalopathy

Diagnosis of hepatic encephalopathy and coma is clinical. While blood ammonia levels may be abnormally increased in severe cases, this is not always so. The estimation is becoming easier to perform, with the development of newer apparatus, but normal results may be obtained in some severe cases.

It is thought that CSF glutamine is useful in the assessment of portal-systemic encephalopathy.

Viral Hepatitis

The virological diagnosis of viral hepatitis has already been considered. Using biochemical, haematological and histological methods, the diagnosis of viral hepatitis is confirmed by histological examination of liver-biopsy material (with electron microscopy for viral demonstration) and the diagnosis is supported by the finding of the following sequential test results:

A. PRE-ICTERIC STAGE

Neutropenia and lymphopenia occur, with atypical lymphocytes seen in stained blood films. The serum bilirubin level is at the upper limit of normal. At this time, bilirubin may be detected in the urine.

B. ICTERIC STAGE

Serum bilirubin levels increase, with both conjugated and unconjugated bilirubin present. There is slight to moderate increase in serum alkaline phosphatase activity. Serum iron is increased, and serum alanine and aspartate aminotransferase activities are increased. The urine contains both bilirubin and urobilinogen at first, but later urobilinogen disappears from the urine. Neutrophils and granular and cellular casts are also seen in the urine. The stools are pale and there is a moderate steatorrhoea.

Many other serum enzyme estimations have been used in the measurement of liver damage, but aspartate and alanine aminotransferases give similar information to other enzymes more tedious to estimate.

Histological examination of liver biopsy material is diagnostic, although the diagnosis can be made clinically in most cases.

TESTS OF PROGRESS

Subsequent tests are useful in detecting recurrence of jaundice with recurrence of hepatitis, and the reappearance of urobilinogen in the urine, with recovery from hepatitis. Serum aspartate and alanine aminotransferase activity measurements are useful in assessing recovery. Faecal urobilinogen (stercobilinogen) reappears in the stools during recovery, and seroflocculation tests gradually become negative once more.

Acute Fulminant Hepatic Failure

Diagnosis is confirmed by histological examination of liver biopsy material. The condition is most frequently due to viral hepatitis, also drug reactions, less commonly due to fungus poisoning, surgical shock with gram-negative septicaemia, or fatty liver of pregnancy.

Serum bilirubin levels rise, with increase in serum aspartate and alanine aminotransferase activities. Serum ferritin levels increase, and can be a very useful indicator of acute hepatocellular damage, with falling serum albumin.

Hypoglycaemia with raised plasma insulin concentrations is rare (except in children). Plasma sodium tends to be low normal or low, with hypokalaemia and hypocalcaemia. Later, with renal failure, plasma potassium levels rise. Bleeding may occur with rising prothrombin ratio (due to falls in the vitamin K-dependent plasma clotting Factors II, VII, IX and X).

TESTS OF PROGRESS

Patient's serum should be tested for hepatitis B urgently and necessary barrier nursing procedures adopted in positive cases, to avoid hazard to staff and patients.

Cholestatic Viral Hepatitis

Diagnosis of this condition is confirmed by histological examination of liver biopsy material, in a hepatitis-like illness, with prolonged jaundice, raised serum bilirubin and moderate-to-marked increase in serum alkaline phosphatase activity.

TESTS OF PROGRESS

Following 30 mg prednisolone daily for 5 days, there is a profound fall in serum bilirubin (cf. obstructive jaundice).

Acute Non-icteric Hepatitis

Diagnosis is confirmed by histological examination of liver biopsy material in suspected cases. The diagnosis is supported by the finding of increased serum alanine and aspartate aminotransferase activities, positive seroflocculation tests, a slight increase in serum bilirubin, increased bromsulphthalein retention, and often positive tests for bilirubin in the urine.

Chronic Hepatitis

1. *CHRONIC PERSISTENT HEPATITIS*

Diagnosis of this condition, characterized by increasing fatigue, with fat and alcohol intolerance plus discomfort over the liver, after an attack of hepatitis, is supported by the finding of markedly raised serum aminotransferase activities which fluctuate with time, and normal serum bilirubin, alkaline phosphatase activity and IgG concentration. Depending on the aetiology, tests for evidence of hepatitis B infection are frequently positive. Liver biopsy material reveals marked cellularity in portal zones with some fibrosis. The limiting plate of liver cells between the portal zones and the liver cell columns is intact, and 'piecemeal' necrosis of liver cells is not seen.

2. *CHRONIC ACTIVE HEPATITIS*

Liver biopsy material reveals lymphocyte and plasma cell infiltration of the portal areas, extending into the liver lobule and causing erosion of the limiting plate of liver cells between the portal zones and the liver cell columns. There is 'piecemeal' necrosis of liver cells, with fibrous septa extending into the liver cell columns, isolating groups of liver cells. Bridging necrosis, often with fibrosis, extends between the portal zone and the central hepatic veins.

Two main clinical forms exist:
  A. 'Lupoid' chronic active hepatitis.
  B. Type B chronic active hepatitis.

A. Lupoid (Non-hepatitis B) Chronic Active Hepatitis

Diagnosis of this condition, affecting usually females, particularly at puberty or the menopause, and characterized by increasing fatigues with attacks resembling acute hepatitis, but which fail to clear completely, is confirmed by the finding of marked increase in serum IgG immunoglobulin (not monoclonal), with serum antibodies against the actin of smooth muscle in 60 per cent and against mitochondria in 25 per cent. ANA antibody may be present in high titre, with LE cells in 15 per cent. Liver biopsy reveals active hepatitis.

There is an association with HLA B8 and HLA DW3.

Moderate anaemia occurs with raised ESR and plasma viscosity. There may be a moderate increase in bone marrow plasma cells, and serum tests for RA factor may be positive.

TESTS OF PROGRESS

Following treatment with prednisolone for at least 2 years, serum tests become less positive, with serum albumin concentration tending to rise towards normal, and liver biopsy revealing less cellular activity.

TESTS PROVIDING USEFUL NEGATIVE RESULTS

Tests for evidence of infection with hepatitis B virus are persistently negative.

B. Hepatitis-B Antigen-positive Chronic Active Hepatitis

Perhaps 10 per cent of patients with hepatitis B fail to clear the HBsAg (surface antigen) from their serum within 6 months of the acute infection. They become:

a. 'Healthy' carriers of the virus.

b. Chronic persistent hepatitis.

c. *Chronic active B-antigen positive hepatitis, followed by cirrhosis.* This last group tend to be patients with high exposure to hepatitis B infection:

    i. Hospital staff in specialized units treating patients with hepatitis B.

    ii. Male homosexuals—B hepatitis is spread as a venereal disease.

    iii. Drug abusers using a common syringe.

    iv. Infants born to hepatitis B-carrier mothers—

        African.

        Mediterranean } especially.

        Far East

Diagnosis is confirmed by the finding of moderately raised serum bilirubin, aminotransferase activities and immunoglobulins. The titre for smooth muscle antibody is low or absent altogether. HBsAg is positive in low titre, with HBeAg positive. IgM antibody to the virus core antigen (HBcAg) is positive. Liver biopsy material reveals chronic active hepatitis, and liver cells stain positive for HBsAg.

TESTS OF PROGRESS

Prednisolone therapy alone is contraindicated. Treatment may consist of a combination of azathioprine with prednisolone, or antiviral agents.

Portal Hepatic Cirrhosis

CLINICAL LATENT STAGE

Diagnosis is confirmed by histological examination of liver-biopsy material. The serum-globulin concentration may be slightly increased, alanine and aspartate aminotransferase activities may be slightly increased, bromsulphthalein retention may be greater than normal, and there is a persistent increased excretion of urobilinogen in the urine. The laboratory tests, other than liver-biopsy examination, are not helpful in confirming the diagnosis.

DECOMPENSATED STAGE

Diagnosis is usually obvious on clinical examination, and is supported by the finding of increased serum bilirubin, moderately increased serum alkaline phosphatase activity, and alanine and aspartate aminotransferase activities, increased serum gammaglobulin and decreased serum albumin. Bromsulphthalein retention in non-jaundiced cases is abnormally increased, the test being pointless in jaundiced patients. There is frequently a moderate normochromic, occasionally macrocytic, anaemia, with a macronormoblastic marrow on aspiration, the white cell count is frequently at the lower end of the normal range, and the platelet count is reduced. The prothrombin time and the activated partial thromboplastin time are increased and do not return to normal after systemic vitamin K. In the presence of massive ascites, the plasma sodium and potassium levels may be at the lower end of the normal range or lower. The ascitic fluid is clear or bloodstained, and contains mainly endothelial cells with a specific gravity of 1·015.

There is persistent increased excretion of urobilinogen in the urine, with bilirubin present in jaundiced cases. The stools also contain increased stercobilinogen (urobilinogen).

Although liver biopsy examination would confirm the diagnosis, it is difficult to get good specimens from the cirrhotic liver, and the diagnosis is already obvious clinically.

TESTS OF PROGRESS

Treatment of ascites and oedema may require sodium restriction, diuretics plus potassium supplements, and fluid restriction, with adequate monitoring of plasma sodium, potassium and chloride levels. Estimation of plasma sodium is especially important after a large paracentesis, since a severe hyponatraemia may result, with a marked fall in plasma proteins. Albumin infusion and its effects can be controlled by laboratory estimation of plasma protein and plasma albumin levels.

With the development of complicating neurological signs, protein intake is cut and wide-spectrum antibiotics are given orally. At this stage, if the estimation is available, blood ammonia is found to be raised.

Primary Biliary Cirrhosis

Diagnosis of this autoimmune condition, characterized by pruritus in 50–70 per cent, with jaundice in 20 per cent, and hepatosplenomegaly, is confirmed by the finding of antimitochondrial antibodies (reacting with the ATP-ase complex on the inner mitochondrial membrane) in 95–99 per cent of cases. Seventy per cent of cases have increased polyclonal serum IgM.

Serum alkaline phosphatase activity is increased by 2–10 × normal, with moderate increase in aminotransferase activities. Serum bilirubin is normal or slightly raised. When serum bilirubin increases later, this indicates a poor prognosis.

Malabsorption results in coagulation factor defects, which respond to vitamin K therapy. Serum lipids are increased. The ESR and plasma viscosity are increased. Serum cholesterol is increased at first, falling with deteriorating liver cell function.

Liver biopsy may confirm the diagnosis. Liver cell copper is increased, localized in the lysosomes (cf. Wilson's disease).

TESTS OF PROGRESS

Vitamin K therapy is indicated when coagulation factor defects are found. Vitamin A and D supplements may be needed to correct defects due to steatorrhoea. Penicillamine therapy, used late in the disease, requires haematological monitoring. Clofibrate is contraindicated, as it causes excessive increase in serum cholesterol and bilirubin. Steroid therapy is also contraindicated.

TESTS PROVIDING USEFUL NEGATIVE RESULTS

Serum albumin and the plasma prothrombin time are normal until late in the disease. Bile is present in the duodenal juice (cf. extrahepatic biliary obstruction).

Portal Hypertension

Cases may be considered suitable for possible operation:
1. Serum albumin more than 3 g/100 ml. Patients with serum-albumin levels below 3 g/100 ml, and in whom the levels cannot be improved and maintained, are probably not suitable for operation.
2. Serum bilirubin below (30 µmol/l).
3. Ascites absent.
4. Normal EEG.
5. Haemoglobin greater than 12·0 g/dl.

Hepatic Venous Obstruction

Diagnosis is supported by the finding of moderately increased serum bilirubin, with gross bromsulphthalein retention, low blood glucose levels, and increased blood urea concentrations. Ascitic fluid has a high protein content, unless the serum albumin level is low.

Venography can be used to demonstrate patency or otherwise of the inferior vena cava, but direct venography of the hepatic veins is not feasible.

Post-portacaval Anastomosis

Following the anastomosis, the blood ammonia level is increased, especially after meals.

Partial Hepatectomy

After partial hepatectomy, the serum aspartate aminotransferase and serum alkaline phosphatase are greatly increased during recovery and regrowth of liver cells.

Pyogenic Liver Abscess

Diagnosis is made by demonstration by scanning. Repeated blood cultures enable the isolation of the infecting organism in many cases (two-thirds yield *Esch. coli* from blood culture and from abscess culture). There is a moderate increase in serum bilirubin, with marked increase in serum alkaline phosphatase activity, falling serum albumin, increased ESR and plasma viscosity, with marked increase in serum vitamin B_{12}, reflecting liver cell destruction. Laboratory tests may reflect changes due to conditions associated with liver abscess, including gallstones, carcinoma, sclerosing cholangitis, or biliary tract anomalies or strictures.

Amoebic Liver Abscess

Diagnosis of amoebic liver abscess can be confirmed at surgical drainage. ELISA techniques enable confirmation of Entamoeba infection in serum, stool, and abscess aspirate. Active, vegetative or cyst forms may be found in the patient's stools.

Hepatic Metastases

Patients complain of malaise, loss of weight, abdominal distension, and often fever and attacks of sweating.

Diagnosis is supported by the finding of increased serum alkaline phosphatase, lactate dehydrogenase and aminotransferase activities, with raised serum alpha-2 and gammaglobulins. There is often mild anaemia with neutrophilia. Serum CEA may be present. Ascitic fluid contains increased protein, with CEA and increased lactate dehydrogenase activity (exceeding LDH activity in the serum).

Diagnosis is confirmed by positive needle biopsy.

Hepatocellular Carcinoma

Diagnosis of this condition can be made by liver biopsy following liver scan. Laboratory tests reveal hypoglycaemia in up to 30 per cent of cases, with raised serum cholesterol in 33 per cent. Hyperlipidaemia is rare. There is often a polyclonal gammopathy with plasmacytosis. Serum alpha-fetoprotein levels are variable, and there may be non-specific increase in serum CEA. Serum ferritin levels are more increased than are serum aminotransferase activities. Serum vitamin B_{12} levels are greatly increased following release from destroyed liver cells.

There is a non-specific anaemia, with neutrophilia and thrombocytosis, with reduced plasma fibrinolytic activity.

TESTS OF PROGRESS

Serum alpha-fetoprotein concentration can be used as a tumour marker in children, for evidence of successful removal of the tumour. Successful surgical removal of such a tumour in adults is very unlikely.

Familial Hyperbilirubinaemia (Dubin–Johnson Type) [R] [?AD ?AR]

Diagnosis of this rare condition associated with persistent hyperbili-rubinaemia, with wide fluctuations in serum bilirubin in an affected patient (50–390 μmol/l, 2·9–23 mg/dl with the majority < 86 μmol/l, 5 mg/dl), is confirmed by the finding of plasma bromsulphthalein levels, after an initial fall, higher at 2 hours than at 45 min after the injection of the dye. Conjugated bromsulphthalein re-enters the plasma after its conjugation in the liver.

Liver biopsy material reveals diffuse greenish-black to chocolate-coloured pigment related to lysosomes (seen on electron microscopy). There is no excess of bile pigment or iron. The pigment is also excreted in the urine during attacks of acute hepatitis in these patients.

The condition may present initially in pregnancy or during the use of oral contraceptives.? There is a defect in transfer of some organic ions from liver to bile.

USEFUL NEGATIVE RESULTS

Serum bile acid levels are normal, and plasma alkaline phosphatase activity is also normal.

Familial Hyperbilirubinaemia (Rotor Syndrome) [R]

Diagnosis of this rare syndrome is supported by the finding of retention of bromsulphthalein at 45 min after injection to a greater degree than in the Dubin–Johnson syndrome, with no subsequent rise in plasma bromsulph-thalein at 90 or 120 min (cf. Dubin–Johnson syndrome). No conjugated dye appears in the plasma, suggesting abnormal transfer of bromsulphthalein from the plasma to the liver, rather than a defect in excretion of the pigment.

USEFUL NEGATIVE RESULTS

Brown pigment is not present in liver biopsy material (cf. Dubin–Johnson type). The gallbladder opacifies normally during cholecystography.

Familial Non-haemolytic Hyperbilirubinaemia [R]

CRIGLER–NAJJAR TYPE [R]

Diagnosis of this rare condition is supported by marked elevation of serum unconjugated bilirubin, deficiency in hepatic bilirubin-conjugating enzyme, with impaired bilirubin tolerance. Abnormally raised serum bilirubin concentration is detected by 1–8 weeks after birth. The major pigment fraction in the bile is the monoglucuronide of bilirubin.

TESTS OF PROGRESS

Type 1: Complete absence of hepatic bilirubin-conjugating enzyme, with absence of conjugated bilirubin in the bile, and death in the first year.
Type 2: Patients respond to phenobarbitone induction of bilirubin-conjugating enzyme activity, and they survive to adult life.

Familial Hyperbilirubinaemia [R] (Gilbert Type) [?AD]

Diagnosis of this condition, thought by some to occur in up to 2–5 per cent of the population, associated with reduced activity of the conjugating enzyme UDP-glucuronyl transferase in the liver (demonstrated on liver biopsy material), and characterized by mild intermittent jaundice without illness, is supported by the finding of inconsistent and minimal increase in serum bilirubin, rarely exceeding 51 μmol/l (3 mg/dl), with isolated rise in unconjugated bilirubin. Bilirubin monoglucuronide is converted to diglucuro-nide with difficulty. Bile contains more bilirubin monoglucuronide than diglucuronide. The bromsulphthalein retention test is only mildly impaired.

TESTS OF PROGRESS

After a 400 calorie diet for 24–72 hours, as serum fasting free fatty acids increase, serum bilirubin increases by 15 μmol/l. Results of this test overlap with normal, and at normal concentrations the coefficient of variation of serum bilirubin estimation is very high. Therefore results may not be clear-cut. When the serum bilirubin is raised, this can be reduced to normal by phenobarbitone 60 mg t.d.s.

Thyrotoxicosis and pregnancy both aggravate any jaundice in this condition. It is important to make the diagnosis of Gilbert's syndrome where it exists, as it is harmless, requires no treatment and patients do not need surgery.

USEFUL NEGATIVE RESULTS

Serum bile acids level is normal, and serum aminotransferase activities are normal. Liver biopsy is normal. The urine does not contain bilirubin.

Primary Shunt Hyperbilirubinaemia (Familial Overproduction Hyperbilirubinaemia) [R]

Diagnosis of this very rare condition is made by the finding of increased serum bilirubin (mainly unconjugated), some spherocytes in the peripheral blood, and a grossly increased output of urinary and faecal urobilinogen not related to any excess haemolysis, but rather ineffective erythropoiesis. There is a moderate reticulocytosis, and plasma iron turnover is increased. Liver biopsy reveals excessive deposition of stainable iron.

TESTS PROVIDING USEFUL NEGATIVE RESULTS

There is no evidence of gross haemolysis proportional to the urinary and faecal urobilinogen output. Splenectomy has no effect on the excretion of urobilinogen.

Familial Hyperbilirubinaemia (Lucy–Driscoll Transient Hyperbilirubinaemia)

Diagnosis of this rare condition in which jaundice appears in the first few days after birth and persists into the second or third week, is made by the demonstration of increased unconjugated bilirubin in the serum, with subsequent complete recovery. (? Inhibitor of bilirubin conjugation present in maternal and infant serum.)

Benign Idiopathic Recurrent Intrahepatic Cholestasis [R]

Diagnosis of this rare condition is supported by the finding of jaundice associated with a 'flu-like' attack, with no demonstrable obstruction of the main biliary ducts.

Electron microscopy of liver biopsy material taken during an attack shows cholestasis only.

TESTS OF PROGRESS

There is no permanent liver damage and liver function tests are normal in remission.

Liver Transplantation

Evidence of successful transplantation is found with restoration of serum pseudocholinesterase activity.

Evidence of rejection and/or cholangitis is associated with fall in serum pseudocholinesterase activity.

DISEASES OF THE GALLBLADDER AND BILE DUCTS

Acute Cholecystitis

Diagnosis of this condition, characterized by abdominal pain precipitated by meals and especially by fatty foods, with flatulence and nausea, with a high proportion of patients having obstruction of the cystic duct by gallstones, others with injury from acute pancreatic enzyme regurgitation, jaundice if a gallstone blocks the common bile duct, and pyrexia, is supported by the finding of marked increase in serum alkaline phosphatase activity (hepatic isoenzyme), with neutrophilia, raised ESR and plasma viscosity.

A few cases are associated with chronic typhoid carrier state, and *S. typhi* can be grown from the bile in these cases.

TESTS OF PROGRESS

Obstruction of one hepatic bile duct is associated with normal serum bilirubin concentration with great increase in serum alkaline phosphatase activity.

Cholangitis

Diagnosis of this condition, characterized by malaise, fever, abdominal pain, vomiting, pruritus and increasing jaundice, is supported by the finding of marked increase in serum alkaline phosphatase activity (biliary), with variable increase in serum bilirubin. Urine urobilinogen output is greatly increased, and the urine is dark, with pale stools.

Septicaemia is found on blood culture, the most frequent organism isolated being *Esch. coli* (Klebsiella sp., Proteus sp., and Pseudomonas sp. being found less frequently).

Primary Sclerosing Cholangitis

Diagnosis of this condition, 75 per cent occurring in patients suffering from ulcerative colitis, more commonly in males, and characterized by intermittent fever, with rigors, jaundice, weight loss and pruritus, is supported by the finding of increased serum alkaline phosphatase activity, increased serum IgM and variable serum bilirubin levels. Diagnosis is confirmed by the characteristic appearances on endoscopic retrograde cholangiography. Liver biopsy is not diagnostic.

TESTS OF PROGRESS

Penicillamine may be used, as there is copper deposition in the biliary tracts, and this treatment requires haematological monitoring.

Cholestasis

Diagnosis of cholestasis, characterized by pruritus, jaundice, xanthomas, loose, pale, bulky stools with steatorrhoea, is confirmed by histological examination of liver biopsy material, and strongly supported by the finding of rising serum bilirubin during the first 3 weeks of obstruction, with increased serum alkaline phosphatase activity (biliary type), 5'-nucleotidase activity and gamma-glutamyl peptidase activity (resulting from increased synthesis of enzymes from liver plasma membranes).

Serum total cholesterol increases, but falls terminally. Serum low-density lipoproteins increase, with increased levels of abnormal lipoprotein-X, and low HDL levels. Trihydroxy-bile salts increase in the serum.

If biliary cirrhosis develops, serum albumin falls. Urine bilirubin increases, with urinary urobilinogen excreted in proportion to the amount of bile reaching the duodenum.

TESTS OF PROGRESS

Following relief of obstruction, the serum bilirubin concentration falls slowly to normal.

OBSTRUCTION OF ONE HEPATIC BILE DUCT

Serum bilirubin levels remain normal, with greatly raised serum alkaline phosphatase activity.

INTRAHEPATIC OBSTRUCTIVE JAUNDICE

The results are very similar to those obtained in extrahepatic biliary obstruction.

Histological examination of liver-biopsy material is often very useful in defining liver damage and its causes.

Congenital Biliary Atresia

Diagnosis of this condition, characterized by jaundice developing by the end of the first week of life, which increases progressively, with the passage of dark urine and pale stools, is clinical. Laboratory findings include very high serum cholesterol levels with xanthomas, steatorrhoea with osteomalacia, and, often, bleeding as a result of vitamin K deficiency. Treatment, when possible, consists of surgical anastomosis of biliary ducts.

TESTS PROVIDING USEFUL NEGATIVE RESULTS

The finding of high normal faecal stercobilinogen (urobilinogen) levels excludes this condition.

Intrahepatic Atresia (Biliary Hypoplasia Syndrome)

Jaundice develops by the third day. 'Biliary' serum alkaline phosphatase activity is greatly increased, with marked increase in serum cholesterol and the development of xanthomas. Serum bile acids, hepatic copper content and urine copper excretion are all increased.

Bile-duct Proliferation

Any condition associated with proliferation of bile ducts, for example after liver resection, with regrowth from remaining liver, results in increase in serum alkaline phosphatase activity which can be shown to be liver alkaline phosphatase by electrophoresis.

Inspissated Bile Syndrome

Inspissated bile may cause obstructive jaundice in a newborn infant, which may persist for more than 10 days. The biochemical findings are of obstructive jaundice and complete recovery is the rule.

Primary Carcinoma of Bile Ducts

Diagnosis of this condition is supported by the finding of progressive obstructive jaundice, with increasing anaemia and positive tests for occult blood in faeces. The site of the growth, and the various ducts it obstructs, may produce various clinical signs and symptoms. Ascending cholangitis may occur, if obstruction to the biliary tree is partial with increased serum alkaline phosphatase activity.

Serum alpha-fetoprotein levels are normal (only very rarely increased).

Haemobilia [R]

Diagnosis of this rare condition is supported by the finding of falling haemoglobin levels, with raised serum amylase activity, serum bilirubin and very great increase in serum alkaline phosphatase activity.

DISEASES OF THE PANCREAS

Acute Pancreatitis

Diagnosis of acute pancreatitis is strongly supported by the finding of marked serum amylase activity during the first 36 hours of acute severe abdominal pain. Serum amylase activity reaches its peak by 5–12 hours, falling to normal by 48 hours. Serum lipase activity increases soon after onset and remains raised for up to 3 days, but the estimation is unsatisfactory technically. In severe cases, with much abdominal fat necrosis, formation of omental calcium soaps, and suppression of PTH secretion, serum calcium falls below normal. Hypoglycaemia often develops. The serum may appear milky. The ratio of amylase clearance to creatinine clearance is abnormal and exceeds 3·0 (amylase activity in iu/l and creatinine in µmol/l), and remains abnormally raised longer than does either serum or urine amylase activity. In severe attacks, methaemalbumin appears in the plasma after 12 hours and reaches peak values by 4–5 days (? associated with release of pancreatic trypsin). Neutrophilia, thrombocytosis, raised ESR and increased plasma viscosity are found, with often a slight increase in serum bilirubin.

TESTS OF PROGRESS

By the fifth day, plasma-activated partial thromboplastin times are shorter than normal, FDPs (fibrin-fibrinogen degradation products), plasma fibrinogen, Factors VIII and V levels, and alpha-1-antitrypsin activity are all increased, and persisting high plasma fibrinogen levels indicate a poor prognosis, as does persistent high serum aspartate aminotransferase activity.

Chronic Pancreatitis

Diagnosis of this condition in the laboratory is difficult without histological evidence or signs of pancreatic calcification. During acute exacerbations the findings are those of acute pancreatitis, including raised serum amylase and lipase activity, and increased urine amylase output. With progressive destruction of the pancreas following repeated attacks, the rise in serum amylase and lipase activities with each fresh exacerbation becomes smaller; at the same time steatorrhoea increases, with daily faecal fat excretion exceeding 7 g/day and nitrogen excretion in the stools exceeding 2·5 g/day.

Following a standard secretin injection, in advanced chronic pancreatitis the volume and bicarbonate content of pancreatic juice fall. Unfortunately, pancreatic provocation tests give disappointing and unreliable results (they mainly detect incomplete obstruction of the pancreatic ducts).

TESTS PROVIDING USEFUL NEGATIVE RESULTS

Xylose tolerance test is normal even when steatorrhoea is due to severe pancreatic disease, unless small intestinal function is also impaired.

Pancreatic-duct Obstruction

Following the development of a major obstruction to the flow of pancreatic secretions, serum amylase and lipase activities are increased after injection of secretin and pancreozymin. With prolonged obstruction, steatorrhoea develops, and it may be possible to demonstrate reduced duodenal juice lipase, trypsin and amylase activities.

Hereditary Pancreatitis [AD with variable penetrance]

Diagnosis of this condition, characterized by attacks of abdominal pain, often with nausea and vomiting and beginning at any time from infancy to old age (average 10–12 years), is supported by biochemical test results of acute pancreatitis. Eventually both endocrine and exocrine pancreatic functions fail, with the development of diabetes mellitus in 10–25 per cent and steatorrhoea. Commonly there is early calcification of the pancreas.

TESTS PROVIDING USEFUL NEGATIVE RESULTS

In quiescent periods, sweat sodium and chloride in sweat tests, serum calcium, phosphate, alpha-1-antitrypsin level and Pi-typing, serum triglycerides and abdominal ultrasound scanning are all normal. Eventually endocrine and exocrine insufficiency of the pancreas develops.

Cystic Fibrosis of Pancreas (Mucoviscidosis)

Diagnosis of this autosomal recessive condition, characterized by meconium ileus, meconium peritonitis or small bowel atresia (meconium is abnormally viscid), unexplained pulmonary disease, oedema, failure to thrive, with malabsorption or rectal prolapse (occurring in 1 in 2000–2500 live Caucasian births) (1 per 17 000 in live black births in the USA) is confirmed by the demonstration of abnormally raised sweat sodium during maximum sweating (after heat or pilocarpine iontopheresis). The sweat sodium excretion exceeds 70 mmol/l in affected homozygote infants. Sweat sodium falls by less than 10 per cent from the maximum rate after 9-alpha-fluorohydrocortisone. Malabsorption affects protein, fat and carbohydrate.

Microscopy of peroral jejunal biopsy material reveals normal small intestinal pattern, except for some inflammatory change and lamellated thick mucus. This thick mucus is also present in sputum, and cases develop emphysema, bronchopneumonia and bronchiectasis in relation to pulmonary cysts.

Rectal biopsy material reveals widely dilated crypts packed with lamellated mucus in some patients.

TESTS OF PROGRESS

These infants are unable to cope with very hot conditions for long. Steatorrhoea varies greatly in the untreated patient, and can be reduced by adding medium-chain triglycerides to the diet. Pancreatic extract may also be given orally. Relatives and siblings should be screened (using sweat or parotid gland secretion). There is no reliable test for heterozygotes.

TESTS PROVIDING USEFUL NEGATIVE RESULTS

The sweat test may be transiently positive in adrenal insufficiency, nephrogenic diabetes insipidus, congestive cardiac failure, fever, dehydration, ectodermal dysplasia, malnutrition, steroid therapy and diuretic therapy.

In infants, if maximum rates of sweating have been induced, and if sweat sodium is less than 50 mmol/l, the diagnosis of cystic fibrosis of the pancreas has been excluded.

Insulinoma

Diagnosis of insulinoma is confirmed by the finding of inappropriate raised serum insulin levels exceeding 15 mU/l in the presence of hypoglycaemia. Symptoms of hypoglycaemia occur most commonly before breakfast, at the end of the afternoon, and after exercise, when a blood sample for insulin and plasma glucose can be taken. Eighty per cent of cases develop hypoglycaemia with inappropriate serum insulin levels after an overnight fast, and 98 per cent have significant hypoglycaemia with inappropriate serum insulin levels after 48 hours of fasting, ending with exercise.

Provocation tests using tolbutamide or glucagon are obsolete and dangerous. Hypoglycaemia can be induced with fish insulin, and endogenous inappropriate insulin can then be measured, at 5 min if insulin is measured, or after 30 min of hypoglycaemia if connecting C-peptide is measured. As an alternative, connecting C-peptide can be measured after 1 hour of hypoglycaemia induced with pork insulin. In all these techniques, when the blood glucose is less than 3 mmol/l (54 mg/100 ml) serum insulin exceeds 4 mU/l, or C-peptide exceeds 0·2 pmol/l (60 pg/100 ml) in the presence of an active insulinoma.

TESTS PROVIDING USEFUL NEGATIVE RESULTS

The fact that commercial insulin contains very little C-peptide is useful in the detection of factitious hyperinsulinism. Blood estimation for the presence of sulphonylureas help to exclude sulphonylurea self-medication.

TESTS OF PROGRESS

After treatment by surgical removal of an insulinoma, inappropriate levels of serum insulin are not found. Diazoxide, 100–600 mg per day, inhibits insulin release from the pancreatic beta cells, and this has been used in the medical treatment of insulinoma. Non-specific ('blind') distal pancreatectomy is carried out on some cases, or beta cell lysis is produced by treatment with streptozotocin, followed by maintenance therapy with diazoxide.

Carcinoma of Pancreas (excluding islet cell tumours)
Laboratory tests in the diagnosis of carcinoma of the pancreas are disappointing. When the diagnosis is known, and either CEA is detected in pancreatic juice aspirate, or if serum CEA levels are high, then successful surgical removal of the tumour is unlikely (similar results found with oncofetal pancreatic antigen).

Serum CEA levels (previously raised) are of use as postoperative markers in confirmed cases of carcinoma of the pancreas.

Non-beta-islet Cell Tumour of the Pancreas ('Pancreatic Cholera'; Watery Diarrhoea Hypokalaemia Achlorhydria (WDHA) Syndrome; Verner–Morrison Syndrome [R])
Diagnosis of this rare condition, characterized by severe watery diarrhoea, with hypokalaemic alkalosis and achlorhydria, is supported by the finding of increased circulating vasoconstrictive intestinal polypeptide (VIP), pancreatic polypeptides or prostaglandins, secreted by an endocrine tumour, usually in the pancreas. The tumour may be localized by catheterization studies.

Rare Pancreatic Disorders

1. CONGENITAL PANCREATIC HYPOPLASIA [R]
Diagnosis of this rare condition is supported by the finding of steatorrhoea, absence of pancreatic lipase in duodenal juice aspirate and increased faecal excretion of bile salts.

2. CONGENITAL PANCREATIC LIPASE DEFICIENCY [R]
Diagnosis of this rare condition is supported by the finding of steatorrhoea

(leakage of free oil from the anus of one case) and absence of pancreatic lipase in duodenal aspirate.

3. ISOLATED COLIPASE DEFICIENCY [R] [AR]

Diagnosis of this rare condition, characterized by steatorrhoea and loose stools, is confirmed by the demonstration of normal activities of amylase, chymotrypsin and trypsin, with normal bile salt concentration, but colipase activity down to 10 per cent of normal in duodenal juice after cholecysto-kinin-pancreozymin stimulation (specialized laboratory required).

TESTS OF PROGRESS

Fat absorption (measured by radio-isotope triiolein breath test) improved after administration of purified colipase.

4. ENTEROKINASE DEFICIENCY [R]

Diagnosis of this condition, characterized by failure to thrive, oedema, hypoproteinaemia, anaemia, neutropenia and steatorrhoea, is supported by the demonstration of the failure of trypsin to convert procolipase to colipase (specialized laboratory required).

5. ZELLWEGER'S (CEREBROHEPATORENAL) SYNDROME [R]

Diagnosis of this metabolic disorder with multiple congenital anomalies, including characteristic facies, renal cortical cysts, progressive liver disease and severe developmental defects of the central nervous system, is supported by the demonstration of the presence of abnormal bile acids in the urine, including dihydroxycoprostanic acid (DHCA) (specialized laboratory required).

6. BILIARY HYPOPLASIA AND ABNORMAL BILE ACID EXCRETION [R]

Diagnosis of 2 cases reported, without congenital anomalies (cf. Zellweger's syndrome), excreting trihydroxycoprostanic acid (THCA) but not DHCA in the urine.

7. PRIMARY BILE ACID MALABSORPTION

Two boys have been investigated and shown to have malabsorption of bile acids.

8. PRIMARY SYNTHETIC DEFECT OF BILE ACIDS [R]

This condition has been described, with chronic diarrhoea, failure to thrive, steatorrhoea, and reduced luminal bile acids.

Following treatment with addition of bile acids to the diet, clinical improvement occurred, which ceased whenever the bile acid supplements were stopped.

Rare Exocrine Pancreatic Deficiency States [R]

1. Lipase deficiency
2. Trypsin deficiency
3. Enterokinin deficiency   have been described.
4. Amylase deficiency

Glucagonoma Syndrome [R]

Diagnosis of this rare syndrome, characterized by necrotizing migratory erythema, ileus, glossitis, angular cheilitis, venous thrombosis and attacks of diarrhoea, is strongly supported by the finding of raised plasma insulin and glucagon levels. The tumour may be localized by catheterization and multiple glucagon estimations on plasma samples from different sites.

TESTS OF PROGRESS

Following surgical removal or suppression by chemotherapy, plasma glucagon levels fall to normal and the skin rash improves.

Somatostatinoma [R]

? A silent non-functioning islet cell tumour of the pancreas. Since it has been described with diabetes mellitus, cholelithiasis, steatorrhoea, indigestion and hypochlorhydria, it is possible that it does have some effects.

10 *Diseases of the Cardiovascular System*

Essential Hypertension

Diagnosis of this condition depends on excluding other known causes of hypertension, e.g. phaeochromocytoma, unilateral renal disease, eclampsia, etc.

Urinary output of catecholamines and VMA may be moderately increased.

TESTS OF PROGRESS

Plasma renin levels, whether high or low, have no prognostic significance. Some patients with raised haemoglobin and haematocrit have a normal red-cell mass (cf. polycythaemia vera) with reduced plasma volume, especially if they have been treated with diuretics.

Constrictive Pericarditis

Diagnosis is supported by the finding of the tests affected by cardiac failure plus increased plasma fibrinogen during periods of acute inflammation. Serum bilirubin may be slightly raised, and the bromsulphthalein test is abnormal in proportion to the cardiac failure. Serum albumin tends to fall.

Acute Pericarditis

This condition is nearly always secondary to some local or general disease:
   Following myocardial infarction
   Post-commissurotomy syndrome
   Active rheumatic fever
   Bacterial infections, including tuberculosis
   Uraemia
   Neoplasia
   Autoimmune conditions (e.g. SLE)
Examination of fluid for cells and culture of fluid for organisms should be undertaken. Predominance of neutrophils suggests a bacterial infective element, predominance of lymphocytes suggests tuberculosis or viral infection.

Congestive Cardiac Failure

Diagnosis of congestive cardiac failure is clinical. The haematocrit may increase, resulting in normal ESR readings, even though plasma protein changes are sufficient to increase plasma viscosity. Nucleated red cells appear in the peripheral blood, with increasing tissue anoxia. Plasma urea (or NPN) increases with increasing failure (due to low GFR and poor elimination of solutes), and is a good measure of failure, falling to normal with recovery.

The urine contains casts and protein, with low sodium output (in the absence of diuretic therapy).

Liver anoxia results in increase in serum alanine aminotransferase activity, and serum bilirubin levels may increase slightly, with increased urinary excretion of urobilinogen.

TESTS OF PROGRESS

Fluid retention results in peripheral oedema, pleural effusion and/or ascites developing. Following fluid and salt restriction with added diuretic therapy, there may be clinical improvement in many cases, but plasma sodium and potassium concentrations (plus chloride, bicarbonate, urea and creatinine) require regular monitoring.

TESTS PROVIDING USEFUL NEGATIVE RESULTS

When assessing results in a given disease in a patient, if the patient is also suffering from cardiac failure, then many test results will reflect cardiac failure effects in addition to the other disease process. For example, after severe pulmonary infarction cardiac failure occurs, and cardiac failure commonly follows after a severe myocardial infarction.

Cyanotic Congenital Heart Disease

In cyanotic congenital heart disease, secondary polycythaemia develops, with increased haemoglobin concentration, increased haematocrit, increased red-cell count, and a tendency for the MCHC to fall below 32 g/100 ml, and reduced MCV. The whole blood arterial oxygen saturation is below normal in severe cases.

There is no special tendency to develop leukaemia as there is in primary polycythaemia vera and although occasional nucleated red cells may be seen in the peripheral blood, other immature cells are not seen.

Acute Rheumatic Fever

Diagnosis of this condition can be strongly supported by the finding of a raised and rising serum antistreptolysin 'O' titre with increased ESR and plasma viscosity, plus positive C-reactive protein test. In many cases in the early stages, *Strept. pyogenes* can be isolated from throat swabs. *Strept. pyogenes* infection stimulates production of antibodies which also cross-react with heart muscle cells. Plasma fibrinogen, serum gamma- and alphaglobulins are increased. Other indicators of acute inflammatory change are increased. The bone marrow plasma cell count is markedly increased (should a bone marrow aspirate be examined for some other diagnosis).

TESTS OF PROGRESS

During treatment, the plasma viscosity should be monitored. If salicylate therapy is given, the ESR will be normal when the serum salicylate concentration is 20 mg/100 ml or more (surface effect on red cells). C-reactive protein disappears from the serum with fall in acute inflammatory state. In pregnancy in a woman with a previous history of rheumatic fever, the erythrocyte sedimentation is a misleading test, as it is increased in normal pregnancy anyway (as is the plasma viscosity) with the normally increased plasma fibrinogen. The serum C-reactive protein is a very useful test of rheumatic activity in these circumstances. Similarly, in the event of cardiac failure developing, as the haematocrit exceeds 50 per cent, so the ESR becomes normal, even though both the plasma viscosity and the serum C-reactive protein tests are abnormal in response to underlying active rheumatic fever. Serum aspartate aminotransferase activity is related to the severity of the attack in the early stages.

There is a high recurrence rate following an attack of sore throat with fever, especially if there has only been a short interval since an attack of rheumatic fever. There appears to be no significant association between recurrence of the disease and a rise in ASO titres. Therefore prophylactic oral penicillin should be maintained for some years after an attack, or indefinitely if there is severe carditis.

TESTS PROVIDING USEFUL NEGATIVE RESULTS

Because of the very definite association of acute rheumatic fever with streptococcal infection and some form of allergic reaction to the infection, the finding of positive ASO titres indicates a recent streptococcal infection and therefore the possibility of rheumatic fever. Negative tests in children who have had rheumatic fever are useful evidence of long-term success in preventing further streptococcal infection. In cases suspected of having acute rheumatic fever, an ASO titre of less than 50 units/ml is generally regarded as excluding the diagnosis of active rheumatic fever.

Although the serum aspartate aminotransferase activity can be used to assess activity of the disease, serum alanine aminotransferase does not also increase unless cardiac failure results in liver anoxia or there is some other condition present.

Acute Myocarditis

Acute myocarditis can develop as part of a generalized infection:
Viral infections:
  Coxsackie B
  Influenza
  Poliomyelitis
  Infectious mononucleosis
Bacterial infections:
  Diphtheria
Protozoal infections:
  Toxoplasmosis
  Trypanosomiasis (Chagas's disease)
Nematode infections:
  Trichinosis
Rheumatic fever

The laboratory findings will depend on the disease and its severity. The diagnosis of myocarditis is clinical and electrocardiography is useful.

Post-infarction Syndrome (Dressler's Syndrome)

Following myocardial infarction, there may be a sudden pyrexia with raised ESR and the presence of antibodies to heart muscle in the serum. The condition rapidly responds to steroid therapy and represents the body's reaction to the temporary circulation of material derived from breaking-down heart muscle.

Post-commissurotomy Syndrome

Recurrent febrile episodes 2–4 weeks after heart surgery, with fever, pleuropericardial pain, pleural effusion, pneumonitis, with or without polyarthralgia may occur. This may be a temporary recurrence of rheumatic activity (but this is unlikely), persistence of normal postoperative sequelae, or, more likely, a reaction to dead muscle tissue or a temporary autoimmune reaction similar to Dressler's post-infarction syndrome.

The serum C-reactive protein test becomes positive, and the ESR is increased, with moderate increases in serum aspartate aminotransferase activity, and positive tests for the presence of anti-heart muscle antibodies.

Myocardial Infarction

TESTS SUPPORTING CLINICAL DIAGNOSIS

Enzymes normally contained in heart muscle are released into the circulation following myocardial infarction. The most commonly used estimations include:

Serum aspartate aminotransferase: serum levels begin to rise 6–8 hours after myocardial damage, reach a peak by 24 hours, and, falling subsequently, become unreliable for diagnosis of this clinical condition after 4 days.

Serum creatine phosphokinase: serum levels begin to rise 3–6 hours after myocardial damage, reach a peak by 24 hours (predominantly the MB isoenzyme) and on average return to normal by the third day after myocardial damage.

Serum lactate dehydrogenase: serum levels begin to rise 12 hours after myocardial damage, reach a peak by 48 hours, and on average return to normal by the eleventh day after myocardial damage. When isoenzymes of lactate dehydrogenase are examined, LD_1 fraction is increased until it is equal to LD_2 fraction or exceeds it. Using 2-oxobutyrate instead of pyruvate as substrate, the faster isoenzymes of lactate dehydrogenase can be measured.

(Other enzymes show a similar pattern, with onset of rise after 6 hours, peak at 24–48 hours, returning to normal by 24–48 hours:

Serum malate dehydrogenase
Serum phosphohexoseisomerase
Serum aldolase
Serum 6-phosphogluconic dehydrogenase)

Plasma fibrinogen (easily estimated by heat-turbidity technique) increases within 48 hours of myocardial infarction, roughly in proportion to the amount of myocardium damaged, returning to normal by 2-3 weeks in the absence of complicating infection or further infarction. This test is useful when a patient is admitted to hospital after a few days have elapsed since infarction.

During tissue repair processes later, the following enzymes have been found to increase:

Serum gamma-glutamyl transferase

Serum 5′-nucleotidase

Serum alkaline phosphatase

but have not been found to be useful clinically.

Evidence of tissue damage and inflammatory response is shown by:

Increased TWBC with neutrophilia, eosinopenia, thrombocytosis, increased ESR and plasma viscosity, increased serum alpha-1- and alpha-2-globulins, serum caeruloplasmin and copper oxidase activity. Heparin tolerance is increased, as shown by increased heparin dosage needed during the first week after infarction to maintain satisfactory anticoagulation. Urine pressor amines increase after an attack.

Following myocardial infarction, the serum cholesterol and total serum lipids fall by the end of the first week, beginning to rise again by the ninth to twelfth days to reach pre-attack levels by 3–8 weeks. There is a significant increase in many patients by 3–5 weeks in the serum pre-beta-lipoprotein level. The timing of these changes is important where lipid profiling is used to determine treatment of abnormalities in serum lipoprotein patterns.

TESTS OF PROGRESS

Serum lactate dehydrogenase and plasma fibrinogen levels should return to normal by 2–3 weeks. Complicating cardiac failure will be reflected by the effects of liver anoxia on serum aspartate and alanine aminotransferases, lactate dehydrogenase, and serum bilirubin.

TESTS PROVIDING USEFUL NEGATIVE RESULTS FOR DIAGNOSIS

Normal serum enzyme activity (aspartate aminotransferase, creatine phosphokinase, lactate dehydrogenase) excludes current myocardial infarction, *if* the timing of the collection of blood samples was correct. Thus, serum aspartate aminotransferase estimation is not useful during the second week after an attack, and serum lactate dehydrogenase estimation is not useful within 6 hours of an attack.

Serum isocitric dehydrogenase activity is markedly increased following liver damage, is not affected by muscle damage, but could reflect liver damage due to heart failure secondary to myocardial infarction.

Infective Endocarditis

1. BACTERIAL ENDOCARDITIS

Diagnosis can be confirmed by blood cultures, taken at intervals over a period of a few days, using aerobic and anaerobic media. Following isolation of the organism, its sensitivity to suitable antibiotics can be determined, and antibiotic therapy given.

Anaerobic bacteria and microaerophilic variants of streptococci may give 'negative' blood cultures unless anaerobic culture techniques are included.

Before treatment, a progressive refactory anaemia develops, with neutrophilia, falling serum albumin, rising globulin (gamma fraction) and plasma fibrinogen, with increasing ESR and plasma viscosity. Microscopic haematuria due to focal glomerulonephritis is almost always found.

TESTS OF PROGRESS

Antibiotic therapy can be monitored by blood antibiotic level estimations, to ensure that adequate continuous antibiotic is given. The blood antibiotic level should be 6 × minimal inhibitory concentration. Following such treatment, blood cultures become negative, and the patient's condition improves, although damage to heart valves may become apparent.

2. NON-BACTERIAL ENDOCARDITIS

A. Endocarditis due to *Coxiella burnetti* (Q fever), or Chlamydia, give routine 'negative' blood cultures, and special techniques are necessary for their detection.

B. Candida endocarditis—'Spontaneous' infection with Candida species is rare. Candida endocarditis rarely complicates open heart surgery, antibiotic therapy (with broad-spectrum antibiotics) for bacterial endocarditis, or in drug addicts (i.e. 'opportunistic' infection).

Unless special techniques for Candida isolation are used, routine blood cultures are 'negative'.

3. NON-BACTERIAL THROMBOTIC ENDOCARDITIS

This condition occurs in association with carcinoma of lung, pancreas, prostate, or breast, and may be associated with cerebral infarction or myocardial infarction in some cases, especially in patients over 50 years of age. Some patients develop thrombocytopenia. Blood cultures are persistently negative.

Mediastinitis

This condition is almost secondary to lung or gastro-oesophageal soiling. Determination of the infecting organisms can be carried out by microscopy and culture of pus or fluid obtained at surgical exploration. There is usually a marked neutrophilia, with raised ESR and plasma viscosity.

Dissecting Aortic Aneurysm

There is neutrophilia. Serum aspartate and alanine aminotransferase activities may be increased, if there is associated congestive cardiac failure plus liver congestion, or extension of the dissection into heart muscle, otherwise these enzymes are not increased.

TESTS PROVIDING USEFUL NEGATIVE RESULTS

Within the first 24–48 hours of the acute dissection serum creatine phosphokinase activity is not increased, unless the dissection extends into the myocardium, excluding a diagnosis of acute myocardial infarction.

Coarctation of Aorta

Diagnosis is made by clinical assessment, aortography and cardiac catheterization. After exercise, with a severe coarctation, increase in plasma haemoglobin can be demonstrated, if a careful venepuncture sample of blood is obtained.

Raynaud's Syndrome

Diagnosis of this condition is clinical. There may be an increased titre of 'cold agglutinins' or cryoglobulin in the serum.

Hereditary Haemorrhagic Telangiectasia (Rendu–Osler–Weber Disease) [AR] [R]

Bleeding occurs from affected areas, which occur in skin, in gastrointestinal tract, or respiratory tract. Loss of blood from bleeding sites results in hypochromic anaemia, with moderate reticulocytosis. Platelet adhesiveness is reduced. The bleeding time is normal when performed in normal skin, but is grossly prolonged in a telangiectatic area.

The condition is familial.

Arterial Thrombosis

Apart from alterations in the blood similar to those occurring after venous thrombosis, if the artery thrombosed was responsible for the blood supply of a large muscle mass, the subsequent muscle necrosis may result in myoglobinuria, with a temporary increase in aspartate aminotransferase, lactate dehydrogenase, creatine phosphokinase, and aldolase activities. When muscle is damaged, serum creatine phosphokinase activity remains increased for up to 15 days.

Mesenteric Thrombosis

Diagnosis is supported by gross neutrophilia, with increased aspartate aminotransferase and amylase activities (but the level of activity is not as great as is found in acute pancreatitis).

Renal Vein Thrombosis

Apart from non-specific evidence of recent venous thrombosis, there may be gross proteinuria, if one renal vein is partially blocked by blood clot.

Splenic Vein Thrombosis

Following non-specific evidence of recent thrombosis, there is a gross increase in the whole blood platelet count after the fourth day.

Deep-vein Thrombosis, Thrombo-embolic Disease

Diagnosis of venous thrombosis is clinical, aided by phlebograms, injection and detection of deposited ^{125}I-tagged fibrinogen, or Doppler techniques.

Following acute thrombosis, there may be neutrophilia, with increased ESR, plasma viscosity and fibrinogen. Plasma antithrombin-III levels fall. There may be a moderate thrombocytosis during the first week. In the absence of anticoagulant therapy, the plasma APTT may be reduced below the normal value, and heparin is partially neutralized in vitro.

TESTS OF PROGRESS

Regular monitoring of heparin infusion, using the activated partial thromboplastin time or thrombin time, and of warfarin using the prothrombin ratio (BCR therapeutic range 2–4) is necessary.

11 *Respiratory Diseases*

Asthma

                    Diagnosis of this condition of reversible bronchoconstriction is essentially clinical. In the extrinsic form of the disease, with sensitivity to known external agents, microscopy of the sputum reveals eosinophilia, with Curschmann's spirals of mucinous fibrils, and sometimes Charcot–Leyden crystals. There may also be an eosinophilia in the peripheral blood.

    In intrinsic forms of the disease, there may be many neutrophils, associated with a precipitating infection. In some cases there may be eosinophils in the sputum, suggesting that the substance to which the patient is sensitive has not been discovered.

    Skin-testing may be used for detection of the allergin. Aerosol testing has also been used, but unless the operator is skilled the tests can be dangerous. Serum immunoglobulin IgE is increased in many asthmatics.

    Cultures of sputum and of upper respiratory tract secretions are useful in the treatment of bronchitis, and also in the detection of fungi causing reactions.

STATUS ASTHMATICUS

During status asthmaticus the blood changes are those of severe respiratory acidosis with anoxaemia. The Po_2 is maintained with a reduced Pco_2 (reflecting the very great difference in solubility in water of oxygen and carbon dioxide, and hence speed of transfer across respiratory membranes). A rising Pco_2 towards normal with a falling Po_2 is ominous. Serum aspartate aminotransferase activity increases as the arterial Po_2 falls in a seriously ill patient. Asthmatic attacks may be provoked by respiratory tract infections.

Hay Fever and Allergic Rhinitis

Nasal secretions contain numerous eosinophils, and there may be an eosinophilia in the peripheral blood as well.

Fibrosing Alveolitis (Diffuse Pulmonary Fibrosis; Idiopathic Interstitial Pulmonary Fibrosis; Hamman–Rich Disease)

A. ALLERGIC ALVEOLITIS (EXTRINSIC)

This condition has been found in certain individuals following exposure to organic dusts in many different situations:

Farmer's lung	Biological detergent workers
Bird fancier's lung	Cheese washers
Poultry breeders	Coffee workers
Sugar-cane strippers	Fish-meal exposure
Mushroom farming	Furriers
Maple-bark stripping	Guinea pig handlers
Grain workers	Pituitary snuff takers
Malting	etc.

Diagnosis is made by the detection of precipitating antibodies against the relevant organic dust. Specific skin tests give positive Type III (Arthus) reactions, and specific inhalation tests give alveolar reactions and impaired gas transfer. In some cases, lung biopsy has revealed the presence of deposits of IgG and complement.

TESTS PROVIDING USEFUL NEGATIVE RESULTS

These include the uncommon findings of non-organ-specific auto-antibodies.

B. INTRINSIC ALVEOLITIS

Diagnosis is made by the finding of non-organ-specific auto-antibodies.

TESTS PROVIDING USEFUL NEGATIVE RESULTS

These include the absence of precipitating antibodies against relevant organic dust materials. With the finding of different organic dusts causing allergic alveolitis, many cases thought at first to be intrinsic in nature have been found to be extrinsic (and hence avoidable).

Pulmonary Aspergilloma (Mycetoma; Fungus Ball)

The detection of a pulmonary cavity is usually carried out by X-ray studies. When the fungus has invaded the cavity (e.g. an old healed tuberculous cavity) precipitating antibodies are present in the serum against *Aspergillus fumigatus* (or less commonly *Aspergillus nidulans*), which persist for weeks after resection of the lesion or after death of the fungus.

Following culture of material from the cavity or of coughed-up material, the fungus can be isolated on culture from up to one-third of the patients.

Emphysema

Plasma sodium, chloride and standard bicarbonate reflect the severity of respiratory acidosis caused by emphysema. A plasma alpha-1-antitrypsin deficiency accounts for 6 per cent of all cases of emphysema, and most cases under 50 years of age in the West.

Heterozygotes as well as homozygotes with abnormal alpha-1-antitrypsin in plasma are liable to early-onset emphysema, with early exertional dyspnoea, affected CO transfer factor, and symmetrical emphysema tending to affect lower lobes rather than upper lobes.

Alpha-1-antitrypsin Deficiency [AR]

This condition is characterized by predisposition to develop lung disease in the homozygote. Fifty to sixty per cent of homozygotes develop emphysema, often with marked cyanosis due to arteriovenous shunting in the lungs, 10–20 per cent develop liver disease, and perhaps 10–20 per cent remain unaffected. Emphysema develops by the fourth decade, and cigarette smoking speeds up the process. Neonate homozygotes may develop cirrhosis and hepatoma may also develop. Heterozygotes inherit the predisposition to develop airways obstructive disease, especially following cigarette smoking.

Diagnosis is confirmed by demonstration of very low specific enzyme deficiency in the serum in homozygotes, with values midway between homozygotes and normal subjects in heterozygotes. There is no treatment, but in affected families, genetic counselling is useful.

Tropical Pulmonary Eosinophilia

Diagnosis is supported by the finding of a total white blood cell count exceeding $15 \times 10^9/l$ (15000 per cmm) with an absolute eosinophilia. The sputum may contain eosinophils, and the stools may contain parasites.

TESTS OF PROGRESS

The initial very high blood eosinophil counts (? hypersensitivity to filarial infestation) responds to diethylcarbamazine therapy.

Simple Pulmonary Eosinophilia (Löffler's Syndrome)

Diagnosis is supported by the finding of a normal or raised total white blood cell count with an absolute eosinophilia. The stools may contain parasites. Pulmonary migration of ascaris larvae (and simple pulmonary eosinophilia) occurs within 2 weeks of infection. Worms only become adult in 2 months, and so only subsequently can ova be found in the stools.

Bronchial Adenoma

If the bronchial adenoma is of the carcinoid type, then, in addition to the local signs and symptoms, the carcinoid syndrome is seen, and there is excessive excretion of 5-HIAA in the urine.

Post-asphyxia

Following recovery, there may be petechial haemorrhages visible in the skin, and there is a temporary increase in the platelet count.

Pulmonary Carcinoma

Diagnosis is strongly supported by the finding of carcinoma cells in the sputum or in lung washings. Haemoptysis is frequently an early sign. Biopsy of enlarged lymph glands may reveal secondary carcinoma. Following partial obstruction to a bronchus, localized bronchopneumonia may develop. Signs and symptoms also reflect the site and size of secondary deposits.

Examination of sputum smears for carcinoma cells is not useful for screening the normal population for unsuspected carcinoma, but it is very useful in confirming the diagnosis in inoperable cases.

TESTS OF PROGRESS

In proven cases of carcinoma of the lung, those with preoperative serum CEA levels above normal die sooner than those with normal low levels of CEA, whether surgery is attempted or not.

Stomatitis, Parotitis, Dental Abscess

Identification of the infecting organism can be determined by microscopy and culture of pus from the affected site. The condition may be secondary to a generalized debilitating disease (e.g. leukaemia).

Sinusitis and Antrum Infections

Identification of the infecting organism can be determined by microscopy and culture of material obtained from the infected cavity. In acute cases, swabs should be taken from the nasal passages near the meatus of the infected cavity. In chronic cases, culture of material obtained by aspiration and wash-outs, or of the lining of the cavity or granulation tissue, should be carried out.

There is usually a neutrophilia and raised ESR and plasma viscosity when there is acute bacterial infection of a sinus.

Tonsillitis and Pharyngitis

Identification of the infecting organism can be determined by microscopy of throat swabs for the demonstration of the organisms of Vincent's angina, and culture of throat swabs for the isolation of haemolytic streptococci, pneumococci, diphtheria, staphylococci, or candida. Swabs for the isolation and identification of viruses are not usually taken in cases of sore throat unless they are part of an epidemiological study.

Neutrophilia commonly occurs, and in severe infections there is also proteinuria.

TESTS OF PROGRESS

Repeat swabs of the throat and nose should be taken after treatment, to determine whether the infecting organism has been eliminated. This is particularly important in closed communities, and especially in hospitals, to prevent cross-infection.

Acute Bronchitis, Bronchiolitis, Tracheitis, Laryngitis

Identification of the infecting organism can be determined by microscopy and culture of sputum, or if the sputum is scanty, of throat swab or laryngeal swab. Throat and nose swabs taken for virus detection should be delivered to the laboratory immediately or transported there on ice (water).

Neutrophilia occurs in association with acute bacterial infections, with increased ESR and plasma viscosity. Neutropenia with moderate lymphocytosis is often found in association with viral infections. When virus infection is possible, paired serum samples should be taken, the first early in the illness and the second 10–12 days later, for the demonstration of a rising antibody titre.

In likely cases, microscopy of sputum for *Mycobacterium tuberculosis* and possibly special culture for the organism should be carried out.

Chronic Bronchitis

Identification of the infecting organisms can be determined by microscopy and culture of samples of sputum. In these cases it is important to be told of any recent antibiotic therapy, since the organisms isolated may be resistant to the antibiotic being administered.

With acute flare-up in a chronic bronchitic patient, there is neutrophilia with increased ESR and plasma viscosity.

In likely cases, special films of sputum should be examined to exclude the presence of *Myobacterium tuberculosis*.

TESTS OF PROGRESS

With successful antibiotic treatment, the volume of sputum coughed up each day and the number of neutrophils in the sputum decrease. Pathogenic organisms may be eliminated from the sputum, and the white cell count returns to normal in the blood.

Bronchiectasis

During acute exacerbations the sputum coughed up becomes more purulent, and there is a peripheral blood neutrophilia with raised ESR and plasma viscosity. The predominant organism from the bronchiectatic cavity may be determined by microscopy and culture of sputum.

In certain cases, special films of sputum should be examined to exclude underlying pulmonary tuberculosis. Also it is worth remembering that *Aspergillus* sp. colonizes healed cavities.

Pneumonia—Bacterial and Fungal

Identification of the infecting organism can be determined by microscopy and culture of sputum, throat swabs, or laryngeal swabs. In acute cases, the infecting organism, e.g. *Streptococcus pneumoniae*, may visibly be the predominant organism in films made from fresh sputum.

Neutrophilia develops rapidly, with very high counts being found, raised ESR and plasma viscosity, and thrombocytosis. There may be respiratory acidosis and the plasma chloride may fall. Blood cultures may be positive, especially useful in diagnosis in the elderly.

TESTS OF PROGRESS

In the elderly, absence of neutrophilia or excessively high leukaemoid counts used to be considered to indicate a poor prognosis. With the very large number of antibiotics available, this method of prognosis is no longer valid.

In pneumonia due to *Strept. pneumoniae*, presence of the capsular antigen in the serum is related to an increased mortality rate.

TESTS PROVIDING USEFUL NEGATIVE RESULTS

In likely cases, a sample of sputum should be examined to exclude the presence of *Mycobacterium tuberculosis*.

Ventilator Pneumonia

It is very important to avoid contamination of mechanical ventilators (used to assist respiration in badly injured or paralysed patients), humidifiers, or suction apparatus with *Pseudomonas aeruginosa* (and *Serratia marcescens*). Subsequent use of the contaminated apparatus on a seriously ill patient (e.g. in intensive care units) may result in necrotizing pneumonia. There is also a serious risk of infection of tracheostomy wounds with *Ps. aeruginosa*.

The organism can be demonstrated by culture of swabs from contaminated apparatus and from infected patients' aspirates, sputum, and wounds.

Primary Atypical Pneumonia (infection with *Mycoplasma pneumoniae*)

In most cases *Mycoplasma pneumoniae* infection is associated either with no symptoms or with upper respiratory tract infection, but in a minority of cases mild bronchitis and pneumonia develop.

Diagnosis of this type of pneumonia is confirmed by the isolation and identification of the organism following special cultural techniques on sputum, throat swab, and upper respiratory tract secretions. Cold agglutinins to the patient's own red cells develop by the end of the first week in 50 per cent of cases and a rising titre from the early stage of the disease to convalescence is diagnostic. Similarly, rising titres against the specific organism can be demonstrated by means of a specific complement-fixation test or by immunofluorescence. In addition, agglutinins to the non-haemolytic *Streptococcus* MG also develop. These three antibody reactions are distinct one from the others.

Neutrophilia is uncommon, but may occur, and also occurs following secondary bacterial invasion. Biological false-positive tests for syphilis are obtained during the illness in many cases.

The organism causes opportunist infections in debilitated patients.

Pneumonia—Virus

Identification of the infecting virus by isolation of culture may be carried out from nose and throat swabs delivered immediately after collection to the laboratory or transported on ice (water). Serum samples should be taken early in the disease and again during convalescence, for the possible demonstration of rising antibody titres.

Neutrophilia is not marked and there may be lymphocytosis. Later, neutrophilia suggests secondary bacterial invasion.

See section on Virus Infections, pp. 3–25 et seq.

Pleurisy with Effusion

This is usually a consequence of some local or general disease, and examination of pleural fluid may be diagnostically helpful:

TRANSUDATES

The protein content of the fluid tends to be 500–1500 mg/100 ml, there are few cells, and the fluid does not clot.

INFLAMMATORY EXUDATES

The protein content of the fluid tends to be 3000–6000 mg/100 ml, and cell counts of 100–10000/cmm are found. As the fluid contains fibrinogen and clots readily, it is important to place some of the fluid in anticoagulant if cell microscopy is required.

In association with pyogenic infections, the cells are predominantly neutrophils, whilst in association with virus infections or tuberculosis, the cells are predominantly lymphocytes.

In cases of carcinoma of the lung or pleural malignancy, malignant cells may be found (if fluid is placed in anticoagulant at the time of aspiration). Erythrocytes are present in increased numbers.

FOLLOWING TRAUMA

Bloodstained fluid is obtained, which may or may not grow organisms on culture, depending on the injury (blood may contaminate any pleural aspirate, from local bleeding at the site of aspiration).

CHYLOUS EFFUSIONS

Milky fluid is aspirated, which is revealed as chyle by microscopy and by chemical demonstration of lipids. In general, aspirated fluid should be examined microscopically, cultured for organisms including *Mycobacterium tuberculosis*, and protein content determined.

Empyema

Identification of the infecting organism in empyema can be determined by microscopy and culture (including culture for *Mycobacterium tuberculosis*) of pus removed by aspiration or during surgery. In chronic empyema, cultures should be made of granulation tissue removed from the cavity walls.

Empyema is associated with neutrophilia, raised ESR and plasma viscosity.

Lung Abscess

Identification of the organism causing a lung abscess may be determined by microscopy and culture of pus expectorated or removed surgically, for pathogenic bacteria and fungi. It should be noted that fungi (e.g. *Aspergillus* sp.)

may be present in an old abscess cavity without invading local tissues but often causing allergic manifestations.

Marked neutrophilia, raised ESR and plasma viscosity, with increasing anaemia, is found in association with an acute lung abscess. Signs of chronic infection and chronic inflammation are associated with a chronic lung abscess.

Pulmonary Infarction, Pulmonary Embolism

Diagnosis of this condition is confirmed by assessment of clinical signs and symptoms, evidence of pulmonary infiltration on X-ray films, pulmonary angiography and pulmonary isotope scanning.

Diagnosis can be supported by the finding of raised ESR and plasma viscosity, neutrophilia and increased serum lactate dehydrogenase activity. Fibrin-fibrinogen degradation products are present in the plasma.

TESTS OF PROGRESS

There is a moderate slow rise in plasma fibrinogen (a much flatter peak than that obtained after myocardial infarction), and heparin tolerance is increased to a maximum by the fifth day (with the result that therapeutic blood levels of infused heparin are difficult to regulate).

TESTS PROVIDING USEFUL NEGATIVE RESULTS

Serum creatine phosphokinase activity is not increased, and serum aspartate aminotransferase activity is moderately increased, but with a much flatter and later peak than after myocardial infarction.

(It is worth noting that spontaneous pulmonary embolism may occur in sickle-cell disease and in homocystinuria.)

Hyaline Membrane Disease

This condition, which is a cause of the respiratory distress syndrome, occurs in newborn infants, and has also been described in adults subjected to total body irradiation. The laboratory findings include: Increased blood P_{CO_2}, falling blood pH, rising plasma potassium and cyanosis (reduced percentage saturation of haemoglobin).

There is a deficiency of plasminogen activator in lung tissue (normally lung contains a high concentration) and this leads to pathological fibrin deposition and hyaline membrane formation, with subsequent pulmonary fibrosis.

Idiopathic Pulmonary Haemosiderosis

Diagnosis is supported by the finding of haemoptysis with numerous haemosiderin-laden macrophages in the sputum. Cells from sputum, gastric washings and lung aspirate give a positive stain for iron. There is a hypochromic, microcytic anaemia which is often severe, with anisocytosis, poikilocytosis and reticulocytosis. Neutrophilia may occur and eosinophilia may also occur. Serum unconjugated bilirubin is intermittently increased, with increased output of urine urobilinogen and faecal urobilinogen (stercobilinogen).

TESTS PROVIDING USEFUL NEGATIVE RESULTS

Even though there is hypochromic anaemia, serum-iron levels are normal, and there is no reduction in serum iron-binding capacity.

Eosinophilic Granuloma of Bone [R]

Twenty per cent of cases with bone disease have lung changes. Frequently there is an associated neutrophilia, and occasionally eosinophilia. The sputum occasionally contains eosinophils or fat-laden histiocytes.

12 *Renal Tract Diseases*

Acute Renal Failure
> **Diagnosis** of acute renal failure is supported by the finding of oliguria, with increasing nitrogen retention. If there is also hypercatabolism (e.g. resulting from burns, trauma, sepsis, starvation or gastrointestinal haemorrhage) the plasma urea/creatinine ratio rises. In uncomplicated cases, the plasma urea rises at a rate of from 5 to 10 mmol/l/day.

Hyponatraemia is caused by water intake and water production from food exceeding excretion. Vomiting may increase hypochloraemia. Plasma potassium tends to rise with the combined failure to excrete potassium adequately in the urine, and loss of potassium from cells. (Plasma potassium may fall in some cases following excessive vomiting or dextrose-rich hyperalimentation.)

With developing metabolic acidosis, due to failure to excrete hydrogen ion adequately, plasma bicarbonate falls with eventual fall in plasma pH. After a few days of failure, moderate anaemia commonly develops. Depending on the cause of renal failure, urine examination gives different results. With acute tubular necrosis, the urine contains large numbers of red blood cells, hyaline, granular and cellular casts with increased protein. Renal biopsy is essential in severe cases for precise diagnosis of the cause of the renal failure.

Favourable signs include urine osmolality > 500 mosm/kg water, urine sodium < 20 mmol/l, urine urea/plasma urea > 8, urine creatinine/plasma creatinine > 40. Unfavourable signs include urine osmolality < 350 mosm/kg water, urine sodium > 40 mmol/l, urine urea/plasma urea < 3, urine creatinine/plasma creatinine < 20.

TESTS OF PROGRESS

Fluid balance studies, with possible use of mannitol or frusemide diuretic therapy, require careful plasma electrolyte estimation. Adequate calorie intake with minimal protein intake reduces the rate of increase in nitrogen retention. Dialysis requires adequate biochemical monitoring.

Following the period of oliguria, during recovery there is often a phase of diuresis, which in part reflects fluid overload during the oliguric phase. This again requires careful monitoring.

Acute Poststreptococcal Glomerulonephritis

Diagnosis of this condition, which is preceded by 7–20 days by a streptococcal infection and which is characterized by oedema (often noted in the face on arising), haematuria or marked reduction in urine flow, with malaise and headache, is supported by the finding of increased urine protein excretion with granular and cellular casts, and variable haematuria. If the urine red cell count exceeds 3000/ml then phase contrast microscopy is useful, as distorted red cells (damaged in the glomeruli) are seen. Renal biopsy may be valuable for confirmation of the diagnosis and for assessment of the degree of damage.

ASO titres are increased and rising (indicating recent streptococcal infection) with a marked fall in serum complement (suggesting nephritogenic immune complexes circulating and becoming deposited). Raised serum complement levels indicate a bad prognosis.

Progressive renal failure is accompanied by increases in plasma urea and creatinine.

TESTS OF PROGRESS

Depending on fluid and dietary intake and severity of oliguria, there may be imbalance of plasma electrolytes and body water. With recovery, a phase of diuresis suggests earlier water overload during an oliguric phase.

Renal Tubular Acidosis Type 1 (Distal, Gradient, Renal Tubular Acidosis)

Diagnosis of this commoner form of renal tubular acidosis, which may be inherited, or secondary to a variety of clinical conditions, and characterized by anorexia, fatigue, muscle weakness, or renal stone formation, is confirmed by the finding of persistent hyperchloraemic acidosis with normal anion gap, and without renal failure. Following an oral load of ammonium chloride (100 mg/kg body weight), normally the urine pH falls below pH 5·5 during the next 5–6 hours. In Type 1 renal tubular acidosis, the urine pH is inappropriately alkaline for the corresponding plasma pH and remains above pH 6·0.

Urine concentrating power is greatly reduced, the urine ammonium secretion rate is normal or reduced and the urine contains bicarbonate.

In incomplete forms, there is a latent inability maximally to acidify urine following an ammonium chloride load.

TESTS OF PROGRESS

The hyperchloraemic acidosis is relieved with greater clinical wellbeing, following daily supplements of 1–3 mmol sodium bicarbonate/kg body weight/day. When muscle weakness is accompanied by hypo-kalaemia, potassium supplements are helpful.

Diuretics and Renal Function

It has been found that both ethacrynic acid and frusemide cause an increased excretion of hyaline casts in the urine without associated proteinuria. Chlorothiazides do not produce casts in this way, but enhance those produced by acidifying agents.

The hyaline casts consist of uromucoid, which is always present in urine, but usually in solution, arising from the ascending limb of the loop of Henle.

Similar casts are passed in the urine after strenuous exercise. In renal disease the casts contain protein.

Renal Tubular Acidosis Type 2 (Proximal Renal Tubular Acidosis; Rate Renal Tubular Acidosis; Bicarbonate-losing Renal Disease)

Diagnosis of this less common form of renal tubular acidosis is confirmed by the finding of persistent hyperchloraemic acidosis with a normal anion gap, which is resistant to therapy with alkali. The urine pH is very low, and after oral ammonium chloride load test, the urine pH is 5·5–6·0 (cf. Type 1 RTA).

In some childhood forms there is bicarbonate wasting, but in adults there is bicarbonate wasting with also loss of excessive amounts of phosphate, glucose, uric acid and amino acids in the urine.

TESTS OF PROGRESS

There is a persistent tendency to rickets and osteomalacia; oral phosphate supplements with vitamin D may be helpful.

Renal Tubular Acidosis Type 4 [R]

In this rare form of tubular acidosis there is a persistent metabolic acidosis, and plasma potassium levels may increase above normal, with impaired clearance of potassium.

Plasma renin and aldosterone levels remain low, and urine ammonium excretion is abnormally low, even though the urine pH is persistently acid.

Hyperglobulinaemic Renal Tubular Acidosis [R]

Diagnosis of this rare condition, in which there is coexisting autoimmune disease, is confirmed by the finding of hypokalaemic, hypochloraemic acidosis, with a urinary pH greater than 6·0. There is inability to acidify the urine after an ammonium chloride load to a pH of less than 5·7. There is also a continued diuresis, which fails to respond to pitressin. The coexisting autoimmune disorder can be detected by increase in serum IgG, IgM, or IgA, with positive serum tests for RA factor, and antibodies present against cell nuclei, smooth muscle, mitochondria and thyroglobulin.

Salt-losing Nephritis [R]

Diagnosis of this very rare condition is confirmed by the finding of poluria with increased sodium output (losing up to 100–200 mmol of sodium/day). Urine potassium output is reduced and urine aldosterone output is increased.

Plasma sodium and bicarbonate concentrations fall and the plasma potassium tends to rise. The plasma chloride concentration is normal or low. The blood urea concentration is increased.

TESTS OF PROGRESS

Parenteral sodium chloride may be required to replace the loss.

TESTS PROVIDING USEFUL NEGATIVE RESULTS

No evidence of adrenal cortical insufficiency is found. There is no increased sodium retention following treatment with aldosterone, DOCA, or with fludro-cortisone.

Potassium-losing Nephritis [R]

Diagnosis of this rare condition is confirmed by the finding of persistent excessive excretion of potassium in the urine, with proteinuria, inability to produce acid urine following oral ammonium chloride, isosthenuria with fixed specific gravity of urine even after fluid restriction and the passage of a neutral or weakly alkaline urine.

The plasma potassium concentration falls below normal, and the blood urea, normal at first, rises later with increasing renal damage. As would be expected, the endogenous creatinine clearance falls as the glomerular filtration rate falls. The plasma chloride concentration falls as the plasma bicarbonate concentration rises. There may also be an increased excretion of sodium in the urine.

TESTS OF PROGRESS

Oral potassium supplements are needed.

TESTS PROVIDING USEFUL NEGATIVE RESULTS

After diamox the urine pH rises normally to a maximum of 8·0, since there is no defect in renal tubular carbonic anhydrase activity. There appears to be an inability to exchange hydrogen ions for potassium ions by the renal tubular cells.

Diabetic Nephropathy

Diagnosis of diabetic nephropathy is supported by the development of progressive renal failure in a diabetic patient. Renal biopsy reveals the presence of insulin and globulin anti-insulin antibodies precipitated in the glomeruli (immunofluorescence). Circulating anti-insulin antibodies have been demonstrated in the serum in patients who have never received insulin.

Goodpasture's Syndrome (Pulmonary Haemorrhage and Glomerulonephritis) [R]

Diagnosis of this rare condition occurring predominantly in males over 16 years of age, and presenting with alveolar lung haemorrhages and haemoptysis, with eventual renal failure, is supported by the finding of haemosiderin-laden macrophages in the sputum or in gastric washings (although this can occur after any pulmonary haemorrhage which persists). The diagnosis is confirmed by the demonstration of linear deposition of IgG and complement on the basement membranes of glomeruli in renal biopsy material, and on the basement membranes of pulmonary alveolar septa and capillaries in lung biopsy material. The presence of an anti-basement membrane antibody has also been demonstrated.

Phenacetin Nephropathy

Diagnosis is supported by the finding of severe impairment of the ability to produce concentrated urine, with a history of phenacetin intake of 2–25 kg over a 2–20-year period. This phenacetin load is sufficient to produce radiological evidence of renal damage, before there is an abnormal fall in the glomerular filtration rate. At the same time, the power to acidify urine is reduced, and there is a tendency to lose sodium in the urine. There may be increased numbers of white blood cells in the urine, without evidence of infection.

Radiation Nephritis

Diagnosis of radiation nephritis is supported by the acute onset of proteinuria with hypertension, and progressive renal failure with oedema and congestive cardiac failure, occurring 6–12 months after the start of radiotherapy treatment.

TESTS OF PROGRESS

It is essential to determine whether the renal damage is bilateral or unilateral. If only one kidney is damaged, then this requires urgent nephrectomy.

Shunt Nephritis

Diagnosis of this condition, in which cerebral intraventricular catheters (ventriculo-atrial) used in the relief of hydrocephalus become infected with *Staphylococcus epidermidis*, and antigen–antibody complexes are deposited in the kidneys, is supported by the finding of rising blood urea, plasma electrolyte disturbances, and the presence of casts and red cells in the urine, plus positive blood cultures growing *Staph. epidermidis*.

TESTS OF PROGRESS

Recovery follows elimination of infection by means of suitable antibiotics, unless there is residual renal damage.

Nephrotic Syndrome

Diagnosis of nephrotic syndrome, characterized by oedema (ranging from periorbital puffiness noticed in the morning to massive pitting oedema), with massive proteinuria ($>$ 3·5 g/1·75 m^2 body surface/day), is confirmed by demonstration of the protein loss. The degree of proteinuria varies from patient to patient, and from day to day, decreasing with bed rest, and increasing with exercise and fever. The presence of red cell casts or of macroscopic haematuria is strong evidence against a minimal change glomerular lesion, and suggests active glomerulonephritis.

Differential protein excretion can be measured by comparison of the clearance of plasma IgG or alpha-2 macroglobulin (high molecular weight proteins) with the clearance of transferrin or albumin (low molecular weight proteins), a low ratio of high MW: low MW suggesting a minimal change lesion in the kidneys. Renal biopsy is essential for accurate diagnosis, and assessment of degree of damage.

Serum cholesterol (free plus ester), triglycerides, beta-lipoproteins and phospholipids are often increased and the plasma has a milky appearance. Serum albumin, alpha-1 globulins and gammaglobulins are reduced. Many of the specific carrying-proteins are lost in the urine, and serum transferrin, caeruloplasmin, and thyroxine-binding proteins are low.

TESTS OF PROGRESS

Urine protein excretion and microscopy, with plasma monitoring of sodium, potassium, urea, etc. can be used to assess response to treatment.

Nephrogenic Diabetes Insipidus

1. ACQUIRED

Associated with:
    glomerulonephritis
    pyelonephritis
    bilateral hydronephrosis
    polyarteritis nodosa
    myelomatosis affecting the kidneys
    primary hyperaldosteronism
    hypercalcaemia
Diagnosis is of the primary condition.

2. INHERITED

Diagnosis of this rare sex-linked condition, characterized by failure to thrive, polydipsia and inability to secrete a concentrated urine, apparent after birth, with failure to respond to vasopressin therapy, is urgent in affected male infants. Female carriers can concentrate their urine specific gravity to 1·019 after 12 hours without fluid.

TESTS OF PROGRESS

Following treatment with diuretics such as chlorothiazide with a low sodium diet plus potassium supplements, the infant's clinical state improves, although acute episodes of uncontrolled diuresis require adequate fluid replacement and monitoring of plasma sodium and potassium concentrations.

TESTS PROVIDING USEFUL NEGATIVE RESULTS

If urine osmolality rises by > 150 mosmol/kg above the value obtained at the end of water deprivation test, when vasopressin is given, nephrogenic diabetes insipidus is excluded.

Acquired Nephrogenic Diabetes Insipidus

Diagnosis of acquired nephrogenic diabetes insipidus associated with acquired renal disease is supported by the finding of polyuria unresponsive to pitressin. The polyuria is associated with hypercalcaemia or hypokalaemia.

TESTS OF PROGRESS

Following correction of the plasma electrolyte imbalance, there is often some functional recovery.

Gordon's Syndrome [R]

Diagnosis of this rare syndrome, in which hypertension is associated with increased extracellular fluid volume, is supported by the finding of increased plasma potassium levels, with reduced plasma aldosterone and renin levels which do not rise following sodium deprivation. There is a high selectivity of proteinuria, with a low IgG/albumin clearance, in the presence of less renal damage than when selectivity is low with an IgG/albumin clearance greater than 0·3.

TESTS OF PROGRESS

Following reduced sodium intake with diuretic treatment, results return towards normal.

Liddle's Syndrome

Diagnosis of this rare syndrome of familial hypertension with increased extracellular fluid volume is supported by the finding of decreased plasma potassium and aldosterone levels.

TESTS OF PROGRESS

Results return towards normal following a low sodium-containing diet and treatment with the diuretic triamterene.

Unilateral Stenosis of the Renal Artery and Hypertension

Intravenous pyelograms and other radiographic tests may be used to detect stenosis of the renal artery. Renal venous plasma renin is increased on the affected side, especially after a period of salt depletion (low salt intake with chlorothiazide for a few days), the concentration of renin being more than +50 per cent of the arterial plasma value. On the unaffected side, the venous/arterial plasma renin difference is nil. Decreased renal plasma flow and glomerular filtration rate may be shown to be reduced in the affected kidney. If decreased function is demonstrated with normal function on the unaffected side, then good surgical results can be predicted. On the other hand, if there are no characteristic changes on the affected side with some depression of function on the apparently unaffected side, then postoperative results are not favourable.

Uraemia

In uraemia there is a marked increase in plasma urea (NPN) and creatinine. The reciprocal of the plasma creatinine concentration decreases in a linear fashion with progressive failure (i.e. plasma creatinine rises increasing rapidly) and is a useful marker. Metabolic acidosis develops with increased plasma phosphate (and sulphate), and falling plasma bicarbonate with secondary fall in P_{CO_2}. Polyuria is present, with inability to dilute or concentrate urine normally, and inability to excrete a water load rapidly. Plasma sodium levels remain within normal limits until late, as does plasma potassium concentration, although after a potassium load, plasma levels may reach dangerous levels. Serum calcium falls below normal.

Moderate anaemia is common, with 'bur' cells to be seen in the peripheral blood film. There is a bleeding tendency, often with thrombocytopenia, with reduced platelet factor 3 availability, and impairment of other platelet functions.

TESTS OF PROGRESS

Treatment by dialysis requires regular plasma electrolyte monitoring.

Renal Glycosuria

Diagnosis of this condition is confirmed by the finding of the appearance of glucose in the urine in abnormal amounts, with blood-glucose concentrations within normal limits. The condition does not appear to be prediabetic.

TESTS PROVIDING USEFUL NEGATIVE RESULTS

Glycosuria increases especially after carbohydrate meals, but there is no associated ketosis. It is important to confirm that there are no other renal defects, and that proteinuria and amino aciduria are present. Plasma sodium, potassium, chloride, bicarbonate and urea are normal.

Orthostatic Proteinuria

Diagnosis of this condition is confirmed by the finding of proteinuria after the subject has been standing for ½–1 hour or more, especially with hyperextension of the back exaggerating lumbar lordosis. The urine does not contain increased numbers of red cells or neutrophils, or casts.

TESTS PROVIDING USEFUL NEGATIVE RESULTS

The early morning urine samples passed as soon as the patient has risen are free of protein, cells and casts. The patients are most frequently young adult males. The condition does not appear to predispose the patient to abnormal hypertension later in life.

Hereditary Haematuria (Alport's Syndrome) [R]

Diagnosis of this rare condition, characterized by progressive nerve deafness and nephritis, is supported by the finding of thrombocytopenia with the presence of giant platelets.

FAMILIAL HYPERPROLINAEMIA

Hereditary nephropathy associated with hyperprolinaemia, hyperprolinuria, deafness, convulsions and mild mental retardation.

FAMILIAL BENIGN HAEMATURIA

Unlike Alport's syndrome, there is no nephritis in the family and a benign clinical course follows.

(Two children have been described, with hereditary haematuria, mental retardation, and abnormal encephalogram patterns.)

MALIGNANCY, SURGERY, AND INFECTIONS, ETC.

Ureterocolic Anastomosis

If the subsequent diet is not carefully regulated by the patient, and if urine is not voided fairly frequently, there is excessive reabsorption of ions from the urine by the colonic mucous membrane. When this occurs, plasma sodium, potassium, bicarbonate and calcium levels fall, and plasma chloride and urea increase.

Renal Tumour

1. WILMS'S TUMOUR

This rare tumour is found predominantly in children under 3 years of age.

2. HYPERNEPHROMA

Renal adenocarcinoma occurs predominantly in adults.
Renal tumours are associated with pain, loin swelling and haematuria, often with proteinuria. The diagnosis of a renal tumour depends on intravenous pyelography.

Renal Vein Thrombosis

Diagnosis is supported by the finding of sudden onset of oliguria, proteinuria and rising blood urea, with severe lower limb oedema, in the absence of either congestive cardiac failure or hypoproteinaemia.

Polycystic Disease

1. INFANTILE POLYCYSTIC DISEASE [AR] [R]

Infants affected by this condition die soon after birth, or are stillborn. A few less severely affected infants survive for a short time, with hepatospleno-megaly also.

2. ADULT POLYCYSTIC DISEASE [AD]

Diagnosis of this condition, characterized by abdominal swelling with loin pain, chronic renal failure, or hypertension, or symptomless proteinuria, is supported by proteinuria appearing by 35–45 years, progressing to renal failure in middle age. Bacterial infection is common, especially in affected women. The diagnosis can be confirmed by excretory urograms and radionuclide imaging, and these tests should also be undertaken in children from 15 years onwards in known families, to enable genetic counselling to be undertaken for affected patients.

Cystic Disease of Renal Medulla [R]

Diagnosis of this rare condition is supported by the finding of progressive renal failure in adolescence or early adult life, with polyuria and excessive sodium loss in the urine.

Sponge Kidney [R]

Diagnosis of this rare condition is supported by the finding of evidence of urine tract infection with haematuria. The findings on intravenous pyelography and retrograde pyelography are different, as the cysts do not fill from below.

Interstitial Cystitis

Diagnosis is made on the cystoscopic appearance. Haematuria may occur, and there may be coexisting autoimmune disease.

TESTS PROVIDING USEFUL NEGATIVE RESULTS

Cultures of urine are sterile and pyelogram studies are normal.

Bladder Carcinoma

Diagnosis is confirmed by identification of carcinoma cells in urine deposits, followed by examination of the growth by cystoscopy. The urine red cell and white cell counts increase with the growth of a bladder carcinoma.

TESTS OF PROGRESS

Bladder carcinoma may be secondary to serious bladder diseases such as schistosomiasis, and ova of the infecting parasite will be seen in the urine.

Workers who are involved in working with various bladder carcinogens, e.g. motor-tyre manufacturers, should undergo regular urine checks for the presence of carcinoma cells in the urine.

Prostatic Carcinoma

Diagnosis is supported by the finding of abnormally raised serum total acid phosphatase, formol-stable, alcohol-labile, or tartrate-labile phosphatase activities (with abnormally raised serum lactate dehydrogenase activity in some cases).

Increased fibrinolytic activity has been reported, but only very rarely has actually caused haemorrhage after surgery.

TESTS OF PROGRESS

In the presence of secondary carcinomatouf deposits in the skeleton, the serum alkaline phosphatase is raised. When successful oestrogen therapy is instituted, the raised serum acid phosphatase activity falls, but with progressive bone repair the serum alkaline phosphatase activity rises, falling later towards normal. With relapse the serum acid phosphatase activity rises once more and can be used as a tumour marker.

Similarly, if secondary carcinomatous deposits are present in the liver, serum alkaline phosphatase activity is increased, and successful oestrogen therapy results in the serum alkaline phosphatase activity falling towards normal.

After stilboestrol therapy and/or orchidectomy, serum lactate dehydrogenase activity falls in parallel with serum alkaline phosphatase activity.

TESTS PROVIDING USEFUL NEGATIVE RESULTS

Absence of increase in serum acid phosphatase activity does not exclude a diagnosis of prostatic carcinoma, since anaplastic tumours may not secrete the enzyme. Similarly in non-metastasizing tumours, less than one-third of cases have raised serum acid-phosphatase activities.

Renal Tract Obstruction

COMPLETE UNILATERAL RENAL TRACT OBSTRUCTION

Following complete obstruction of one ureter, with no interference with the other ureter, or bladder or urethra, there is no increase in the blood urea or blood NPN unless renal function was already reduced before the obstruction.

COMPLETE BILATERAL RENAL TRACT OBSTRUCTION

There is progressive rise in the blood urea with developing uraemia, and complete suppression of urinary flow.

PARTIAL UNILATERAL RENAL TRACT OBSTRUCTION

At first, there is no increase in blood urea or blood NPN, but later there may develop very severe progressive hypertension, with its associated effects ('Goldblatt kidney').

Kidney Transplant Rejection Syndrome

Diagnosis of impending rejection is suggested by progressive decrease in renal blood flow, urine volume and urea and creatinine clearances, with increased uptake of ^{125}I-labelled fibrinogen and hence increased counts over the kidney area.

In addition, the urine sodium concentration falls, and protein and cellular casts increase in the urine. Finally, if the estimation is available, the serum complement activity is decreased.

Falling urinary β-microglobulin excretion relative to albumin excretion is a favourable sign of acceptance of a grafted kidney.

Perfusion studies of cadaver kidneys have not enabled prediction of delayed function or non-function to be made.

Dialysis Dementia and Encephalitis

Following a prolonged period of repeated dialysis (e.g. more than 15 months), attacks of dementia and encephalitis have occurred. In these cases, severe phosphate depletion with high plasma aluminium concentrations have been found, derived from the dialysis apparatus, or from high aluminium content of domestic water supply.

The condition is cured by desferrioxamine therapy, but there is little change in bone aluminium content.

Urinary Tract Infections (including Cystitis, Pyelitis, and Pyelonephritis)

Diagnosis of infection in the urinary tract is confirmed by the isolation of the infecting bacteria on culture from the urine. With the availability of dip-inoculum techniques, an accurate bacterial count can be made, and bacterial counts of more than 100 000/ml (or, better, of more than 10 000 clones passed/min) confirm that the bacteria present are infecting organisms and not contaminants.

Proteinuria is also found, but in the early stages of urinary tract infection may not be present when bacteria are first isolated in significant numbers, e.g. screening of newborn infants and of women during pregnancy has revealed significant bacteriuria indicating early infection, in the absence of significantly increased proteinuria, and, untreated, many of these may progress to serious renal damage.

Erythrocytes are present in the urine in cases of infection, especially in acute infection of the bladder.

Neutrophils are present in increased numbers in both acute and chronic renal tract infections. In chronic pyelonephritis, the excretion of neutrophils in the urine is frequently intermittent.

Casts may be present in acute and chronic pyelonephritis, indicating that infection has extended into or close to the renal tubules. Pure pus-cell casts are regarded as diagnostic of chronic pyelonephritis by some.

In tuberculous infections, using ordinary methods of culture, there is apparently a sterile pyuria. Repeated examinations of overnight urine should be made, with microscopy of specifically stained deposits for acid-alcohol-fast bacilli, cultures on special media, and inoculation of treated urine deposits into laboratory animals.

Unilateral renal infection can be demonstrated by examination of urine samples collected separately from each ureter during cystoscopy.

When chronic pyelonephritis is suspected, some authorities use provocation tests, injecting pyrogens, or giving steroids, to demonstrate a subsequent increase in urine neutrophil excretion. The value of these is debatable, although, if such treatment releases pockets of bacteria which can be isolated on culture, the procedure is then useful.

During acute pyelitis, and in acute or chronic pyelonephritis, there is impairment in renal ability to concentrate urine after water restriction, and also there is impairment in the ability to eliminate a water load rapidly. Similarly the ability to acidify the urine after an ammonium chloride load is lost.

TESTS OF PROGRESS

Following successful treatment of acute pyelitis and acute pyelonephritis, there is recovery of the renal ability to dilute, concentrate and acidify urine, if renal function was normal before the attack.

Antibiotics in Renal Failure

The following antibiotics should never be used when there is renal failure:
  Tetracyclines
  Chloramphenicol
  Nitrofurantin
The following antibiotics are excreted by the kidney, and in the presence of renal failure, the dose should be reduced, and blood levels of the antibiotic monitored:

Streptomycin	Colistin
Gentamicin	Vancomycin
Kanamycin	PAS

The following antibiotics are excreted by the kidney, but are not highly toxic:

Penicillins	Lincomycin
Cephalosporins	Isoniazid
Cephaloridine	Trimethoprim
Cephalothin	

The following antibiotics are excreted by routes other than via the kidney, and are safe for use in the presence of renal failure:

Sodium fusidate	Sulphamethazole
Sulphadimidine	Nalidixic acid

Epididymo-orchitis

Identification of an infecting organism can be made by microscopy and culture of pus removed either directly during surgery or via the urethra.

Since this condition is frequently secondary to urinary infection, microscopy and culture of the urine are useful. Repeated examinations, with collections of overnight or 24-hour urine samples, should be made if underlying tuberculous infection is suspected, with injection of suitably prepared material into laboratory animals if necessary. If the condition is a complication of gonococcal infection, in addition to isolation of the organism on culture and provisional identification of the organism in pus, the gonococcal complement-fixation test is positive.

When the condition is a complication of mumps, then it is not suppurative. Serological tests may assist diagnosis, if these are needed.

Urethral Syndrome

Diagnosis of an infective variety of this syndrome in adult women is confirmed by the isolation of slow-growing carbon dioxide-dependent gram-positive organisms from urethral swabs, including *Lactobacillus* sp. (commonest), *Corynebacterium* sp. and *Streptococcus milleri*.

Renal Calculus

Renal calculi containing calcium may develop in patients with primary diseases associated either with normal serum calcium levels or with hypercalcaemia.

Renal calcium-containing stones associated with hypercalcaemia:
    Primary hyperparathyroidism
    Sarcoidosis
    Milk-alkali syndrome
    Vitamin-D excess
    Idiopathic hypercalcaemia of infants
    Chronic pulmonary berylliosis (very rare)
Renal calcium-containing stones without associated hypercalcaemia:
    Bone fractures with subsequent immobilization
    Idiopathic hypercalciuria
    Idiopathic hypercalciuria plus hypophosphataemia
    Primary renal tubular acidosis
    'Over-absorbers of calcium'
    'Renal leakers of calcium'
    Renal tract infection
    Primary hyperoxaluria

It is important to appreciate that the formation of renal calculi in these conditions are indicators of an underlying disease process. The results of tests will reflect the response to the underlying disease.

Nephrolithiasis

URIC ACID CALCULI

a. Gouty subjects: 'overproducers' of uric acid.
b. Hypoxanthine-guanine pyrophosphoribosyl transferase deficiency (Lesch–Nyhan).
c. Phosphoribosyl pyrophosphate synthetase overactivity.
d. Type 1 glycogen storage disease (glucose 6-phosphatase deficiency)
    (b), (c) and (d) are rare causes of renal stone.
e. Secondary hyperuricaemia with hyperuricosuria.
f. (Idiopathic uric acid stone formation associated with lithium therapy?)

MAGNESIUM AMMONIUM PHOSPHATE CALCULI

Occurring in young boys, middle-aged females and the elderly, in association with anatomical and/or functional abnormality and/or infection of the urinary tract, and/or antecedent metabolic stone.

CALCIUM PHOSPHATE CALCULI

Renal tubular acidosis Type I.

CALCIUM OXALATE AND MIXED CALCIUM STONES

a. Recurrent stone-formers (often with family history)
b. Hypercalciuria
   i. Idiopathic   — absorptive type
                        — renal type
   ii. Secondary, including
                        — sarcoidosis
                        — primary hyperparathyroidism
c. Hyperoxaluria
   i. Primary hyperoxaluria [R] — Type I
                        — Type II
   ii. Secondary

MEDULLARY SPONGE KIDNEY

Congenital anomaly with cyst formation and dilatation of collecting ducts in the renal pyramids. Cases develop pure calcium phosphate stones, or mixed stones (with a minority with infection of the urinary tract developing magnesium ammonium phosphate stones).

Cystinuria [R]

Homozygotes develop cystine stones in middle age.

Perinephric Abscess

Identification of the infecting organism can be made by microscopy and culture of pus at operation. Systemic non-specific changes associated with infection are found, including neutrophilia, raised ESR and plasma viscosity.

13 *Blood Disorders*

HAEMOLYTIC ANAEMIA

Haemolytic Anaemia due to Intrinsic Red Cell Faults

Apart from:
- A. Congenital spherocytic haemolytic anaemia,
- B. Paroxysmal nocturnal haemoglobinuria,
- C. Glucose-6-phosphate dehydrogenase deficiency,
- D. Puruvate kinase deficiency,

which are described individually, after this list of haemolytic anaemias associated with intrinsic biochemical faults, the remainder are very rare, the number of cases of each condition ranging from one to a very few.

1. *Red cell membrane defects with abnormal red cell shape:*
   - *a.* Congenital spherocytic haemolytic anaemia (*see later*).
   - *b.* Elliptocytosis.
   - *c.* Stomatocytosis.
   - *d.* Severe microcytosis.
   - *e.* 'Spur cell' anaemia.
   - *f.* Haemolytic anaemia with dessicytes.

2. *Normal red cell shape:*
   - A. *Associated with glycolytic enzyme deficiency:*
     - *a.* Glucose-6-phosphate dehydrogenase deficiency (*see later*).
     - *b.* Pyruvate kinase deficiency.
     - *c.* Hexokinase deficiency.
     - *d.* Phosphohexoseisomerase deficiency.
     - *e.* Phosphofructokinase deficiency (*see also* Glycogen Storage Disease Type VIII).
     - *f.* Aldolase deficiency.
     - *g.* Triosephosphate isomerase deficiency.
     - *h.* Glyceraldehyde-3-phosphate dehydrogenase deficiency.
     - *i.* 2,3-Diphosphoglycerate mutase deficiency.
     - *j.* Phosphoglycerate kinase deficiency.
     - *k.* Enolase deficiency.
   - B. *Associated with red cell membrane defects:*
     - *a.* Paroxysmal nocturnal haemoglobinuria (*see later*).
     - *b.* Phosphatidyl choline excess.
     - *c.* Vitamin E deficiency.
     - *d.* Sialic acid deficiency.

C. *Associated with deficiency in maintenance of membrane ATP:*
   a. Adenylate kinase deficiency.
   b. Adenosine triphosphatase deficiency.
   c. ATP deficiency with normal adenylate kinase and adenosine triphosphatase.
   d. Ribose phosphate pyrophosphokinase deficiency.

D. *Associated with abnormalities of glutathione metabolism:*
   a. Gamma-glutamyl cysteine synthetase deficiency.
   b. Glutathione synthetase deficiency.
   c. Glutathione reductase deficiency.
   d. Glutathione peroxidase deficiency.
   e. Glutathione deficiency.

E. *Pyrimidine-5′-nucleotidase deficiency.*

Autoimmune Haemolytic Anaemia

Diagnosis is confirmed by the finding of normochromic anaemia with increased reticulocyte counts, variable moderate increase in serum bilirubin which is predominantly unconjugated, increased peripheral blood neutrophils often with thrombocytopenia. Plasma haemoglobin levels are increased with disappearance of plasma haptoglobins. Erythrophagocytosis may be observed.

Two main clinical groups of this condition are found.

'WARM' ANTIBODY *(active at or near 37 °C)*

Eighty per cent of the idiopathic autoimmune haemolytic anaemia cases are due to the development of 'warm' auto-antibodies, which are incomplete, with positive anti-gamma G Coombs' test, and which are not complement-dependent. Antibodies may develop against the Rhesus blood-group system (e.g. against the patient's own 'D').

TESTS OF PROGRESS

This condition improves when large doses of steroids are given in the early stages, and also may respond favourably to splenectomy, heparin therapy and cytotoxic drugs.

'COLD' ANTIBODY *(active at or near room temperature)*

Twenty per cent of the idiopathic autoimmune haemolytic anaemia cases are due to the development of 'cold' auto-antibodies, which are complete, cause visible auto-agglutination in blood samples, especially at low temperatures (cold agglutinins), and are anti-gamma M positive, anti-gamma G Coombs' tests being negative. The 'cold' antibody is complement-dependent.

TESTS OF PROGRESS

Treatment is difficult, but cytotoxic agents are effective in some cases, and depolymerizing agents may also be useful.

A. Hereditary Spherocytosis (Acholuric Jaundice) [AD]

Diagnosis of this commonest hereditary red-cell defect of Northern Caucasians, characterized by a persistent variable haemolytic state, with splenomegaly and often jaundice, and attacks of haemolysis precipitated by infection, is confirmed by the finding of spherocytes in the peripheral blood films with slightly reduced or normal MCV, and increased red-cell saline osmotic fragility (Mean Cell Fragility exceeds 0·45 per cent). In cases with spherocytosis but with only slightly increased saline osmotic fragility, incubation of the blood samples at 37 °C for 24 hours exaggerates the abnormal saline fragility (when compared with normal incubated control blood samples). The autohaemolysis test (rarely performed nowadays) is abnormal, and partially correctable by added glucose.

Red-cell survival studies reveal sequestration of red cells almost exclusively in the spleen, with a greatly reduced red-cell survival. The abnormality of the red cell has been shown to be due to a deficiency of normal spectrin in the red-cell membrane. The peripheral blood shows increased reticulocyte count, with a moderate increase in serum bilirubin. Bone marrow aspirates show active erythropoiesis with increased stores of stainable iron. During haemolytic attacks nucleated red cells appear in the peripheral blood, with marked increase in urinary and faecal urobilinogen excretion. Marrow aplasia may occur during such attacks, with severe fall in haemoglobin, thrombocytopenia and neutropenia.

TESTS OF PROGRESS

Splenectomy reduces the excessive destruction of the abnormal red cells, and should be undertaken after 5 years of age. There is a serious risk of infection following splenectomy before this age, and inoculation with polyvalent pneumococcal vaccine should probably be given following any splenectomy, since infection with *Strept. pneumoniae* is a risk. Splenectomy is also associated with a risk of thrombosis for the first few weeks afterwards. Following splenectomy, although the red-cell abnormality is unchanged, the red-cell survival is increased.

If splenectomy is not undertaken, or if the condition is mild and not detected until middle age, there is a serious risk of complications due to the inevitable formation of pigment biliary stonds.

TESTS PROVIDING USEFUL NEGATIVE RESULTS

The Coombs' test is negative, methaemalbumin is not detected, and haemoglobinuria does not occur.

B. Paroxysmal Nocturnal Haemoglobinuria [R]

Diagnosis of this rare acquired chronic variable haemolytic anaemia, characterized by episodes of haemoglobinuria (especially after sleep), attacks of thrombosis and abdominal pain, and weakness with fatigue, is confirmed by the demonstration of abnormal sensitivity of a clone of red cells to lysis by complement. The abnormal cells are 50–100 × as sensitive to lysis by complement as normal red cells, and the Ham acid lysis test, cane-sugar water test (for screening) and sucrose-haemolysis test are all positive.

The affected red cells have high titres of both i and I antigen, with greatly increased sensitivity to lysis by anti-I. The peripheral blood reveals a hypochromic anaemia, with variably increased reticulocytes (frequently much lower than expected for the low whole blood haemoglobin level). Thrombocytopenia and neutropenia occur, in relation to periods of marrow hypoplasia, and the neutrophils often contain less alkaline phosphatase activity than normal.

Bone marrow iron stores are depleted or even nil. Urine cell deposits contain haemosiderin, and free haemoglobin in solution is found after attacks of haemolysis.

TESTS OF PROGRESS

Patients require repeated blood transfusions with washed red cells (to avoid infusion of complement). Some cases terminate as acute leukaemia.

C. Glucose-6-phosphate Dehydrogenase (G-6-PD) Deficiency [XR]

Perhaps 100 000 000 people have this red-cell deficiency throughout the world as a sex-linked inherited condition. Various clinical presentations have been defined:

1. DRUG-INDUCED ATTACKS OF HAEMOLYSIS

Attacks are associated with oxidant-type drugs. Acute attacks of abdominal or back pain with haemoglobinuria follow 2–3 days after administration of the drug (subject being normal before the drug). This type of attack occurs especially in Negroes of West African origin.

2. HAEMOLYTIC ATTACKS OCCURRING DURING INFECTION

These can occur in any type of the deficiency.

3. FAVISM

Acute intravenous haemolysis occurs following the eating of broad beans (*Vicia fava*), developing 6–24 hours after the meal, with gross reticulocytosis. This type of attack occurs in Mediterranean people and in Cantonese Chinese, who are also sensitive to oxidant drugs and react to infections.

4. HEREDITARY NON-SPHEROCYTIC HAEMOLYTIC ANAEMIA DUE TO G-6-PD DEFICIENCY

This variety occurs in Northern Europe, is severe and develops in infancy or childhood, haemolysis being continuous, but worse during infections, and exacerbated by infections. There is a later risk of gallstones.

G-6-PD ACTIVITY LEVELS

Northern Europe variety—4–10%
Mediterranean variety—0–7%
Negroes—8–20% (subject normal until oxidant drug given)

Cantonese Chinese—2–24%

Sephardic Jews—25–40%

Varieties of the enzyme can be demonstrated by their different electrophoretic mobilities.

Diagnosis of G-6-PD deficiency is confirmed by demonstration of reduced activity of the enzyme in the patient's red cells. During attacks of haemolysis, the peripheral blood shows increased reticulocytes, and haemoglobinuria in severe attacks.

TESTS OF PROGRESS

Avoidance of drugs known to cause attacks, avoidance of broad beans if these cause attacks, and the rapid treatment of any infection reduce the number and severity of attacks.

Blood transfusion may be life-saving during acute severe attacks, especially in infants.

There is a tendency to salmonellosis, especially in West Africans.

D. Pyruvate Kinase Deficiency [AR]

Diagnosis of this uncommon non-spherocytic congenital haemolytic anaemia, characterized by wide variations in severity of chronic haemolytic anaemia with acute exacerbations, associated especially with infection or pregnancy, is confirmed by demonstration of abnormally reduced red-cell pyruvate kinase activity, the level of activity varying from affected family to family. The autohaemolysis test is positive, and is poorly corrected by added glucose or adenosine.

The red-cell 2,3-diphosphoglycerate concentration is high, with decreased haemoglobin affinity for oxygen, and therefore tissues easily obtain oxygen from the blood, even though the haemoglobin concentration may be maintained at levels as low as 8 g/dl, without any need for transfusion.

TESTS OF PROGRESS

The patient's state may be improved by splenectomy. Folate supplements are necessary, because of the rapid red-cell turnover. Gallstones develop after many years.

TESTS PROVIDING USEFUL NEGATIVE RESULTS

The Coombs' antihuman globulin test is negative.

Postsplenectomy Effects

Following splenectomy, the platelet count rises excessively during the following three weeks, counts often exceeding 1 000 000/cmm with a risk of thrombosis. Similarly, there is a neutrophilia and lymphocytosis during the first week after operation.

Later it can be noted that the red cells are thinner, and target cells are present in increased numbers in the peripheral blood. Many red cells contain Howell–Jolly bodies and Heinz bodies, and Heinz bodies are more easily produced artificially (e.g. Heinz body provocation test). A few siderocytes may be found in the peripheral blood.

TESTS OF PROGRESS

It appears that the spleen plays a part in resistance to infection in infants and young children, as after splenectomy they are more susceptible to infection. Polyvalent pneumococcal vaccine should be given.

Congenital Absence of Spleen

Diagnosis of this very rare condition is suggested by the finding of moderate numbers of nucleated red cells and red cells containing Howell–Jolly bodies in the peripheral blood. Heinz bodies may be present in up to 10 per cent of the red cells.

TESTS PROVIDING USEFUL NEGATIVE RESULTS

There is no anaemia and there are no excessive numbers of abnormal or primitive white blood cells in the peripheral blood. The platelet count is normal.

Splenic Atrophy

Findings similar to those of postsplenectomy.

Hypersplenism

Diagnosis of hypersplenism is supported by the finding of one or more of the following: anaemia, neutropenia, thrombocytopenia, in association with splenomegaly, and a normal cellular bone marrow aspirate.

The diagnosis of hyperplenism is confirmed if the blood count returns to normal after splenectomy.

Haemolytic-uraemic Syndrome in Infants

Diagnosis of this rare condition is confirmed by the finding of acute haemolytic anaemia with thrombocytopenia and increasing uraemia. Blood films reveal bur and fragmented red cells. Fibrin-fibrinogen degradation products are present in the plasma.

The condition is thought to be associated with virus infection.

TESTS OF PROGRESS

Treatment with heparin and steroids is effective in many cases, with supportive treatment of renal failure and hypertension during the acute illness.

Auto-erythrocyte Sensitization (Painful Bruising Syndrome) [R]

Diagnosis of this rare condition, characterized by tissue sensitivity to extravasated red blood cells in women, with formation of painful ecchymoses, is confirmed by positive intradermal skin test results to injection of the patient's own red blood cells or red cell stroma.

Paroxysmal Cold Haemoglobinuria [R]

Diagnosis of this rare condition, occurring mainly in children, and in many cases related to recent virus infections, characterized by attacks of haemoglobinuria in very cold weather, is confirmed by the finding of complement-binding IgG antibody (Donath–Landsteiner), which causes haemolysis after the patient's red cells and serum have been chilled to 4 °C, and then warmed to 37 °C. The direct Coombs' antihuman globulin test may also be positive.

TESTS OF PROGRESS

No special treatment, other than the avoidance of cold, is necessary.

Chronic Cold Haemagglutin Disease (CHAD) [R]

Diagnosis of this disorder affecting elderly people, characterized by anaemia which is worse in cold weather, with attacks of jaundice and Raynaud's phenomenon, is diagnosed by the appearance of gross agglutination of red cells in blood at room temperature, the blood appearing normal when warmed to 37 °C and mixed.

The direct Coombs' human antiglobulin test is positive (the antibody binding with complement to the red cell antigen). Titres of 'complete' cold agglutinins are high, and are almost always monoclonal IgM. Most antibodies are anti-I, with a few anti-i.

TESTS OF PROGRESS

Intermittent courses of treatment with chlorambucil, combined with avoidance of exposure to extreme cold, is usually effective.

SECONDARY CHAD

About 16 per cent of patients with CHAD are suffering from a malignant lymphoma, with an auto-antibody of the same specificity. The older textbooks mention syphilis as a cause of this condition, but this must be a very rare cause now.

March (Exertional) Haemoglobinuria

Diagnosis of this condition is confirmed by the finding of haemoglobinuria following prolonged running or marching on hard surfaces. Plasma-haemoglobin levels may be increased after such exercise, and the plasma haptoglobins are reduced or absent. (Casts may be found in the urine after severe exercise in normal subjects.)

TESTS OF PROGRESS

Change to running on grass, or with padded soles to the shoes, may prevent the condition.

Tests for the presence of myoglobinuria are negative.

Artificial Heart-valve Anaemia

Before the design and the nature of the materials used were improved, following replacement of a damaged aortic heart valve by an artificial prosthesis, or, less frequently, following replacement of damaged mitral and tricuspid heart valves, a microangiopathic haemolytic anaemia resulted, with fragmented red cells visible in stained blood films. Urine haemosiderin excretion was detectable. The newer prostheses do not cause this trouble. Unfortunately, pig heart valve replacement may be followed eventually by calcification of the animal valve.

BLOOD DISEASES

Iron-deficiency Anaemia

Diagnosis of iron-deficiency anaemia is confirmed by the finding of reduced haemoglobin concentration, MCV at the lower limit of normal or less, MCH reduced to below 27 pg, and MCD reduced also. Stained blood films show obvious hypochromia, with anisocytosis and increasing poikilocytosis in severe anaemia. Oval erythrocytes and target cells are seen frequently. Reticulocyte counts are normal or low, although they may increase after haemorrhage. Similarly, the white-cell count and platelet count are normal, but rise following haemorrhage.

Serum iron tends to be reduced, with increased serum total iron-binding capacity and reduced percentage saturation. Bone-marrow aspirates show erythroid hyperplasia with smaller nucleated red cells than normal. Stainable iron is markedly reduced or absent and iron stores are reflected by serum ferritin levels.

TESTS OF PROGRESS

Following satisfactory treatment with iron (oral or parenteral) plus elimination of loss of iron from the body (e.g. via haemorrhages), there is a reticulocyte increase about the fifth to seventh day, and a subsequent rise in haemoglobin concentration to normal.

Following treatment, stainable iron is detectable in the bone-marrow aspirate.

TESTS PROVIDING USEFUL NEGATIVE RESULTS

It is important to exclude other causes of hypochromic anaemia, which do not respond to iron therapy alone:

Refractory anaemia associated with renal disease, malignancy, renal disease or chronic infection and/or inflammation.

Thalassaemia

Sideroblastic anaemias

Hereditary Sideroblastic Anaemia [R]

Diagnosis of this rare sex-linked recessive anaemia is confirmed in affected male patients by the finding of moderate anaemia with both normochromic and hypochromic red cells in stained blood films (dimorphic picture). The MCHC is low (22–28 g/100 ml), with normal or reduced MCV. The serum iron is raised and the normal total iron-binding capacity is almost completely saturated.

In bone-marrow aspirates the nucleated red cells tend to be smaller than normal (micronormoblasts) and on staining for the presence of iron, many normoblasts are found to be 'ring sideroblasts' with iron deposited in the perinuclear mitochondria.

TESTS OF PROGRESS

A few cases respond to prolonged treatment with pyridoxine. Chelation therapy may be useful.

Primary Acquired Sideroblastic Anaemia

Diagnosis of this condition causing insidious increasing anaemia in predominantly middle-aged or older patients is confirmed by the finding of haemoglobin concentrations of about 6–7 g/100 ml with apparently both hypochromic and normochromic red cells in stained films (dimorphic picture). A few macrocytic cells are seen, with some poikilocytosis, schistocytes and target cells. The mean red-cell volume may be increased, and the reticulocyte count is normal or moderately increased (up to 5 per cent). The MCHC is normal or slightly decreased (30–34 g/100 ml), and serum-iron values may be normal or raised, with normal iron-binding capacity.

The white-cell count and platelet count may both be low.

Bone-marrow aspirates show erythroid hyperplasia, with increased stainable iron in nucleated red cells. This stainable iron is present in increased numbers of granules in the cells, and many cells have siderotic granules ringing around the nuclei ('ring sideroblasts'—evidence of damaged mitochondria). Megaloblastic change may be seen in some cases, and vacuoles in the cytoplasm are seen in some late normoblasts. There is evidence of ineffective haemopoiesis.

TESTS OF PROGRESS

Following prolonged treatment with pyridoxine (over 6 weeks) about one-third of cases can be maintained with nearly normal haemoglobin levels in continuing pyridoxine supplements.

Secondary Sideroblastic Anaemia

Diagnosis of this complication of drug therapy, or of primary haemopoietic disorders, is confirmed by the finding of anaemia with a dimorphic blood-film appearance (hypochromic cells and normochromic cells) with increased stainable iron in marrow nucleated red-cell precursors.

The primary cause of this complication should be discovered including:
Antituberculous treatment with isoniazid, cycloserine, pyrazinamide
Lead poisoning
Alcoholism
di Guglielmo's disease
Thalassaemia
Chloramphenicol

Congenital Atransferrinaemia [R]

Diagnosis of this extremely rare condition is confirmed by the demonstration of extremely low TIBC (20 µg/100 ml) and very low serum-iron concentrations (20 µg/100 ml), with severe hypochromic anaemia. Target cells are seen in the peripheral blood and the bone-marrow aspirate contains increased numbers of nucleated red cells with complete absence of stainable iron.

Megaloblastic Anaemia (Vitamin B_{12} Deficiency)

1. ADULT ADDISONIAN PERNICIOUS ANAEMIA

Diagnosis of this condition, with highest incidence about 60 years of age, and most frequent in Northern Europeans, caused by severe malabsorption of vitamin B_{12}, due to lack of gastric intrinsic factor as a result of atrophic gastritis, characterized by insidious development of severe anaemia with sore tongue, mild jaundice, and neurological damage in some cases, is confirmed by demonstration of a macrocytic anaemia, with low serum vitamin B_{12} levels, and inability to absorb oral vitamin B_{12} without added intrinsic factor.

The MCV rises to between 100–140 fl. Nucleated red cells appear in the peripheral blood, and megaloblasts may be seen in 'buffy layer' preparations. The leucocyte count falls (both neutrophils and lymphocytes), and hypersegmented neutrophils are seen. The platelet count also falls, and on occasion severe thrombocytopia is found.

The bone marrow is hypercellular with increased erythroid series, and with many mitotic figures present. Giant metamyelocytes may also be seen.

Serum lactate dehydrogenase levels are markedly increased before treatment (indicating dyserythropoiesis), and serum albumin and globulin levels fall. Parietal cell antibodies (IgG) are present in 90 per cent of cases, blocking intrinsic factor (IF) antibodies occur in 55 per cent with binding IF antibodies in 37 per cent of cases. Schilling (or Dicopac) radio-isotope absorption tests can be used to demonstrate the fault in vitamin B_{12} absorption, whether the patient is already being treated or not.

TESTS OF PROGRESS

Regular blood tests are useful in the assessment of the adequacy and frequency of vitamin B_{12} injections necessary for the rest of the patient's life.

TESTS PROVIDING USEFUL NEGATIVE RESULTS

Red cell folate activity is normal.

2. CONGENITAL INTRINSIC FACTOR DEFICIENCY [R]

Diagnosis of this rare condition, characterized by irritability, gastrointestinal disturbance, vomiting, emaciation, loss of reflexes and vibration sense, and severe megaloblastic anaemia, is confirmed by the demonstration of severe megaloblastic anaemia with raised MCV, low serum vitamin B_{12}, and very poor absorption of vitamin B_{12} orally, the absorption being corrected by added intrinsic factor (e.g. Dicopac test).

TESTS OF PROGRESS

Following 250 µg hydrocobalamin 4-weekly for life, recovery is complete. If the diagnosis is made early enough and treatment started at once, mental retardation can be avoided.

USEFUL NEGATIVE RESULTS

Gastric biopsy is normal in appearance, and both hydrochloric acid and pepsin secretions are normal. Parietal cell antibodies are absent. No intrinsic factor is detectable. (*Variant*: 1 boy has been described, in whom intrinsic factor was present, but inactive and abnormal in structure.)

3. CHILDHOOD 'AUTOIMMUNE' PERNICIOUS ANAEMIA [R]

There is a high incidence of IF antibody (90 per cent) titres with only 10 per cent of cases having parietal cell antibodies. The condition is often associated with myxoedema (or adrenal atrophy) in siblings.

4. CONGENITAL (SELECTIVE) VITAMIN B_{12} MALABSORPTION (IMERSLUND–GRÄSBECK SYNDROME) [R] [AR]

Diagnosis of this condition, characterized by pallor, weakness, irritability, loss of appetite, glossitis, constipation, mild jaundice, diminished vibration sense, extensor plantar responses, mental retardation and symptoms of anaemia, is confirmed by the demonstration of severe megaloblastic anaemia, with low serum vitamin B_{12}, poor absorption of vitamin B_{12} with, or without, added IF orally.

TESTS OF PROGRESS

Since the ileal B_{12}-receptor sites are absent or defective in this condition, patients must be treated with 250 µg hydrocobalamin by injection every 2–4 weeks for life. The earlier the diagnosis can be made, the less severe will be any mental retardation.

TESTS WHICH PROVIDE USEFUL NEGATIVE RESULTS

Gastric pepsin and free hydrochloric acid secretion is normal.

Inherited Transcobalamin I Deficiency [R]

Diagnosis of this rare condition is confirmed by the finding of abnormally low serum vitamin B_{12} levels, but few or no signs of deficiency.

Deficiency of the specific deficiency of transcobalamin I can be demonstrated by specialized techniques. It appears that this protein acts as a temporary circulating store of vitamin B_{12}.

Inherited Transcobalamin II Deficiency [R]

Diagnosis of this rare condition is confirmed by the finding of severe megaloblastic anaemia in affected infants, with thrombocytopenia, leucopenia, but with serum vitamin B_{12} levels not grossly reduced.

Deficiency of the specific deficiency of transcobalamin II can be demonstrated by specialized techniques.

TESTS OF PROGRESS

Remission of the severe megaloblastic anaemia only occurs if large weekly doses of vitamin B_{12} are given for maintenance therapy. It appears that transcobalamin II is essential for the transport of vitamin B_{12} in the body.

Nutritional Megaloblastic Anaemia

Diagnosis of megaloblastic anaemia due to inadequate intake of either vitamin B_{12} or folic acid, or both, is confirmed by the demonstration of either low serum vitamin B_{12} levels or low serum and red-cell folate activity, with the exclusion of other causes of megaloblastic anaemia.

Nutritional megaloblastic anaemia of infancy is due to inadequate intake of folic acid in the diet. It is possible for vitamin-B_{12} deficiency to develop in an infant, if its mother is breast-feeding it and she is also suffering from vitamin-B_{12} deficiency.

Megaloblastic Anaemia of Pregnancy

Diagnosis of megaloblastic anaemia of pregnancy, which tends to be detected clinically during the last trimester of pregnancy in multigravidae and in multiple pregnancies, is confirmed by the finding of moderate to severe anaemia with less obvious macrocytosis than in Addisonian megaloblastic anaemia. Red cells show anisocytosis and poikilocytosis, often with some hypochromic cells (dimorphic picture). The white-cell count varies, but the neutrophils are multilobed with many hypersegmented forms. The platelet count may be normal or moderately reduced. Serum and red-cell folate activity is reduced below normal.

Megaloblasts can often be found in carefully prepared 'buffy layers' from peripheral blood, avoiding the need for marrow puncture.

Bone-marrow aspirate reveals some normoblastic activity and also megaloblastic cells. Giant metamyelocytes and multilobed megakaryocytes are also seen.

TESTS OF PROGRESS

With the routine supplements of iron and folic acid given to antenatal patients nowadays, this form of anaemia is unusual. If it is suspected that the patient is suffering from Addisonian megaloblastic anaemia, then the patient should be treated with both vitamin B_{12} and folic acid, after blood specimens have been collected for serum vitamin-B_{12} and red-cell folate estimations. Fuller investigation of the patient is then possible after the puerperium (e.g. Schilling or Dicopac Test).

TESTS PROVIDING USEFUL NEGATIVE RESULTS

Serum vitamin-B_{12} concentrations are normal.

Megaloblastic Anaemia and Anticonvulsant Drugs

During long-term therapy with anticonvulsant drugs moderate folate deficiency may be demonstrated by estimation of red-cell folate activity. Anticonvulsant drugs, including phenytoin sodium, primidone, phenobarbitone, etc. interfere with the efficient absorption of folate from the diet. If large doses of folic acid are given to repair such deficiency, then absorption of anticonvulsants is interfered with by the excess of folic acid.

It is possible to maintain the body folate levels satisfactorily without interfering with anticonvulsant control by giving yeast tablets (2 tablets t.d.s.).

Anticonvulsant therapy, even in the absence of anaemia, is associated with a moderate normochromic macrocytosis.

Rare Causes of Megaloblastic Anaemia due to Faults in Folate Metabolism

1. FORMIMINOTRANSFERASE DEFICIENCY [R]

Diagnosis of this rare condition is made by the finding of mental retardation associated with excessively high serum folate activity with hypersegmented neutrophils in the peripheral blood, excessive excretion of formiminoglutamic acid (FIGLU) in the urine after oral histidine, and ultimately demonstration of marked deficiency in activity of the enzyme formiminotransferase in both erythrocytes and liver-biopsy material.

Serum-folate levels are found to be above normal in maternal relatives.

2. CYCLOHYDROLASE DEFICIENCY [R]

Diagnosis of this rare condition is made by the finding in association with mental retardation, of grossly increased serum folate activity and no increase in urinary excretion of formiminoglutamic acid (FIGLU) following a histidine load. There is a gross reduction in activity of the enzyme methenyltetrahydrofolate cyclohydrolase in both red cells and liver-biopsy material.

3. N^5-METHYLTETRAHYDROFOLATE TRANSFERASE DEFICIENCY [R]

Diagnosis of this very rare condition is confirmed by the finding of megaloblastic anaemia in an infant with excessively raised serum folate activity. The specific enzyme deficiency is demonstrated in liver-biopsy material.

4. CONGENITAL MALABSORPTION OF FOLATE [R]

Diagnosis of megaloblastic anaemia with mental retardation and cerebral calcification due to an isolated defect in folate absorption from the gut and in transfer of folate from the blood to the CSF is confirmed by the finding of a severe megaloblastic anaemia with low plasma-folate and very low CSF-folate levels, which fail to respond to treatment with folic acid derivatives.

TESTS OF PROGRESS

Given very large doses of folic acid daily, megaloblastic anaemia is converted to normoblastic formation with normal haemoglobin levels, but the CSF-folate activity does not increase.

TESTS PROVIDING USEFUL NEGATIVE RESULTS

Serum vitamin-B_{12} levels are normal. No evidence of malabsorption.

ABNORMAL HAEMOGLOBIN METABOLISM

Thalassaemia

1. β-THALASSAEMIA

A. *β-Thalassaemia major*

Diagnosis of the homozygous state, characterized by anaemia developing about the 3rd month of life, with increasing hepatosplenomegaly and retardation of growth, with characteristic changes in the bones, is confirmed by the demonstration of severe hypochromic, microcytic anaemia with numerous target cells and nucleated red cells in the peripheral blood, only moderately increased reticulocyte count, with erythroid hyperplasia in the bone marrow. The red cells contain many irregular inclusion bodies (seen using methyl violet stain), and the red-cell half-life is reduced to about 25 days, with increased serum iron.

Haemoglobin F is increased (20–90 per cent of the total) and electrophoresis of haemolysate on starch gel reveals excess of free haemoglobin alpha chains.

TESTS OF PROGRESS

There are two main varieties of β-thalassaemia, thalassaemia major in which many children die before puberty, and thalassaemia intermedia which is less severe. Thalassaemia minor is found in both parents.

Repeated blood transfusions at intervals of 6–8 weeks are given to maintain the haemoglobin at 10–12 g/dl. The patient should be ascorbic acid-replete, and folic acid supplements should be given. Iron therapy must be avoided. Splenectomy after 5 years of age can be considered if splenomegaly with leucopenia and thrombocytopenia develop. Regular slow subcutaneous desferrioxamine may be given to reduce the degree of siderosis, inevitable after repeated transfusions.

Although β-thalassaemia major can be diagnosed antenatally, the severity of the resulting thalassaemia (major or intermedia) cannot be accurately forecast.

B. β-*Thalassaemia minor*

Diagnosis of heterozygous β-thalassaemia, characterized by mild hypochromic anaemia, with low MCV and MCH (the discriminant factor will distinguish this condition from simple iron-deficiency anaemia) is supporterd by the finding of increased haemoglobin A₂ (up to about 5 per cent) and slight increase in haemoglobin F (2–5 per cent) in about 50 per cent of cases.

TESTS OF PROGRESS

No treatment is required. Genetic counselling may be indicated.

2. α-*THALASSAEMIA*

A. *Haemoglobin Bart's Hydrops Syndrome*

Diagnosis of the homozygous state of α-thalassaemia, characterized by intrauterine death about the 34th week of pregnancy, is confirmed by the demonsoration that the haemoglobin pattern consists almost entirely of Hb Barts (Hb γ₄) with gross abnormalities in the size and shape of the red cells, and numerous nucleated red cells in the peripheral blood.

TESTS OF PROGRESS

Parents show mild abnormalities in size and shape of their red cells, but no abnormality on haemoglobin electrophoresis.

B. *Haemoglobin H Disease*

Diagnosis of the milder α-thalassaemia haemoglobin H disease, characterized by hypochromic anaemia and microcytic anaemia, is confirmed by the finding of numerous peripheral blood nucleated red cells and precipitated HbH (β₄) in red cells (stained with brilliant cresyl blue stain) with HbH on haemoglobin electrophoresis.

TESTS OF PROGRESS

Splenectomy can be considered, if signs of hypersplenism develop. Oxidant drugs, which precipitate HbH in the red cells, should be avoided.

C. α-*Thalassaemia Minor*

Diagnosis of the heterozygous carrier state for α-thalassaemia is supported by the finding of mild thalassaemic changes in the blood, in some cases, with normal electrophoretic patterns of levels of HbA₂ and HbF. Such carriers have up to 5 per cent Hb Barts in the neonatal period only. There are many varieties of α-thalassaemia.

F-Thalassaemia (Δ-β-Thalassaemia)

Diagnosis of this condition is confirmed by the finding of only haemoglobin F in the homozygote state (since no beta- or delta-chains are produced). The clinical condition is similar to that of homozygous β-thalassaemia.

Diagnosis of the heterozygote state is suggested by the finding of haemoglobin F levels of 5–30 per cent without increases in haemoglobin A_2.

Δ-Thalassaemia

This rare condition has been diagnosed by the demonstration of complete absence of haemoglobin A_2.

Hereditary Persistence of Haemoglobin F [AD]

Diagnosis of this harmless dominant condition, characterized by a tendency to an increased packed cell volume, and genetic production of fetal haemoglobin (HbF) beyond the neonatal period, occurring in some West African Negroes, Greeks, Swiss and a few northern Europeans, is of no clinical importance, except that it should not be mistaken for thalassaemia.

Sickle-cell Anaemia

Diagnosis of this inherited homozygous disease, occurring particularly in Africa, with a much lower incidence in Saudi Arabia, Italy, Greece, the Middle East and India, characterized by the early onset of chronic anaemia (by the third month), with splenomegaly, recurrent leg ulcers and episodes of infarction, is confirmed by the demonstration of haemoglobin S without any haemoglobin A in the peripheral blood by electrophoresis. Various screening kits are available for detection of the presence of HbS, but the final proof is electrophoresis.

The peripheral blood reveals sickled red cells, with increased serum bilirubin and no serum haptoglobin. During crises there is a neutrophilia with a moderate thrombocytosis.

In the deoxygenated state, red cells form sickle shapes, which can revert to normal an oxygenation. If sickling is severe, or the red cell has repeatedly sickled, then irreversible sickle cells (ISC) are formed, which block small blood vessels causing increasing peripheral anoxia (and incidentally increasing further sickling of red cells).

The concentration of haemoglobin F affects the severity of the condition, the higher the HbF concentration in the red cells the lesser the severity of sickling. Saudi Arabian sickle-cell anaemia is not as severe as the African variety, as HbF concentrations are 15–20 per cent.

Plasma haemoglobin is increased, following intravascular destruction of distorted red cells. Serum lactate dehydrogenase activity is increased. Bone-marrow trephines show intense erythropoiesis, with areas of infarction. Aplasia may occur during periods of marrow exhaustion, or related to infection. The haemoglobin–oxygen dissociation curve is shifted to the right, increasing release of oxygen to tissues peripherally, but paradoxically increasing the tendency to peripheral sickling.

TESTS OF PROGRESS

Repeated attacks of infarction may occur. Leg ulcers develop, and infection with salmonella, *Esch. coli* and *Strept. pneumoniae* occur, and there is reduced complement-mediated serum opsonization of salmonella.

Progressive damage occurs in the kidneys, resulting in decreasing ability to produce a concentrated urine, with resulting polyuria. Excretion of hydrogen ion is impaired, with tendency to metabolic acidosis. Finally, there is reduced excretion of serum uric acid.

No satisfactory specific treatment is available. Infections should be treated as emergencies. Surgical operations require thorough oxygenation during the entire operation, and exchange transfusion before major surgery has been carried out to avoid sickling. 'Bloodless field' surgery is impossible. Flying at altitude or incompletely pressurized is dangerous.

Antenatal diagnosis of HbS disease is possible at 8–14 weeks of pregnancy, using DNA from fetal white blood cells or amniotic fluid cells.

TESTS PROVIDING USEFUL NEGATIVE RESULTS

In the absence of electrophoresis, inability to produce sickling of red cells by deoxygenation (rubber band tight round the finger, or *Esch. coli* added to a sealed cell of red blood cell suspension) virtually excludes the diagnosis. (The marked variability found in homozygote sickle-cell anaemia may be explained by the possibility that cases may also be homozygous for α-thalassaemia, heterozygous for α-thalassaemia, or normal. α-thalassaemia inhibits in-vivo sickling, and HbA_2 levels are raised in α-thalassaemia.)

Sickle-cell–Hereditary Persistence of Haemoglobin F

This combination is beneficial, since the presence of haemoglobin F in all the red cells counteracts the sickling tendency.

Sickle-cell Thalassaemia

Diagnosis is confirmed by the finding of very large numbers of target cells in the peripheral blood, with haemoglobin S present on electrophoresis. Plasma haemoglobin is increased to 5–10 mg/100 ml and serum lactate dehydrogenase activity is increased in some cases. The clinical effects of thalassaemia minor and heterozygote sickle-cell disease are additive, and this is a serious condition.

Thalassaemia Minor Plus Heterozygous Abnormal Haemoglobinopathy

Diagnosis is confirmed by the finding of very large numbers of target cells in the peripheral blood, with decreased red-cell saline osmotic fragility, and an abnormal haemoglobin detected by electrophoresis. Thalassaemia-haemoglobin C, -haemoglobin D, -haemoglobin E, -haemoglobin G, and -haemoglobin H have been described.

Sickle-cell Trait (Heterozygote)

Diagnosis of this condition is confirmed by the demonstration of the presence of haemoglobin S (< 50 per cent) and haemoglobin A in the peripheral blood on electrophoresis. Red cells can be made to sickle by reducing the oxygen tension in vitro. Sickle cells are not seen in the peripheral blood.

TESTS OF PROGRESS

In AS heterozygotes during infection with malaria (*Plasmodium falciparum*) the parasitized cells apparently become sickled and are removed from the circulation before the malarial parasite has time to multiply in the red cell. Pressurized air flight or flying at over 5000 ft, without oxygen is dangerous. Surgical operations require adequate oxygenation. Orthopaedic 'bloodless' surgical operations are dangerous.

Haemoglobin C Disease

Diagnosis of this rare condition is confirmed by the finding of a mild chronic, microcytic, normochromic, haemolytic anaemia, with up to 80 per cent of the peripheral blood erythrocytes in the form of 'target' cells. The red-cell saline osmotic fragility is reduced below normal, and attacks of mild jaundice may occur. Haemoglobin electrophoresis reveals the presence of haemoglobin C only, with no increase in haemoglobin F.

Haemoglobin C Trait

This condition is asymptomatic, and may be detected by the finding of numerous target cells in the peripheral blood, and haemoglobin C and haemoglobin A on electrophoresis of haemolysates.

Sickle-cell Haemoglobin C Disease

Diagnosis of this condition, which is thought to be included in approximately 15–20 per cent of clinical sickle-cell disease, is confirmed by the finding of numerous target cells with anisocytosis and poikilocytosis in the peripheral blood, and haemoglobin S plus haemoglobin C on electrophoresis of haemolysates. There is a moderate normochromic haemolytic anaemia, with moderately raised plasma-haemoglobin levels of 10–25 mg/dl.

Haemoglobin D Disease

Diagnosis of this rare condition is confirmed by the finding of slight normochromic anaemia with numerous 'target' cells in the peripheral blood and with reduced red-cell saline osmotic fragility. Haemoglobin electrophoresis of haemolysate reveals the presence of haemoglobin D.

Haemoglobin D Trait

The condition is symptom-free and is detected by the demonstration of the presence of haemoglobin A and haemoglobin D on electrophoresis of haemolysate.

Sickle-cell Haemoglobin D Disease

Diagnosis of this condition, which is rare and which resembles mild sickle-cell anaemia, is confirmed by the finding of target cells in the peripheral blood, and haemoglobin S and haemoglobin D on electrophoresis of haemolysate.

Haemoglobin E Disease

Diagnosis of this disease is confirmed by the finding of a chronic, normo-chromic, microcytic, haemolytic anaemia, with numerous target cells in the peripheral blood and reduced red-cell saline osmotic fragility. Two clinical forms of the disease are found, one which resembles severe thalassaemia and the other which is much milder. Diagnosis is confirmed by the finding of haemoglobin E on electrophoresis of haemolysate.

Haemoglobin E Trait

This condition is symptom-free. The diagnosis can be confirmed by the demonstration of haemoglobin A and haemoglobin E on electrophoresis of haemolysate.

Haemoglobin M Disease

Diagnosis of this dominant haemoglobinopathy, which is associated with methaemoglobinaemia, is confirmed by the demonstration of the presence of the abnormal haemoglobin (various different forms of abnormal haemoglobin M exist) on electrophoresis of lysed red cells. The presence of abnormally increased amounts of methaemoglobin in the circulating red cells can be demonstrated, 15 per cent of the total haemoglobin being present in this abnormal form.

TESTS OF PROGRESS

There is no improvement in cyanosis with either methylene blue or ascorbic acid.

TESTS PROVIDING USEFUL NEGATIVE RESULTS

There is no deficiency in the red-cell reducing enzyme system. The abnormality is due to a defective haemoglobin.

APLASTIC ANAEMIA, ETC.

Refractory Anaemia

Refractory anaemia occurs in association with:
Aplastic or hypoplastic anaemia
Thalassaemias
Infection
Rheumatoid arthritis
Uraemia
There may be a normochromic, normocytic anaemia or the red cells may be hypochromic. Serum iron results are variable, being normal, increased, or

low. The serum total iron binding capacity (TIBC) tends to fall, but stained marrow aspirates contain stainable iron, especially after repeated blood transfusions.

Anaemia Associated with Infection

Moderate anaemia (haemoglobin 9–12 g/dl) is often found in association with infection. The findings are not diagnostic. The anaemia is normochromic and normocytic at first, but may progress to become mildly hypochromic and microcytic. The reticulocyte count is usually normal. Bone-marrow aspirates appear normal, but there may be an increased M/E ratio, with reduced sideroblasts, with normal or increased stainable iron stores.

It appears that the incorporation of iron into haemoglobin is interfered with.

Aplastic Anaemia

Diagnosis of aplastic anaemia is supported by the finding of normochromic, normocytic or moderately macrocytic anaemia, with falling haemoglobin and anisocytosis and some poikilocytosis in stained blood films. The reticulocyte count is low, unless there are islands of surviving active marrow still present. The white blood-cell count is at the lower end of the normal range or less, with a neutropenia. Thrombocytopenia of varying degree is also found. Commonly the ESR and plasma viscosity are increased. ^{59}Fe is only slowly cleared from the plasma after injection, and iron incorporation is reduced.

Bone-marrow aspirates may contain visible fat globules, and the nucleated cell content is low. Aspiration of marrow may be unsuccessful.

Diagnosis is confirmed by a bone-marrow trephine. Marrow sections reveal depression of erythroid series, myeloid series, and reduced numbers of megakaryocytes.

Distorted nucleated red cells (especially late normoblasts) may be seen.

TESTS OF PROGRESS

Evidence of red-cell regeneration indicates at least temporary recovery, and the steady maintenance of a moderately reduced haemoglobin concentration in the absence of repeated blood transfusion is encouraging.

Cases with severe thrombocytopenia, even without evidence of bruising and bleeding, have a bad prognosis, often dying from sudden severe haemorrhage.

Cases considered potential candidates for bone-marrow transplantation should receive as few blood transfusions as possible, to reduce the risk of development of HLA antibodies.

Children suffering from aplastic anaemia, in whom HbF production persists, have a better prognosis than those children in whom HbF is not detectable.

Treatment with steroids such as prednisone, or anabolic steroids such as oxymethalone, may be effective, if the treatment is continuous for at least 6 weeks to 3 months before it is rejected as not effective. (Experimental work suggests that those patients who excrete excessive amounts of erythropoietin in their urine are the patients likely to respond favourably to this latter treatment.) A positive response to anabolic steroids may be detected by an increase in ^{59}Fe incorporation.

In cases with depressed platelet production, during recovery, erythropoietic and granulocytopoietic activity often returns before platelet production recovers.

Occasional cases develop myeloid leukaemia terminally.

TESTS PROVIDING USEFUL NEGATIVE RESULTS

Progressive fall in haemoglobin levels of up to 1 per cent (0.15 g/dl) per day (on average) in the absence of evidence of either haemolysis or bleeding makes this diagnosis a possibility only after deficiency anaemias have been excluded.

Congenital Dyserythropoietic Anaemia [R]

Diagnosis of this rare group of conditions is made by the demonstration of moderate normochromic anaemia beginning in infancy or adolescence. Serum bilirubin, predominantly unconjugated, is moderately raised (1·4–3·5 mg/dl), with relatively low reticulocyte counts. Evidence of active but faulty erythropoiesis is found, with increased urine urobilinogen excretion, and greatly increased plasma-iron turnover. Peripheral iron utilization is reduced below normal. Serum-iron levels are raised, but the total iron binding capacity (TIBC) is reduced. Red-cell life is slightly shorter than normal, but evidence of increased intravascular red-cell destruction is shown by greatly reduced serum-haptoglobin concentrations.

The peripheral blood white-cell count and differential are normal and the platelet count is normal.

Bone-marrow biopsy enables one to distinguish between three types of this condition.

TYPE I

The red-cell series in the bone marrow shows megaloblastic changes in the absence of either vitamin-B_{12} or folic-acid deficiency and in the absence of excessive urine orotic acid excretion. Internuclear chromatin bridges are seen between the nucleated red-cell precursors. In this Type I, the peripheral red cells are macrocytic.

TYPE II

Normoblasts are found with bi- and multinuclear forms. Many mitoses are pluripolar and karyorrhexis is seen. In the peripheral blood red cells agglutinate with anti-i antiserum. The erythrocytes also undergo lysis in the acid serum (Ham) test, but do not lyse in sucrose solution. They are susceptible to lysis in the presence of anti-i and anti-I antisera.

TYPE III

Erythroblasts are characterized by multinuclearity, with up to a dozen nuclei in a single cell, gigantoblasts and peripheral blood macrocytosis.

TESTS OF PROGRESS

Treatment with vitamin B_{12}, folic acid, riboflavin, pyridoxine, or steroids has no effect. Iron therapy is contraindicated and splenectomy is ineffective. Since the anaemia is usually only mild, there is no need for regular transfusion. Later effects from iron deposition in skin, liver, or kidney have not yet been described.

TESTS PROVIDING USEFUL NEGATIVE RESULTS

Increased urine-urobilinogen output does not support a diagnosis of hypoplastic anaemia. Absence of lysis in sucrose solution, with lysis of erythrocytes in acidified serum (Ham test) excludes a diagnosis of paroxysmal nocturnal haemoglobinuria.

Familial Hypoplastic Anaemia in Infants (Fanconi Syndrome) [R]

Diagnosis of this very rare condition is confirmed by the finding of insidious anaemia developing in infancy, with thrombocytopenia, leucopenia, marrow hypoplasia and chromosomal abnormalities.

TESTS OF PROGRESS

Steroid therapy may cause a moderate remission, but growth is stunted. Repeated blood transfusions may lead rapidly to severe haemosiderosis.

Pure Red-cell Aplasia (Diamond–Blackfan Syndrome) [R]

Diagnosis of this very rare condition is confirmed by the finding of the development of a normochromic, normocytic anaemia in infancy, with marked reduction in erythroid-cell production in the bone marrow.

TESTS OF PROGRESS

Steroid therapy may produce some remission. Transfusion haemosiderosis develops following repeated transfusions.

TESTS PROVIDING USEFUL NEGATIVE RESULTS

Both the white-cell count and the platelet count are normal.

Post-acute Haemorrhage

Immediately after acute haemorrhage the blood volume is reduced. Fluid enters the circulation rapidly from the extracellular space, and the blood volume is partially restored, with reduction in the haemoglobin concentration and the haematocrit. There are neutrophilia and thrombocytosis, with many 'stab' cells.

After very severe acute haemorrhage, nucleated red cells appear in the peripheral blood with megakaryocyte fragments and great variation in the size of the platelets.

Fibrinolytic activity is increased and the plasma-activated partial thrombo-plastin time is reduced below the lower normal limit.

Post-chronic Haemorrhage

There is evidence of increased red-cell formation (i.e. reticulocytosis) and progressive iron deficiency with falling MCHC. The platelet count may be normal or slightly increased and the white-cell count is normal. The blood volume is normal.

Bone-marrow aspirates reveal active erythroid hyperplasia with low or absent stores of stainable iron.

Incompatible Blood Transfusion

The findings depend on the severity of the reaction and can range from a moderate reduction in survival time of the transfused red cells to immediate destruction in the circulation of the transfused red cells. In severe immediate reactions plasma haemoglobin levels increase, and plasma methaemalbumin is detectable with disappearance of plasma haptoglobins. This is followed by haemoglobinuria and increase in serum bilirubin (unconjugated) with peak values at 3–6 hours. At first, there is leucopenia with thrombocytopenia, and in some cases a defibrination syndrome develops, with persisting thrombo-cytopenia, depressed plasma fibrinogen and increased fibrinolytic activity, with detectable fibrin- and fibrinogen-degradation products in the plasma. The prothrombin time and the activated partial thromboplastin time may also be prolonged (i.e. disseminated intravascular coagulopathy, DIC).

Urine urobilinogen is greatly increased, and the urine, in addition to haemoglobin, may also contain many casts and increased protein. In severe cases, oliguria follows, with rising blood urea, due to severe renal tubular damage.

Abnormal iso-antibodies appear in the serum, and ABO iso-antibodies are active haemolysins. The Coombs' test may become positive, and other blood-group antibodies may be detected by means of enzyme-treated red cells (e.g. ficin, bromelin, etc.).

TESTS OF PROGRESS

It is essential for the investigation of such cases that the following specimens are available for analysis:

1. The pre-transfusion blood sample from the recipient, which was used for the original blood grouping and cross-matching procedures.

2. The blood bottles with any remaining blood plus the corresponding pilot tubes, which were cross-matched for the recipient.

3. All urine passed by the patient since the reaction was noticed.

4. Post-transfusion sample of blood from the recipient.

HAEMORRHAGIC DISORDERS

Congenital Afibrinogenaemia [AR] [R]

Diagnosis of this rare condition, characterized by bleeding which may start in the first year, with haematomas, gastrointestinal and mucous membrane bleeding, and haemarthroses in 20 per cent of cases, is confirmed by the demonstration of the virtual absence of plasma fibrinogen (when assayed by clotting, chemical, or immunological estimations).

The prothrombin time, thrombin clotting time, reptilase time and APTT, are all abnormally prolonged, and are all corrected to normal by the addition of fibrinogen.

TESTS OF PROGRESS

Plasma fibrinogen concentrate can be used to treat haemorrhage and to cover surgery. Plasma fibrinogen concentrations of about 1 g/l are adequate for normal haemostasis.

TESTS PROVIDING USEFUL NEGATIVE RESULTS ·

There is no evidence of increased fibrinolysis, disseminated coagulopathy, or circulating anticoagulants.

Congenital Hypofibrinogenaemia [R]

Diagnosis of this rare condition, which is probably the heterozygous state of congenital afibrinogenaemia, occurring in apparently symptom-free normal subjects, is confirmed by the demonstration of a markedly reduced plasma fibrinogen, with normal clotting tests.

Congenital Dysfibrinogenaemia [R]

Diagnosis of this rare condition, characterized by bleeding from mucous membranes, wound dehiscence and excessive bleeding after surgery or trauma, haemorrhagic and spontaneous abortions, or a tendency to thrombosis, is confirmed by the demonstration of a qualitatively defective fibrinogen.

The thrombin time is mostly abnormally prolonged, as is the reptilase clotting time (which releases only fibrinopeptide A). The thrombin clotting time is abnormally shortened in those cases of dysfibrinogenaemia with a thrombotic tendency.

Methods using clotting techniques to estimate plasma fibrinogen concentration give low results, while the corresponding tests using immunological techniques give normal fibrinogen concentration results.

TESTS OF PROGRESS

Acquired dysfibrinogenaemia occurs in hepatocellular disease, and therefore this needs to be excluded before the diagnosis of inherited dysfibrinogenaemia can be made.

Congenital Factor V Deficiency

Diagnosis of this rare condition, characterized by bruising, bleeding from mucous membranes, menorrhagia and excessive bleeding after dental extraction, surgery or trauma, is confirmed by the demonstration of deficiency of Factor V. The prothrombin clotting time, activated and non-activated APTT, are all abnormally prolonged, and are corrected by the addition of normal absorbed plasma, but not by aged serum or Russell's viper venom.

TESTS OF PROGRESS

Fresh frozen plasma can be used to cover bleeding or surgery.

TESTS PROVIDING USEFUL NEGATIVE RESULTS

Platelet function tests are normal.

Congenital Prothrombin Deficiency (Factor II Deficiency) [R]

Diagnosis of this rare condition, characterized by excessive bruising, mucous membrane bleeding, menorrhagia and postoperative bleeding, is confirmed by the demonstration of a prolonged prothrombin clotting time, not corrected by adsorbed normal plasma, aged serum, or Russell's viper venom. Estimation of plasma prothrombin using Taipan or *Echis carinatus* venoms, reveals a true low plasma prothrombin coagulation activity.

In cases of failure to synthesize prothrombin, plasma prothrombin antigen levels are correspondingly low, whereas prothrombin antigen levels are not reduced in cases of dysprothrombinaemia.

Heterozygotes are symptom-free, or have only a mild bleeding tendency.

TESTS OF PROGRESS

Fresh frozen plasma can be used to treat bleeding episodes, or to cover surgery or trauma.

Congenital Factor VII Deficiency [R]

Diagnosis of this rare condition, characterized by epistaxis, haemarthroses, gastrointestinal bleeding, menorrhagia and sometimes dangerous neonatal intracranial haemorrhage, is confirmed by the demonstration of plasma Factor VII deficiency. The one-stage prothrombin time is abnormally prolonged, and is corrected by addition of Russell's viper venom.

The defect can consist of (*a*) VII^-: virtually unmeasurable VII_c and VII_{Ag}. (the majority of cases). (*b*) VII^+: very low VII_c with normal VII_{Ag}. (*c*) VII^R: low VII_c and low VII_{Ag}.

TESTS PROVIDING USEFUL NEGATIVE RESULTS

The APTT is normal.

TESTS OF PROGRESS

Small transfusions of fresh frozen plasma can be used to cover bleeding episodes or surgery.

Congenital Factor VIII Deficiency (Haemophilia A) [XR]

Diagnosis of this sex-linked recessive condition, characterized by episodes of abnormal bleeding with haematoma, haemarthroses, and/or deep tissue bleeding, in inverse proportion to the circulating Factor VIIIC level (which varies from family to family) is confirmed by the demonstration of abnormally low levels of plasma Factor VIIIC (normal = 50–200 u/dl) with normal or raised levels of Factor VIIIRAg.

Severe haemophiliacs have levels of 0–1 u/dl of Factor VIIIC. Moderate haemophiliacs have 2–5 u/dl, and mild cases have more than 5 u/dl. The whole blood clotting time may be prolonged (but may not be, and cannot be used to detect cases). The plasma-activated partial thromboplastin time is abnormally prolonged (if reagents sensitive to Factor VIIIC deficiency are used).

TESTS OF PROGRESS

Treatment with cryoprecipitate or Factor VIII concentrate is used to:

a. Prevent bleeding episodes (including self-administration at home after bumps).

b. Treatment of haemarthroses or bleeding episodes.

c. Cover for surgery. For major surgery, plasma Factor VIII levels should be kept above 30 u/dl with 12-hourly infusions. For minor surgery, levels require to be maintained above 20 u/dl, and DDAVP plus tranexamic acid (or epsilon-aminocaproic acid) should be given to mild cases to reduce their Factor VIII requirement, when, for instance, they undergo tooth extraction.

Haemophiliacs are liable to develop chronic active liver disease (post-transfusion hepatitis). Drugs affecting platelet function (e.g. aspirin) should be avoided. Antibodies neutralizing Factor VIIIC may develop with time, requiring saturation with high doses of Factor VIII, exchange transfusion, or if these measures fail, the use of activated prothrombin complex (bypassing the clotting deficiency). Carriers can be detected by demonstrating reduced plasma Factor VIIIC activity with normal or slightly raised VIIIRAg (e.g. in daughters of a haemophiliac father, or in a mother with at least one affected son). Prenatal diagnosis of haemophilia in the male fetus can be made about the 14th–15th week of pregnancy, on fetal blood samples.

Congenital Factor IX Deficiency (Christmas Disease; Haemophilia B) [XR]

Diagnosis of this sex-linked recessive condition (with an incidence in the United Kingdom one-tenth of true haemophilia), characterized by episodes of bleeding with haematoma, haemarthroses, and/or deep tissue bleeding, in inverse proportion to the circulating plasma Factor IX level (which varies from family to family), is confirmed by the demonstration of prolonged plasma-activated partial thromboplastin time and reduced plasma Factor IX concentration in the plasma. There are four different varieties, but this is not of direct clinical value.

TESTS OF PROGRESS

Bleeding episodes should be treated with Factor IX concentrate, and patients should be taught self treatment at home with concentrate. Factor IX concentrate is needed to cover surgery. Mild cases should be given tranexamic acid (or epsilon-aminocaproic acid) to reduce the requirement for Factor IX concentrate to cover minor surgery (e.g. tooth extraction).

Antibodies to Factor IX develop rarely (much less frequently than antibody development in true haemophilia).

The platelet count and platelet function tests are normal. The whole blood clotting time is normal in the majority of cases. The prothrombin time is normal, except in one variety, B_m, which gives a markedly prolonged ox-brain prothrombin time.

Congenital Factor X Deficiency [R] [AR]

Diagnosis of this rare disease, characterized by a bleeding diathesis in homozygotes and a mild tendency to bleed in heterozygotes, is confirmed by the demonstration of reduced plasma Factor X clotting activity, with very low, low or normal Factor X antigen levels, depending on the molecular variant form inherited.

The prothrombin time is prolonged, and the prolonged time is corrected by the addition of normal plasma, or aged serum, but not by the addition of alumina-adsorbed plasma. The activated partial thromboplastin time is prolonged.

TESTS PROVIDING USEFUL NEGATIVE RESULTS

Other plasma clotting factors are present in normal concentration. There is no improvement in plasma Factor X clotting activity following vitamin K therapy, and there is no evidence of amyloidosis (a rare association with isolated Factor X deficiency). Whole blood or plasma transfusion rapidly corrects the Factor X deficiency for a day or more.

Russell's viper venom corrects the prothrombin time in some cases but not in others, and is therefore not a reliable test for detection of this deficiency.

Congenital Factor XI Deficiency [R] [AR]

Diagnosis of this rare condition, characterized by a bleeding tendency, with excessive bruising and menorrhagia in women, epistaxis, postoperative and post-tooth extraction bleeding, occurring particularly in Ashkenazi Jews, is confirmed by demonstration of prolonged activated partial thromboplastin time. Reduced plasma Factor XI activity can be detected using artificially produced Factor XI-depleted plasma.

TESTS OF PROGRESS

The 'wasted' plasma recovered after preparation of cryoprecipitate from plasma is rich in Factor XI and can be used to treat known cases to cover surgery, trauma, or excessive bleeding.

TESTS PROVIDING USEFUL NEGATIVE RESULTS

Other plasma clotting factors are present in normal concentration. The prothrombin time is normal.

Congenital Factor XII Deficiency (Hageman Deficiency) [AR]

Diagnosis of this rare condition, rarely associated with mild bleeding problems, is diagnosed by the demonstration of a greatly prolonged whole blood clotting time, with a markedly prolonged APTT. Specific estimation of plasma Factor XII has shown reduced concentrations.

TESTS OF PROGRESS

In rare postoperative bleeding, fresh-frozen plasma rapidly restores haemostasis to normal.

TESTS PROVIDING USEFUL NEGATIVE RESULTS

Platelet numbers and functions are normal. No other plasma clotting factor is deficient.

Congenital Factor XIII Deficiency (Fibrin Stabilizing Substance (FSS) Deficiency) [R] [AR]

Diagnosis of this rare condition, characterized by prolonged bleeding after surgery or trauma, often starting up to 36–48 hours after the injury, with delayed wound healing and keloid scar formation, is confirmed by the demonstration of persistent abnormally reduced Factor XIII activity, with abnormally rapid clot lysis in 5 M urea solution, 1 per cent monochloracetic acid or in 2 per cent acetic acid. Prolonged haemorrhage from the umbilical cord stump may occur after birth, and there is a higher incidence of intracranial haemorrhage than normal.

TESTS OF PROGRESS

Haemostasis is easily restored to normal by transfusion of fresh frozen plasma, cryoprecipitate or purified Factor XIII, and prophylactic therapy is also easy, since Factor XIII has a transfused half-life of 6–10 days.

TESTS PROVIDING USEFUL NEGATIVE RESULTS

The bleeding time, prothrombin time, activated partial thromboplastin time, serum prothrombin consumption, platelet count and platelet function, and plasma fibrinogen concentration, are all normal.

Congenital Fitzgerald, Williams, Flaujeac Factor Deficiency (Kininogen Deficiency) [AR] [R]

Diagnosis of this rare asymptomatic abnormality is supported by the demonstration of a prolonged activated partial thromboplastin time, which is not corrected by prolonged surface contact activation. Confirmation is only possible using cross-correction studies with known cases. The deficiency and prolongation of the APTT are not of clinical significance.

TESTS PROVIDING USEFUL NEGATIVE RESULTS

The prothrombin time is normal. Plasma Factors VIII and IX are present in normal concentration.

Congenital Prekallikrein (Fletcher Factor) Deficiency [AR] [R]

Diagnosis of this rare asymptomatic coagulation abnormality is confirmed by the demonstration that prolonged surface contact activation of plasma shortens the prolonged activated partial thromboplastin.

The deficiency is not of clinical significance.

TESTS PROVIDING USEFUL NEGATIVE RESULTS

The prothrombin time is normal. Plasma Factors VIII and IX are present in normal concentration.

Haemorrhagic Disease of the Newborn

Diagnosis of this condition is confirmed by the finding of blood in vomit, stool and sputum of a newborn infant, with a greatly prolonged prothrombin time and prolonged activated partial thromboplastin time. Plasma Factors II, VII, IX and X are abnormally reduced.

TESTS OF PROGRESS

Following treatment with vitamin K_1 plus fresh blood transfusion (if necessary), the prothrombin time and activated partial thromboplastin time return to normal.

TESTS PROVIDING USEFUL NEGATIVE RESULTS

The bleeding time is normal or only slightly prolonged. The platelet count is normal.

Inhibitors of Blood Coagulation

1. FACTOR VIII INHIBITORS

Haemophiliacs become unresponsive to replacement therapy with Factor VIII. The affected cases are usually severe. Inhibitors may also develop in non-haemophiliacs, for example, rarely postpartum, also in various auto-immune disorders, and very occasionally in apparently healthy individuals. **Diagnosis** is supported by demonstration of failure of normal plasma to correct the abnormally prolonged activated partial thromboplastin time.

2. FACTOR IX INHIBITORS [R]

Inhibitors may rarely develop in postpartum women, in autoimmune disease and in inherited Factor IX deficiency (Christmas disease).

3. VON WILLEBRAND FACTOR INHIBITOR [R]

Replacement therapy with Factor VIII material is not followed by the typical delayed increase in Factor VIII activity usually seen in von Willebrand's disease.

4. INHIBITORS AGAINST FACTORS I, II, V, VII, X AND XIII [R]

Such inhibitors against individual factors have been rarely described. The abnormal clotting test found, is not restored to normal by the addition of normal plasma.

TESTS PROVIDING USEFUL NEGATIVE RESULTS

Addition of polybrene to the prothrombin test or APTT will eliminate unsuspected heparin activity.

Disseminated Intravascular Coagulopathy (Consumptive Coagulopathy, DIC)

Diagnosis of the occurrence of disseminated intravascular coagulopathy is confirmed by the demonstration of:
 a. Fragmented red cells visible in peripheral blood films.
 b. Thrombocytopenia.
 c. Abnormally reduced plasma fibrinogen (less than 1 g/l).
 d. Abnormally increased circulating fibrin/fibrinogen degradation products.
 e. Abnormally reduced plasma Factor V and Factor VIII levels, with abnormally prolonged prothrombin time and plasma-activated partial thromboplastin time, and thrombin time.
 (*f.* Secondarily increased fibrinolysis—this is not essential for diagnosis.)
In acute decompensated DIC all these results are abnormal.

In subacute partially compensated DIC platelet counts may be normal or reduced, and plasma fibrinogen levels are not grossly reduced.

In low-grade hypercompensated DIC, platelet counts are variable, plasma fibrinogen levels are raised above normal, the APTT may be shorter than normal, and the prothrombin time is normal.

TESTS OF PROGRESS

Reptilase clotting times are useful, if heparin therapy is started, as this test (cf. thrombin time) is unaffected by the presence of heparin.

Congenital Alpha-2 Plasmin Inhibitor Deficiency [R]

Diagnosis of this rare condition associated with a bleeding tendency is confirmed by the demonstration of rapid spontaneous lysis of freshly taken blood, after initial clotting, with a high concentration of FRA (fibrin/fibrinogen-related antigen in the serum. The defect is corrected by the addition of alpha-2 antiplasmin.

TESTS PROVIDING USEFUL NEGATIVE RESULTS

Plasma clotting factors, platelet numbers and functions are normal. There is no abnormal increase in FDPs in freshly collected blood with added plasmin inhibitor, i.e. although fibrinolysis is accelerated, there is no abnormal excessive fibrinogenolysis.

TESTS OF PROGRESS

Tranexamic acid corrects the abnormal fibrinolytic system and also the bleeding tendency.

BLEEDING DUE TO PLATELET OR VESSEL DEFICIENCIES

Primary Idiopathic Thrombocytopenic Purpura (Werlhof's Disease)

This condition can present as an acute disease, self-limiting in a large proportion of cases, and affecting children predominantly between the ages of 2 and 6 years, 50 per cent being preceded by virus infections, including rubella and rubeola. It can also present in young adults (three females to every male) as a more chronic condition, and in adults of any age, less frequently. **Diagnosis** is supported by the finding of platelet counts below $20 \times 10^9/1$ in the acute variety, and below $50–100 \times 10^9/1$ in the chronic variety, with haemorrhages from mucous membranes, nose bleeds, and occasionally haematuria and intracranial haemorrhage in the initial phase of the acute variety. Menorrhagia is common in young adult females with the chronic variety. The bleeding time may be prolonged and the Hess tourniquet test is positive. Specialized laboratories can demonstrate the presence of antibodies on the surface of platelets, and reduced platelet half-life in the circulation. The diagnosis is confirmed by the demonstration of bone marrow aspirate or trephines with normal red cell and white blood cell precursors, but with an increased number of megakaryocytes, which are immature, and which show less platelet budding than normal. Red cell hyperplasia follows persistent bleeding.

TESTS OF PROGRESS

The acute variety in children is usually self-limiting, but steroid therapy does reduce the risk of serious intracranial haemorrhage. In adults, steroid therapy may result in an increase in the platelet count. If the dose of steroids required to produce this response is too large, then splenectomy can be considered. After splenectomy, a proportion recover, a proportion can maintain a satisfactory platelet count on a moderate steroid dose, and a proportion do not improve. This latter group will require immunosuppressive therapy. Platelet transfusions can be used to cover splenectomy or other operations.

TESTS PROVIDING USEFUL NEGATIVE RESULTS

Diagnosis depends on the exclusion of other causes of thrombocytopenia, including acute leukaemia, and response to drugs causing thrombocytopenia.

Thrombotic Thrombocytopenic Purpura (Thrombotic Microangiopathic Haemolytic Anaemia) [R]

Diagnosis of this rare condition, characterized by anaemia, neurological abnormalities, microangiopathic haemolytic anaemia, thrombocytopenia with bruising and bleeding, renal abnormalities and fever, presenting as an acute illness, is supported by the finding of anaemia with bur cells and 'helmet' red cells in the peripheral blood, thrombocytopenia, reticulocytosis, with circulating nucleated red cells, neutrophilia, increased plasma haemoglobin, and serum bilirubin. A small proportion of cases have frank disseminated intravascular coagulopathy. Recently it has been found that these cases have a complete absence of circulating plasminogen activator and impaired vessel wall release of prostacyclin.

TESTS OF PROGRESS

Treatment with heparin and steroids cause improvement in some cases. Plasmapheresis with plasma exchange (not with albumin) causes satisfactory response in others, but greater benefit follows simple transfusion with fresh frozen plasma (suggesting a deficiency state). Vincristine 2 mg i.v. followed by 1 mg i.v. every other day, has caused remission in cases not responding to other treatment, in this condition which used to be fatal.

Treatment with low-dose aspirin (less than 40 mg/day) plus dipyridamol (100 mg t.d.s.), dextran-70 every 12 hours i.v. has also been tried. Success of treatment or remission of the condition can be monitored by platelet counts (which rise towards normal) and serum LDH levels (which fall towards normal).

TESTS WHICH PROVIDE USEFUL NEGATIVE RESULTS

Bone marrow aspirates show erythroid hyperplasia and myeloid hyperplasia. There is no evidence of acute leukaemia. Fibrinolytic activity in the plasma is nil. The prothrombin ratio, activated partial thromboplastin time and fibrinogen concentration are normal, unless disseminated intravascular coagulopathy has developed.

Von Willebrand's Disease

This inherited bleeding condition, which affects both sexes, occurs in two clinical forms:

1. COMMON HETEROZYGOUS FORM [AD]

These patients present in childhood with bleeding from mucous membranes, easy bruising, severe haemorrhage after trauma, gastrointestinal haemorrhage and, later, severe menorrhagia in females.

2. LESS COMMON VERY SEVERE HOMOZYGOUS RECESSIVE FORM [AR]

These patients present with severe haemophilic type of bleeding (including haemarthroses) and purpura. The heterozygous subjects are symptom-free.
Diagnosis of von Willebrand's disease is confirmed by the demonstration of a prolonged bleeding time, with reduced plasma Factor VIIIC and Factor VIIIRAg, defective ristocetin-induced platelet aggregation corrected by normal plasma, and defective platelet adhesion in glass bead columns (Salzman's test).

TESTS OF PROGRESS

Unlike haemophilia, following transfusion with fresh plasma or cryoprecipitate, the plasma Factor VIIIC activity is variably increased for up to 36 hours, after an initial delay of a few hours after infusion.

USEFUL NEGATIVE RESULTS

The platelet count is normal. Platelet aggregation, induced by ADP, epinephrine, collagen, thrombin and arachidonate, is normal.

PLATELET MEMBRANE ABNORMALITIES

1. Bernard–Soulier Syndrome [AR]

Diagnosis of this rare hereditary bleeding disorder, characterized by superficial bruising and ecchymoses, mucosal bleeding and excessive prolonged post-traumatic haemorrhage, is confirmed by the demonstration of defective ristocetin-induced platelet aggregation which is not corrected by normal plasma. (The primary defect is a gross deficiency of platelet membrane glycoproteins (GP) I_b and I_s.)

There is thrombocytopenia with giant platelets visible in stained films. The bleeding time is prolonged, and platelet adhesion measured by passage through glass bead columns (Salzman's test) is below normal.

TESTS OF PROGRESS

Affected patients need platelet transfusions to cover surgical operations. Heterozygotes are clinically normal, but giant platelets can be seen in their blood.

USEFUL NEGATIVE RESULTS

Platelets clump normally on native blood smears. Platelet aggregation, induced by ADP, adrenaline, thrombin, collagen and arachidonate, is normal. Clot retraction is also normal. Normal plasma corrects ristocetin-induced platelet aggregation in von Willebrand's disease.

2. Thrombasthenia (Glanzmann's Disease) [AR]

This hereditary bleeding disorder is characterized by superficial bruising, epistaxis, menorrhagia, and prolonged bleeding from superficial cuts, and it occurs in two varieties:

a. Type I: More severe symptoms, with low platelet fibrinogen and very poor clot retraction.

b. Type II: Moderate symptoms, with nearly normal platelet fibrinogen and only moderately defective clot retraction.

Diagnosis is confirmed by a prolonged bleeding time, absence of platelet clumping on native blood smear, defective clot retraction, absence of platelet aggregation with ADP, and impaired aggregation with adrenaline, collagen, thrombin and arachidonate. There is also diminished platelet adhesion in glass bead columns (Salzman's test). The primary defect is reduced or absent platelet glycoproteins (GP) II_b and III_c.

TESTS OF PROGRESS

Platelet transfusion will be necessary to cover trauma or surgery. Steroids and splenectomy are contraindicated.

Heterozygotes are symptomless, and can only be detected by demonstration of reduced GP II_b and III_c in the platelet membrane.

3. Platelet Factor 3 Deficiency [R]

Diagnosis of this very rare primary bleeding disorder, characterized by moderately severe bleeding episodes, is confirmed by demonstration of reduced prothrombin consumption and reduced platelet Factor 3 availability. Patients require platelet transfusion to cover surgery or trauma.

INTRACELL PLATELET ABNORMALITY

Dense-body (Storage Pool) Deficiency

These syndromes are characterized by abnormal deficiency of dense bodies in platelets, demonstrated on electron microscopy.

A. HERMANSKY–PUDLAK SYNDROME [AR]

This condition, characterized by life-long bleeding tendency, oculocutaneous albinism (tyrosinase-positive), bruising and epistaxes, is diagnosed by the finding of pigmented macrophages in the bone marrow, increased bleeding time, reduced platelet Factor 3 availability, absence of secondary aggregation with ADP and adrenaline, and no aggregation with collagen, plus marked reduction in platelet ADP and 5-HT content.

The platelet count is normal.

B. WISKOTT–ALDRICH SYNDROME [XR]

This condition is not characterized by a bleeding tendency. There is eczema, increased susceptibility to infection, thrombocytopenia ($5–150 \times 10^9/1$) with reduced platelet survival.

C. CHEDIAK–HIGASHI SYNDROME [AR]

This condition is not characterized by a bleeding tendency. Symptoms include photophobia, nystagmus, pseudoalbinism, increased susceptibility to infection, hepatosplenomegaly, lymphadenopathy, a high incidence of lymphoreticular malignancy and early death.

Thrombocytopenia occurs, with giant organelles present in most leucocytes.

D. THROMBOCYTOPENIA WITH ABSENT RADII [AR]

This syndrome is characterized by the bilateral absence of radii, cardiac malformation in one-third of cases, thrombocytopenia from early infancy, a leukaemoid blood picture in one-half of cases, and death of two-thirds of cases in the first year. Severe haemorrhages are rare in survivors, who may require platelet transfusions to cover surgery.

E. IDIOPATHIC STORAGE POOL DISEASE [R] [AD]

Dense body deficiency demonstrated by electron microscopy is associated with only a mild bleeding tendency. Dense body material appears to be necessary for second wave aggregation of platelets. Platelet aggregation with ADP, adrenaline and collagen, is usually defective.

Alpha-granule Deficiency (Gray Platelet Syndrome) [AD] [R]

Diagnosis of this rare hereditary bleeding disease, characterized by mucous membrane haemorrhages and ecchymoses, is supported by the finding of a prolonged bleeding time, platelets which vary more than normal in size, with a normal or moderately reduced total platelet count.

The diagnosis is confirmed by the demonstration of the presence of very few granules in the platelets on electron microscopy. Platelet Factor 4, beta-thromboglobulin and platelet fibrinogen content are reduced. Aggregations of platelets with collagen, ADP, adrenaline are nearly normal, but there is a defect in release with collagen, thrombin and adrenaline.

Combined Alpha- and Beta-granule Deficiency [R]

A congenital bleeding tendency with deficiency of both alpha- and beta-granules has been described. Electron microscopy is required for its diagnosis.

Abnormal Platelet Structure

1. A condition with microthrombocytes has been described. The newer blood counting machines measure platelet volume.

2. 'Swiss-cheese' platelets [R]—a condition with structurally abnormal platelets has been described.

3. Alport's syndrome [R]—the combination of deafness, nephritis and macrothrombocytopathia has been described.

Cyclo-oxygenase Deficiency [R]

Diagnosis of this rare mild bleeding disorder is confirmed by the demonstration of primary wave platelet aggregation with ADP, without a secondary wave, and absence of response to arachidonate. The absence of secondary aggregation with ADP is restored by the addition of normal or storage-pool platelets, but not by 'aspirinated' platelets.

Hereditary Aspirin-like Defect

Diagnosis of this mild bleeding tendency is supported by the demonstration of a prolonged bleeding time, reduced aggregation with collagen, absence of secondary wave aggregation with ADP, and absence of platelet aggregation with arachidonic acid.

Enhanced Sensitivity to Aspirin

Diagnosis of this condition, characterized by 'oozing and bruising' after taking aspirin, in an otherwise haematologically normal subject, is supported by the combination of the clinical history and the finding of normal platelet function tests in the absence of aspirin intake, and grossly reduced response to collagen aggregation of platelets after aspirin ingestion.

Lipoxygenase Deficiency [R]

Diagnosis of this rare condition, characterized by hypercoagulability, is supported by increased spontaneous platelet aggregation in vitro, and platelet aggregation occurring at very low concentrations of arachidonic acid. (The condition may (*a*) be familial; (*b*) occur in myeloproliferative disorders.)

Thromboxane A₂ Synthetase Deficiency [R]

Diagnosis of this rare mild-to-severe bleeding diathesis, is confirmed by the demonstration of lack of secondary aggregation with ADP or adrenaline restored to normal with 'aspirinated' platelets or platelets from storage-pool disorder. When platelet-rich plasmas (PRPs) are mixed, and platelet aggregation examined, thromboxane A_2-deficient and cyclo-oxygenase-deficient PRPs mutually correct. Thromboxane A_2-deficient PRP corrects normal 'aspirinated' PRP, whereas cyclo-oxygenase-deficient PRP does not.

USEFUL NEGATIVE RESULTS

Platelets fail to respond to arachidonic acid, have normal 5-HT uptake and normal nucleotide content (cf. storage-pool disease).

Hereditary Capillary Fragility (Vascular Pseudohaemophilia)

Diagnosis of this rare dominant condition is confirmed by the finding of a history of abnormally excessive bleeding following trauma, with abnormalities in nail-bed capillaries and bulbar conjunctival capillaries, the capillaries showing excessive tortuosity and irregularities. The bleeding time is usually prolonged.

TESTS PROVIDING USEFUL NEGATIVE RESULTS

The platelet count and platelet function tests are normal. There is no plasma coagulation factor defect, as measured by the prothrombin time and the activated partial thromboplastin time. In particular, plasma Factor VIII is within normal limits, excluding the diagnosis of von Willebrand's disease.

Purpura Simplex

Bruising in response to slight injury is found in otherwise normal subjects, predominantly women, and no abnormality of plasma clotting factors, platelet count or platelet function, or capillary structure is found.

It is worth noting that up to 10 per cent of normal subjects give positive results with the Hess capillary fragility test.

Henoch–Schönlein Purpura (Anaphylactoid Purpura)

Diagnosis of this condition, the commonest vasculitic syndrome of childhood, characterized by a rash with purpura, migrating joint involvement, abdominal pain (occasionally with melaena), renal involvement with haematuria in 50 per cent (severe renal damage in 10 per cent), is aided by the finding of deposits of IgA, C3 and C4 in the capillary walls in skin and renal biopsy material. The Hess capillary fragility test is positive and cryoglobulin may be detected in the serum.

TESTS PROVIDING USEFUL NEGATIVE RESULTS

Platelet counts and platelet function tests are normal. The prothrombin time, plasma-activated partial thromboplastin time and plasma clotting factors are normal.

Benign Purpura Hyperglobulinaemica of Waldenström [R]

Diagnosis of this rare condition is supported by the finding of increased gammaglobulin in the serum presenting as a broad band on electrophoresis, in association with irregular attacks of purpura, in women. Capillary fragility is greatly increased. There is a normochromic anaemia, and the ESR and plasma viscosity are increased.

TESTS PROVIDING USEFUL NEGATIVE RESULTS

No abnormality of the platelet count or of platelet function is found, unless the macroglobulin coats the platelets and thus causes a prolonged bleeding time and reduced adhesive platelet count. The one-stage prothrombin clotting time may also be increased.

LEUKAEMIAS

Acute Leukaemia

Diagnosis of acute leukaemia is supported by the finding of severe increasing anaemia, with anisocytosis, poikilocytosis and some polychromasia of the red cells, thrombocytopenia which is commonly severe, and a total white-cell count of less than $10 \times 10^9/l$ in up to one-third of cases, or more commonly from $20–50 \times 10^9/l$ per cmm. In stained blood films, in addition to the presence of nucleated red cells, it is found that the predominant white cells are 'blast' cells. The bleeding time is prolonged if the platelet count is low, and various non-specific changes occur in serum-enzyme levels of activity, including serum lactate dehydrogenase, alanine and aspartate aminotransferases, aldolase, but these are of negligible diagnostic value.

The bone marrow is very cellular, and 'blast' cells predominate with more mature cells of the same series (e.g. myeloblasts plus promyelocytes). The ʳythroid series is severely depressed, and megakaryocytes are scanty. Auer ˡies may be found in the cytoplasm of myeloblasts, myelocytes, mono-ˢs, or monocytes (depending on the type of the leukaemia).

Acute Myeloid Leukaemia

Various types of acute myeloid leukaemia occur:

ACUTE MYELOBLASTIC LEUKAEMIA

Diagnosis is confirmed by the finding that the peripheral blood white-cell count may not be greatly increased, and only a few myeloblasts may be seen in stained films. The myeloblasts tend to be small and may be mistaken for lymphocytes. The bone-marrow aspirate enables the diagnosis to be confirmed, since the marrow is hyperplastic and the majority of the cells are myeloblasts.

ACUTE MYELOID LEUKAEMIA

Diagnosis is confirmed by the finding that the peripheral stained blood films reveal a mixture of myeloblasts, promyelocytes and myelocytes with few adult neutrophils. The marrow aspirate enables the diagnosis to be confirmed, since the marrow is hyperplastic and the majority of the cells are myeloblasts.

ACUTE MYELOCYTIC LEUKAEMIA

Diagnosis is confirmed by the finding that the peripheral stained blood films reveal numerous promyelocytes with undifferentiated cytoplasmic granules, and often no obvious myeloblasts. The marrow aspirate enables the diagnosis of this rare variety to be confirmed, since the marrow is hyperplastic and the majority of the cells are myeloblasts. Disseminated intravascular coagulopathy may develop.

STEM-CELL LEUKAEMIA

The predominant cells both in the peripheral blood and bone marrow are primitive and undifferentiated. On tissue culture, they do not develop into typical myeloid, lymphoid, or monocytoid cells.

TESTS OF PROGRESS IN ACUTE MYELOID LEUKAEMIA

Chemotherapy is difficult in patients over the age of 60 years. In the less common acute myeloid leukaemia in children, there is more response to chemotherapy.

Acute Lymphatic Leukaemia

Diagnosis is confirmed by the finding that painful, enlarged lymph glands are associated with a high peripheral blood white-cell count, of which 90 per cent or more are lymphocytes or lymphoblasts. Both mature and immature lymphocytes are seen. The marrow aspirate enables the diagnosis to be confirmed since the majority of the cells in the marrow are lymphocytes or lymphoblasts.

TESTS OF PROGRESS

The non-T, non-B cell variety responds to chemotherapy better than does the B-cell variety. The T-cell variety is initially responsive, but remission is short. Acute lymphatic leukaemia is less common in adults, but does respond to chemotherapy. One-half of affected children can expect a long-term remission following treatment.

TESTS PROVIDING USEFUL NEGATIVE RESULTS

There is often thrombocytopenia in severe infectious mononucleosis (glandular fever), but in leukaemia the Paul–Bunnell test is negative.

Acute Reticulum-cell Leukaemia

Diagnosis is confirmed by the finding that enlarged lymph glands plus splenomegaly are associated with a moderately raised white-cell count. In stained blood films there is seen a relative lymphocytosis, but the lymphocytes are abnormal in appearance. In bone-marrow aspirates clumps of these cells are seen in large numbers.

Acute Plasma-cell Leukaemia

Diagnosis of this very rare condition is not acceptable until the absence of any increase in serum IgD or IgE has been excluded and no Bence Jones protein has been found in the urine (excluding the diagnosis of myeloma). Large numbers of plasma cells are found in stained blood films.

Monocytic Leukaemia

NAEGELI TYPE

Diagnosis of myelomonocytic leukaemia is confirmed by the finding of paramyeloblasts, resembling monocytes and monoblasts, in the peripheral blood and in bone-marrow aspirates in cases of clinically acute leukaemia. Frequently these cases show a progressive change to a more obvious myeloblastic leukaemia.

SCHILLING TYPE

Diagnosis of this rare form of true monocytic leukaemia is confirmed by the finding of predominantly promonocytes in the peripheral blood, with very few neutrophils or lymphocytes, and with a few myelocytes present. Similar cells are the commonest cells present in bone-marrow aspirates.

Chronic Lymphatic Leukaemia (Chronic Lymphocytic Leukaemia)

Diagnosis of this condition with slowly proliferating and long-surviving lymphocytes is confirmed by the finding of increased white blood-cell counts, usually from 50 to 90 × 10^9/l although higher counts are found. The predominant cells are mature lymphocytes (90–95 per cent of the white cells), but some lymphoblasts may also be found. In the early stages the haemoglobin is normal or slightly below normal, with a normal platelet count. Following rogressive development of the condition, anaemia is found (and acquired 'oimmune 'warm' or 'cold' haemolytic anaemia may occur, with reticulo- ɩis, positive Coombs' test and circulating nucleated red cells). Later, the ɩt count falls.

Bone-marrow aspirates contain an abnormally increased proportion of lymphocytes, but the relative number of lymphoblasts in proportion to lymphocytes does not appear to be a useful prognostic guide.

Lymph-gland biopsy may be useful to confirm the diagnosis. Various staging systems to assess the extent and severity of the disease have been devised.

TESTS OF PROGRESS

In the absence of anaemia or symptoms, in the presence of an abnormally high white-cell count, probably only supportive treatment accompanied by regular blood count is all that should be given.

With the development of anaemia, with pressure exerted by enlarging lymph glands, treatment with X-ray irradiation and/or chemotherapy with chlorambucil is indicated. The massive release of uric acid following such treatment needs special control.

Hairy-cell Leukaemia (Leukaemic Reticulo-endotheliosis)

Diagnosis of this B-cell malignancy, characterized by progressive debility, purpura and/or bleeding, in middle age or later (7 males : 1 female), with splenomegaly in most cases, is confirmed by the demonstration of 'hairy cells' on electron microscopy of bone-marrow aspirate. These cells contain acid phosphatase, which is resistant to tartrate. There is pancytopenia, and the 'hairy cells' can be seen in the peripheral blood film.

TESTS OF PROGRESS

This condition responds poorly to intensive chemotherapy. Blood transfusions are required at intervals to maintain the whole blood haemoglobin level.

TESTS PROVIDING USEFUL NEGATIVE RESULTS

The 'hairy cells' do not stain for the presence of esterase, and do not form 'rosettes' with sheep red cells.

Chronic Myeloid Leukaemia

Diagnosis of this condition is confirmed by the finding of moderate normochromic, normocytic anaemia, with a markedly raised white blood-cell count (usually more than $100 \times 10^9/l$). White cells consist of neutrophils, metamyelocytes and myelocytes predominantly, with up to 5 per cent of myeloblasts present. Rarely, the predominant cells may be eosinophilic or basophilic. The platelet count may be normal, but is frequently greatly increased, counts of over $1000 \times 10^9/l$ being found. Atypical large platelets and megakaryocyte fragments are also seen when the platelet count is very high. The neutrophil alkaline phosphatase activity is reduced almost to nil.

Bone-marrow aspirates are hyperplastic with myeloid hyperplasia, the predominant cell being the myelocyte. Myeloblasts are also abnormally increased in number, and later in the disease the erythroid cells are reduced in number. Megakaryocytes are plentiful. Examination of blood and bone-marrow reveals the presence of an abnormal chromosome, the so-called 'Philadelphia chromosome'.

TESTS OF PROGRESS

Prognosis is poor in cases with initially:

a. Increased peripheral blood basophils

b. Increased myeloblasts in peripheral blood

c. Thrombocytopenia

Following successful treatment with busulphan, 6-mercaptopurine, or X-ray irradiation, the peripheral blood white-cell count falls towards normal, the bone-marrow myeloblast count falls towards normal, the Philadelphia chromosome is no longer detectable, and the neutrophil alkaline phosphatase activity returns to normal. The massive excretion of uric acid may need special control. With relapse, the white-cell count climbs once more, with increasing numbers of myeloblasts, and with depression of neutrophil alkaline phosphatase activity and reappearance of the Philadelphia chromosome (i.e. malignant clone activity). Neither chemotherapy nor splenectomy delays metamorphosis. Once acute metamorphosis has occurred, 50 per cent remission occurs only if the 'blasts' are lymphoid.

Eosinophilic Leukaemia [R]

Diagnosis of this rare condition behaving clinically as a haematological malignancy, and which is probably a distinct entity, is confirmed by the finding of a high persistent eosinophil count in the peripheral blood, with marked eosinophil infiltration of the bone marrow.

The eosinophils stain strongly with PAS (i.e. rich in glycogen), stain strongly for acid phosphatase, and contain no alkaline phosphatase.

Polycythaemia Vera, Erythraemia

Diagnosis of this myeloproliferative disease is confirmed by the finding of haemoglobin concentrations of over 17 g/dl, with packed cell volumes exceeding 0·55, and red-cell counts of over 8×10^9/l. The MCV tends to be at the lower limit of normal. There is an increase in the white-cell count in many cases, and platelet counts are also above normal in many cases. Occasionally, megakaryocytes or fragments of megakaryocytes may be seen in peripheral blood films. Occasional nucleated red cells may be seen.

The total blood volume is increased to 83–133 ml/kg body weight and the red-cell mass is increased to 36–110 ml/kg body weight.

With the very great increase in circulating red cells, the ESR is virtually nil, but plasma-viscosity readings are normal in the absence of secondary disease. Coagulation studies on plasma may be misleading, unless the citrate concentration in samples is adjusted. (Excess citrate may cause some prolongation in prothrombin clotting times, and marked prolongation of activated partial thromboplastin times, spuriously suggesting a coagulation defect.)

Bone-marrow aspirates reveal active red cell, myeloid cell and megakaryocyte development, but are not diagnostic.

Neutrophil alkaline phosphatase activity is increased in many cases and serum uric acid may also be increased.

TESTS OF PROGRESS

Repeated venesections should be carried out to reduce the haematocrit to below 0·5 (preferably below 0·45). When this is achieved, with accompanying hypochromia and microcytosis, the blood count parameters will resemble those of thalassaemia (e.g. negative Discriminatory Factor). Unlike secondary polycythaemia, iron supplements should not be given, or haematopoiesis is again stimulated.

Subsequently, if venesection alone is insufficient to maintain the haematocrit below 0·45, therapy with ^{32}P or busulphan must be considered. Platelet counts should be kept below 400 × $10^9/l$. Regular haematological monitoring is essential.

Some cases terminate as myeloid leukaemia.

Pseudopolycythaemia, Benign Polycythaemia, Relative Polycythaemia

Abnormally increased haemoglobin concentration, with increased haematocrit, occurs in these cases, in whom it is found that the red-cell mass is normal, whereas the plasma volume is reduced. Many of the patients with this condition have essential hypertension and are on treatment with diuretics.

Erythraemic Myelosis, Erythroleukaemia (Di Guglielmo's Disease)

Diagnosis of this rare condition is confirmed by the finding of leuco-erythroblastic anaemia, with large numbers of nucleated red cells in the peripheral blood. In the acute form the nucleated red cells are predominantly basophilic whereas in the more chronic form the nucleated red cells have orthochromic cytoplasm and pyknotic nuclei. The reticulocyte count may also be increased and varies greatly from day to day. Thrombocytopenia is usual, and the white-cell count is normal or low, with some early myeloid forms present. The neutrophil alkaline phosphatase activity is low.

In bone-marrow aspirates, there is marked hyperplasia and dysplasia of the red-cell series. Ring sideroblasts are found, and in many cases megaloblastoid change is apparent. The nucleated red cells give a positive reaction to PAS staining (a negative reaction being found in true megaloblastic change). There may be a moderate increase in marrow myeloblasts and megakaryocytes are reduced in number. Chromosomal abnormalities are frequently found.

TESTS OF PROGRESS

Cytotoxic drugs may delay the progress of this disease, which often terminates as acute myeloblastic leukaemia.

Essential (Primary) Thrombocythaemia (Idiopathic Haemorrhagic Thrombocythaemia)

Diagnosis of this myeloproliferative disease, which may present with either gastrointestinal haemorrhage or peripheral vascular occlusion, is confirmed by the finding of persistent gross increase in the platelet count, exceeding $1000 \times 10^9/l$ with increased numbers of apparently normal megakaryocytes in the bone marrow aspirate.

Platelet function tests give variable results, and are not clinically useful. The bleeding time may be prolonged. If splenic vein thrombosis occurs, a fairly common complication, Howell–Jolly bodies appear in the peripheral blood.

TESTS OF PROGRESS

Following treatment with ^{32}P, the platelet count begins to fall by the end of the first week, whereas following treatment with busulphan, 2–6 mg/day, the platelet count falls by 4–6 weeks. Treatment should not be continued after the platelet count has fallen to $300 \times 10^9/l$.

Later, haemorrhages or thrombosis may occur, or myelosclerosis or polycythaemia may develop.

TESTS PROVIDING USEFUL NEGATIVE RESULTS

Other causes of persistent high platelet counts are excluded, e.g. chronic myeloid leukaemia, myelosclerosis, malignancy.

Myelosclerosis, Myelofibrosis (Agnogenic Myeloid Metaplasia)

Diagnosis of this condition occurring in the older age group (two-thirds are 50–70 years of age), characterized by insidious onset of anaemia, or of abdominal discomfort due to enlargement of the spleen, is made by examination of trephine biopsy of bone marrow (e.g. rib, iliac crest), with evidence of fibroblastic proliferation and evidence of disruption of the normal red-marrow architecture by fibrosis. Reticulin density alone in biopsy material is not helpful.

Three varieties have been described, based on histological appearance:
a. Megakaryocytic myelosis
b. Myelofibrosis
c. Osteomyelosclerosis

The condition results in a slowly progressive anaemia. The peripheral blood erythrocytes show increasing anisocytosis and poikilocytosis, and nucleated red cells are seen in increasing numbers. The reticulocyte count is frequently increased and fluctuates excessively from day to day. The TWBC may be normal, increased, or reduced, and 'stab' cells, myelocytes and moderate numbers of myeloblasts may be seen. Although this condition may terminate in frank myeloid leukaemia, the neutrophil alkaline phosphatase activity is often increased above normal. The platelet count may be normal, increased, or reduced, large platelets and even megakaryocytes being seen in stained films.

Bone-marrow aspirates may be 'dry taps' or suggest hypoplasia. Splenic punctures have been reported as revealing active haemopoiesis.

Acute Malignant Myelofibrosis (Megakaryocytic Leukaemia) [R]

These patients present with pancytopenia, and 'blast' cells are seen in the peripheral blood films. There is absence of overt hepatosplenomegaly. Bone-marrow trephine reveals a myelofibrotic picture with excessive numbers of megakaryocytes.

Patients die after a few months in a phase of acute leukaemia with high peripheral 'blast' counts. The serum lactate dehydrogenase activity is abnormally increased.

RARE CONDITIONS

Familial Polycythaemia (Benign Primary Polycythaemia) [R]

Diagnosis of this rare, possibly dominant, condition is supported by the finding of a family history of benign polycythaemia and the finding of polycythaemia without leucocytosis or thrombocytosis presenting in childhood or in young adults. Some cases may be due to a haemoglobinopathy or red-cell enzyme deficiency, associated with increased haemoglobin affinity for oxygen, in which case the PO_{50} is a useful estimation.

TESTS OF PROGRESS

No treatment has been recommended for this relatively benign condition.

Chronic Idiopathic Neutropenia (Agranulocytosis)

Diagnosis of this rare condition, which is seen most commonly in young women, and which is complicated by repeated attacks of infection in some, is confirmed by the finding of persistently low peripheral blood neutrophil counts $2–0 \cdot 5 \times 10^9/l$ with no response to infection, relative lymphocytosis in some cases, and normal haemoglobin and platelet counts or slight anaemia or slight thrombocytopia. The ESR may be increased.

In bone-marrow aspirates, the red-cell series and megakaryocyte formation are normal. On the one hand, the myeloid series may be hypoplastic and, on the other hand, the myeloid series may be hyperplastic with arrest at the stage of myelocytes, very few 'stab' cells or adult neutrophils being seen.

TESTS OF PROGRESS

In cases with hypoplasia of the myeloid series, it is important both to prevent infection and to treat infection with suitable antibiotic therapy.

In cases with hyperplasia of the myeloid series with 'maturation arrest', it may be worth trying the effect of a short course of steroid therapy, and if this results in a significant increase in peripheral blood neutrophils then splenectomy may be indicated.

TESTS PROVIDING USEFUL NEGATIVE RESULTS

There is no evidence of aleukaemic leukaemia or lymphoma.

Periodic Neutropenia (Cyclical Agranulocytosis)

Diagnosis of this rare condition is confirmed by the finding of periodic recurrence of neutropenia occurring at intervals of 14–30 days, with bouts of infection and malaise at the time of the neutropenia. Between attacks, the white-cell count returns to normal.

The bone-marrow aspirate shows selective myeloid hypoplasia during an attack of agranulocytosis.

TESTS OF PROGRESS

There may be improvement in some cases after splenectomy.

Infantile Genetic Agranulocytosis (Kostmann's Syndrome) [R]

Diagnosis of this very rare condition is confirmed by the finding of persistent severe neutropenia, with increased circulating eosinophils, lymphocytes, and monocytes. There may be increased platelet counts and there may be increased serum gammaglobulins in response to associated infection.

Bone-marrow aspirate reveals severe depression in myeloid cell production with only scanty myelocytes and promyelocytes.

TESTS OF PROGRESS

Family histories may reveal the mode of inheritance of the condition, and repeated blood counts will reveal any periodicity in the neutrophil counts.

Chronic Granulomatous Disease [R]

Diagnosis of this rare condition is confirmed by the finding of repeated attacks of relapsing infection, with neutrophilia related to infection. The neutrophils are unable to reduce nitroblue tetrazolium (NBTZ test) and are unable to ingest and destroy *Staphylococcus pyogenes*. Phagocytosis of *Candida albicans* may be normal, but the ability to lyse *Candida* in the cell is lost. Antibody responses are normal. Serum immunoglobulins IgA, IgG and IgM are all increased. A variant of this condition has been described, affecting fair-haired and red-haired patients, in which neutrophils can ingest and destroy streptococci normally, but are unable to destroy *Staph. pyogenes*. The patients suffer from repeated attacks of staphylococcal boils and abscesses, and the condition is appropriately named Job's syndrome.

Other Leucocyte Dysfunctions [R]

Diagnosis of these very rare conditions associated with repeated bacterial infection is confirmed by the finding of:

1. Lack of myeloperoxidase activity in neutrophils.
2. 'Lazy leucocyte' syndrome. Morphologically normal neutrophils in marrow, but defective release into peripheral blood in response to infection.
3. Abnormally reduced neutrophil chemotaxis in response to bacteria.

ANOMALIES

Acanthocytosis

Acanthocytes ('bur' cells) are seen in peripheral blood films in the more severe forms of a-beta-lipoproteinaemia.

Blood from uraemic patients contains numerous crenated cells which resemble 'bur' cells. In a-beta-lipoproteinaemia, the blood-urea concentration is not raised.

Blood which has taken many days to reach the laboratory since its collection contains numerous crenated cells.

Hereditary Hypersegmentation of Neutrophils

Diagnosis of this harmless inherited anomaly is confirmed by the finding that the neutrophils in the peripheral blood contain more nuclear lobes than normal.

TESTS PROVIDING USEFUL NEGATIVE RESULTS

The blood count is otherwise normal, with no evidence of underlying vitamin-B_{12} or folic-acid deficiency, or of iron deficiency, all conditions in which hypersegmentation of neutrophil nuclear lobes may be found.

Alder's Anomaly

Diagnosis of this rare harmless inherited anomaly is confirmed by the finding of coarse, dark azurophile granules in the cytoplasm of white cells in stained blood films.

Chédiak–Higashi–Steinbrinck Anomaly

Diagnosis of this autosomal recessive condition is confirmed by the finding of large abnormal cytoplasmic granules in peripheral blood neutrophils and inclusion bodies in tissue cultures of skin fibroblasts. Heterozygotes are otherwise clinically normal. Homozygotes are liable to repeated infections which they are unable to resist. These latter affected infants do not survive beyond 5 years.

May–Hegglin Anomaly

Diagnosis of this rare dominant condition is confirmed by the finding of Döhle (? Amato) bodies in the neutrophils, consisting of fusiform or crescentic bodies in the cytoplasm near the cell periphery. Thrombocytopenia occurs in over a third of cases, and platelets are frequently large and poorly granulated, with irregular shapes. Platelet function is normal.

There is maturation failure of the megakaryocytes in the bone marrow.

Clinically the condition appears to occur either in a completely symptomless form or as a severe and fatal purpuric state.

Pelger–Huet Anomaly

Diagnosis of this autosomal dominant condition is confirmed by the finding of markedly hyposegmented peripheral blood neutrophils, which have only one or two nuclear lobes. Heterozygotes are otherwise clinically normal. Homozygotes do not survive long.

Hereditary Angioneurotic Oedema [R]

Diagnosis of this very rare autosomal dominant condition is confirmed by the demonstration of deficiency in serum inhibitor of C1 esterase. Excessive swelling follows minor injury in these patients. Persistent action of C1 esterase might be the cause of persistently lowered serum concentrations of the C4 component of complement in these patients.

Inherited Deficiencies of Components of Complement [R]

A. HEREDITARY C2 DEFICIENCY

There is no increased liability to infection but there is an increased tendency to develop collagen diseases.

B. HEREDITARY C3 DEFICIENCY

Recurrent pyogenic infections.

C. HEREDITARY C5 DEFICIENCY

Liability to eczema with increased susceptibility to staphylococcal infection.

RETICULO-ENDOTHELIAL DISEASES

Hodgkin's Disease (Lymphadenoma)

Diagnosis of this malignant disease, characterized by multiple symptomatology, including the appearance of a painless and enlarging mass, or of unexplained persistent fever with fatigue and weight loss, is confirmed by histological examination of affected enlarged lymph glands. Biopsy material from bone marrow, skin, liver, or spleen, is diagnostic only in the late stages of the disease. The findings in the peripheral blood are non-specific. A normochromic, normocytic anaemia develops, with anisocytosis and poikilocytosis of the red cells, and occasionally circulating nucleated red cells. Occasionally, haemolytic anaemia develops, of the autoimmune type, with positive Coombs' test. The white-cell count may be normal, increased, or decreased. Similarly, the platelet count may be normal, increased, or decreased. An absolute eosinophilia develops in up to 10 per cent of cases, especially in cases with skin involvement.

Bone-marrow findings are non-specific, although occasionally Reed–Sternberg cells may be identified in marrow aspirate. Marrow reticulum cells and plasma cells may be increased.

With bone involvement, serum alkaline phosphatase activity may be increased.

TESTS OF PROGRESS

Various methods of classification of the extent of the disease have been used, poor prognosis being associated with widespread disease, and with certain histological features.

Treatment with radiotherapy and/or chemotherapy on a long-term basis has greatly improved the outlook in this disease, but frequent regular haematological monitoring is necessary.

Non-Hodgkin's Lymphoma

Diagnosis is made by lymph-gland biopsy, bone-marrow biopsy, splenic biopsy and/or liver biopsy, and careful histological examination enables such lymphomes to be classified.

TESTS OF PROGRESS

In general terms, prognosis of diffuse varieties is less good than for nodular forms, and regional disease has a less favourable prognosis than localized disease.

Diffuse undifferentiated < diffuse histiocytic < diffuse mixed < diffuse lymphocytic poorly differentiated < diffuse lymphocytic well differentiated.

Nodular histiocytic < nodular mixed < nodular lymphocytic poorly differentiated < nodular lymphocytic well differentiated.

During and following treatment with radiation/chemotherapy/? immunotherapy, monitoring of haemoglobin, white blood cells and platelets is necessary.

Letterer–Siwe Disease

Diagnosis of this rare disease may be supported by the finding of numerous large histiocytes in bone-marrow aspirate or in lymph-gland biopsy material. Spleen, liver, lymph glands, lungs and bone marrow are infiltrated with sheets of histiocytes. Rarely haemohistiocytes may be seen in peripheral blood films. A normocytic, normochromic anaemia may develop, and thrombocytopenia occurs in some cases. The reticulocyte count may be increased. There may be neutrophilia, eosinophilia, or lymphocytosis, and nucleated red cells may occur in the peripheral blood.

Sézary's Syndrome

Diagnosis of this rare disease of the reticulo-endothelial system is confirmed by the finding of Sézary giant cells in the peripheral blood or in marrow-aspirate films.

Hand–Schüller–Christian Disease

Diagnosis of this rare disease is confirmed by histological examination of bone biopsy of bony erosions. Occasionally positive biopsy material can be obtained from liver, spleen, or lymph glands. Foamy histiocytes may be seen in films of bone-marrow aspirate.

Severe leuco-erythroblastic anaemia develops later in the disease.

14 *Endocrine Disorders*

PITUITARY DISEASES

Acromegaly

Diagnosis is suspected by the finding of a random fasting morning Human Growth Hormone (HGH) level exceeding 10 mU/l (μg/l), but random tests may produce false positive results. The normal diurnal variation in plasma cortisol is lost, with higher results being found at midnight.

To confirm the diagnosis, with an intravenous cannula set up 1 hour before the start of the test (to avoid increase in serum HGH due to stress) a 50-g oral glucose tolerance test is carried out on the fasting patient, with initial HGH, TSH, T4, T3, thyroxine index (free T4 and T3 if available) and plasma cortisol levels being taken at the start, and HGH and cortisol levels being measured with each blood glucose sample throughout the glucose tolerance test. In acromegaly HGH levels fail to fall below 2 mU/l and may show a paradoxical rise following glucose. (HGH may also fail to be depressed normally following oral glucose in severe renal or liver disease.)

The fasting blood glucose level may be increased and the blood glucose curve is 'diabetic', with insulin resistance. Glycosuria is found in up to 40 per cent of cases. The HGH level does not fall following intravenous insulin (0·3 units per kg body weight) with blood glucose falling below 2·2 mmol/l (40 mg/100 ml), when plasma cortisol and HGH levels are measured every 30 minutes for 2 hours. Urine calcium and hydroxyproline output may be increased and serum calcium is raised in some cases, reflecting increased bone turnover. Plasma inorganic phosphate may be increased with reduced renal phosphate clearance.

TESTS OF PROGRESS

The thyroid function tests are necessary to exclude throtoxicosis, and a TRH test injection is followed by TSH estimations. Plasma prolactin and gonadotrophins in females, and serum testosterone in males, are useful in cases of acromegaly in the assessment of failure of pituitary function, giving useful baseline levels prior to treatment, and indicating the need for specific replacement therapy. Low plasma cortisol levels at 9.00 a.m. falling below 200 nmol/l (7 μg/dl), or after glucose or insulin stress, indicate need for replacement therapy. In cases treated by irradiation of the pituitary gland, implantation of radioactive pellets in the pituitary fossa, surgical removal of discrete adenomas, or ablation of a diffuse hyperplasia of the anterior pituitary gland, plasma HGH estimations can be used to demonstrate success of the treatment. Ideally plasma HGH levels should fall to 10 mU/l or less without associated deficiency in pituitary trophic hormones. Estimation of thyroid function, plasma cortisol, gonadotrophin in females and serum testosterone in males can be used to assess specific replacement therapy.

TESTS PROVIDING USEFUL NEGATIVE RESULTS

Fasting morning basal HGH levels of less than 5 mU/l virtually exclude the diagnosis of acromegaly. Plasma cortisol levels exceeding 550 nmol/l during glucose or insulin tolerance tests indicate an adequate hypothalamic–adrenal axis.

Pituitary Gigantism [R]

Diagnosis of gigantism in adults (height exceeding 80 inches), and in children (height more than + 3 sd. above the mean height for coevals) resulting from excessive secretion of HGH by the pituitary in patients before the epiphyseal plates of the long bones and the vertebrae have fused, is confirmed by the finding of raised plasma HGH levels, which remain raised after an oral glucose load, or after insulin-induced hypoglycaemia.

Patients in whom the tumour is confined to the sella turcica have low HGH levels in the CSF; raised CSF levels indicating suprasellar extension.

USEFUL NEGATIVE RESULTS

Other anterior pituitary hormone levels in the serum are low, including FSH, LH, TSH, and ACTH. Serum TSH levels may not respond to TRH injection, and serum prolactin levels may also be low with no response to TRH. Hypogonadism is frequently found in these cases.

In patients who are constitutionally tall, the serum HGH level is normal, and an oral glucose load causes HGH suppression to less than 2 mU/l.

TESTS OF PROGRESS

After successful surgical ablation of the tumour, serum HGH levels fall to normal.

Pituitary Tumour

Diagnosis of the presence of a pituitary tumour, characterized by the early signs of amenorrhoea in women, or loss of body and facial hair with increasing impotence in men, with subsequent headache and loss of visual fields, is supported by the finding of loss of endocrine function (chromophobe adenoma). Some tumours are initially associated with hypersecretion of anterior pituitary hormones, resulting in gigantism before puberty, or acromegaly after puberty, followed later by progressive pituitary failure.

TESTS OF PROGRESS

Following successful surgical removal of a pituitary tumour, replacement therapy can be successfully monitored by regular estimations of plasma cortisol and serum T4 levels.

Hypopituitarism (Anterior Lobe)

Diagnosis of hypopituitarism, characterized by early failure of gonadotrophin and growth hormone secretion, with failure of ACTH and/or TSH production later, is supported by the finding of:

1. Low levels of plasma T4 and cortisol (and testosterone in men).
2. Low levels of plasma LH, TSH, FSH and prolactin.
3. Low response levels of GH (growth hormone), ACTH (releasing cortisol) and prolactin to insulin tolerance test.
4. Low response of TSH and prolactin to TRH.
5. Demonstration of intact adrenals by normal adrenocortical response to ACTH injection.
6. Abnormal response to clomiphene test in adults (with reduced secretion of LH and gonadal steroids).
7. Reduced release of GH after arginine infusion.
8. Metyrapone test can be used to assess the hypothalamic–pituitary–adrenal axis.

Nelson's Syndrome [R]

Diagnosis of ACTH-secreting pituitary tumours, which are rarely malignant and which appear 6 months–16 years after bilateral adrenalectomy for adrenal hyperplasia associated with Cushing's syndrome, and which are accompanied by extreme hyperpigmentation of the skin is confirmed by the demonstration of very high plasma ACTH and MSH levels.

Prolactin-secreting Pituitary Adenoma (Microadenoma)

Diagnosis of this condition associated with amenorrhoea, with/or without galactorrhoea, and infertility in women, or sterility with impotence and/or gynaecomastia in men, is supported by the finding of raised serum prolactin levels, with low serum testosterone levels in men.

TESTS OF PROGRESS

Surgical removal or pharmacological suppression with bromocriptine is only necessary, if relief of sterility or infertility is required, otherwise no treatment is indicated.

TESTS PROVIDING USEFUL NEGATIVE RESULTS

It is important to ascertain that the patient is not taking any drug capable of causing galactorrhoea.

Pituitary Dwarfism

Diagnosis of this condition of reduced stature without disproportion, which is not manifest at birth, and with normal intelligence but delayed puberty, is confirmed by the demonstration of absence of serum growth hormone, even after insulin-induced hypoglycaemia. Further tests may reveal secondary hypothyroidism and secondary hypoadrenal function, consequences of hypopituitarism.

Follicular stimulating hormone (FSH) output in the urine is abnormally low after puberty.

Short stature without disproportion manifest at birth, may also be due to:

Constitutional delay in growth and adolescence

Congenital dwarfism

Association with primary hypothyroidism

Turner's syndrome

Pituitary Infantilism

Diagnosis is supported by the finding of low output of 17-oxosteroids in the urine.

Fröhlich's Syndrome (Juvenile Dystrophia Adiposogenitalis)

Diagnosis of this rare condition, characterized by dwarfism, hypothyroidism, and adiposity (rarely attacks of hypoglycaemia), is supported by the finding of deficiency of pituitary trophic hormone following a combined insulin tolerance test (HGH, ACTH, TSH and prolactin responses are reduced).

TESTS PROVIDING USEFUL NEGATIVE RESULTS

Laurence–Moon–Biedl syndrome (a rare congenital familial condition characterized by obesity, hypogonadism, dwarfism, mental retardation, polydactyly and retinitis pigmentosa) does not give the same response to the combined insulin tolerance test.

Diabetes Insipidus

Diagnosis is indicated clinically by the finding of massive and persistent polyuria, rarely less than 3 litres per day, with fixed low specific gravity of the urine, and loss of the normal diurnal variation in urine flow. Increased fluid intake, if available, enables the patient to maintain a normal plasma osmolality. The diagnosis is confirmed by results obtained following water deprivation. Without previous overnight fluid restriction, and after initial weighing, the patient is deprived of all fluids, being weighed every 4 hours. If the body weight falls by more than 3 per cent the test must be stopped. In diabetes insipidus the urine osmolality remains less than 300 mosmol/kg (specific gravity less than 1·010), with persistent high volume, while the plasma osmolality, initially high-normal, rises above 300 mosmol/kg. The patient is then allowed unrestricted fluid and food, and either 2 µg desmopressin i.m. or 20 µg desmopressin nasally is given. Urine samples are collected and tested hourly. Following desmopressin, urine osmolality rises above 600 mosmol/kg and the patient's sense of thirst is relieved within the next 4 hours, with a fall in urine volume.

If plasma vasopressin estimations are available they are only useful in diagnosis in dehydrated patients or during infusion of hypertonic saline, and in the context of concurrent plasma and urine osmolalities and basal urine flow.

TESTS PROVIDING USEFUL NEGATIVE RESULTS

Renal function, assessed by blood urea, and microscopy and culture of the urine, is normal. There must be no evidence of diabetes mellitus with glycosuria, nor should there be evidence of hypercalcaemia with associated renal damage, nor hypokalaemia. A positive response to desmopressin excludes nephrogenic diabetes insipidus.

During fluid deprivation, normal subjects have a reduction in urine flow to 0·5 ml/min with increase in urine osmolality to more than 800 mosmol/kg. In 8 hours the plasma osmolality in normal subjects does not rise above 300 mosmol/kg.

TESTS OF PROGRESS

Treatment with 0·1–0·2 ml (10–20 μg) desmopressin intranasally (or 1–2 μg i.m. daily) gives satisfactory water balance control. Chlorpropamide and carbamazepine both sensitize the kidneys to the action of vasopressin.

Compulsive Water Drinking [R]

Diagnosis of this rare condition is confirmed by the finding of normal plasma osmolality following water deprivation for 8 hours, with a normal rise in urine osmolality above 600 mosmol/kg—although some chronic cases only concentrate their urine to the lower limits of normal. In these latter cases, it is found that urine concentration following water deprivation exceeds urine concentration following desmopressin (cf. diabetes insipidus).

USEFUL NEGATIVE RESULTS

Water deprivation results in urine osmolality ≥ 450 mosmol/kg in most cases, and desmopressin at the end of the water deprivation test has little effect on urine osmolality. If the urine concentration does not rise before plasma osmolality reaches 295 mosmol/kg and/or plasma sodium reaches 143 mmol/l, primary polydipsia is excluded. Also plasma osmolality remains in the normal range. With free access to water, if plasma osmolality exceeds 295 mosmol/kg and plasma sodium exceeds 143 mmol/l then primary poly-dipsia is excluded.

Syndrome of Inappropriate Antidiuretic Hormone Secretion (SIADH)

This clinical state, with a variety of causes, ranges from symptomless dilutional hypnatraemia with water retention to acute water intoxication with fatigue, nausea, vomiting, mental confusion, usually without oedema; the symptoms being related to the severity of hyponatraemia and water retention but more to the rate of development of the syndrome.

Plasma sodium concentration falls (weakness being common at 120 mmol/l, and neurological changes occurring at 110 mmol/l, but urine sodium excretion continues at a level inappropriate for the corresponding plasma sodium concentration, urine osmolality being persistently high for the plasma osmolality. Plasma urea concentration tends to be low.

TESTS OF PROGRESS

Apart from specific treatment of its cause, fluid restriction results in return of plasma sodium towards normal in mild cases. In more severe cases, fluid restriction plus therapy with demeclocycline and small doses of fludrocortisone is necessary. Therapy with large doses of oral urea shows promise, and there is an inverse relationship between urine urea excretion and urine sodium excretion.

Emergency treatment with frusemide bolus, followed by intravenous hypertonic saline when diuresis has started, is potentially dangerous (with risks of changes in plasma potassium and too rapid transfer of water from cells to ECF) and is unnecessary in most cases.

TESTS PROVIDING USEFUL NEGATIVE RESULTS

There is no evidence of diabetes mellitus, no hypercalcaemia, adrenal function is normal and renal function is normal, apart from the inability (due to ADH action) to form a dilute urine.

Pituitary Hypogonadotrophinism

Diagnosis is supported by the finding of reduced or absent excretion of gonadotrophins in the urine. Females are infertile, and males do not produce spermatozoa and are also therefore infertile.

TESTS PROVIDING USEFUL NEGATIVE RESULTS

In primary hypogonadism the urinary output of gonadotrophins is increased. Adrenal and thyroid functions are normal.

(Gonadotrophins are not detectable in the urine until puberty in normal people.)

Essential Hypernatraemia [R]

Diagnosis of this rare condition, characterized by episodic muscle weakness, and normotensive hypernatraemia with hyperosmolality, thought to be due to absence of release of ADH in response to increase in osmolality, but normal ADH release in response to blood volume variation, is supported by the finding of persistent hypernatraemia with hyperosmolality.

TESTS PROVIDING USEFUL NEGATIVE RESULTS

Renal function is normal. Response to vasopressin is normal. The plasma sodium concentration remains high after prolonged water loading with low sodium intake.

ADRENAL DISORDERS

Cushing's Syndrome (Preliminary Screen)

Diagnosis of Cushing's syndrome is strongly suggested by the finding of absence of suppression of plasma cortisol overnight after 1 mg oral dexamethasone, at bedtime on the previous evening. The morning plasma cortisol at 0800–0900 hrs exceeds 180 nmol/l. The normal plasma cortisol rhythm is lost, and either raised morning and midnight, or normal morning and raised midnight plasma cortisol levels are found (the patient not being stressed by blood sampling). A further initial screening test, the 2-day dexamethasone suppression test is also found to be abnormal. Plasma cortisol remains above 350 nmol/l, and there is adequate suppression of 17-oxogenic steroid excretion in the urine. A fourth test, the insulin tolerance test, is also abnormal. This latter test is potentially dangerous, and can only be carried out under careful supervision in hospital. After insulin-induced hypoglycaemia (severe enough to be associated with sweating, hunger and drowsiness), there is an impaired increase in plasma cortisol. If these preliminary screening tests for Cushing's syndrome are positive, then further special tests are required to define the cause of Cushing's syndrome, and to exclude the effects of obesity, alcoholism, etc.

USEFUL NEGATIVE RESULTS

Following the 1 mg dexamethasone suppression test, morning plasma cortisol levels below 180 nmol/l virtually exclude the possibility of Cushing's syndrome.

Normal levels of plasma cortisol, with the normal circadian rhythm are strongly against a diagnosis of Cushing's syndrome.

Following the 2-day dexamethasone suppression test (0·5 mg dexamethasone 6-hourly for 8 doses), the finding of plasma cortisol levels below 180 nmol/l, and urine 17-oxogenic steroid excretion below 25 μmol/24 hours are normal responses.

After hypoglycaemia induced by insulin injection, the plasma cortisol increases by more than +220 nmol/l.

MORE SPECIFIC DIAGNOSTIC TESTS

A. INCREASED GLUCOCORTICOID AND ANDROGEN SECRETION BY ADRENAL ADENOMA OR CARCINOMA

Diagnosis is supported by the finding of no detectable ACTH in the patient's plasma, and an impaired plasma cortisol response to the Synacthen test. There is no suppression by the high-dose dexamethasone suppression test of either plasma cortisol or of urinary 17-oxogenic steroid excretion (except for a few cases of obesity, etc.).

Following injection of metyrapone, there is no rise in plasma ACTH or increase in urine excretion of 17-oxogenic steroids.

In cases of Cushing's syndrome due to adrenal carcinoma, urine 17-oxo-steroids are markedly increased (more than 150 μmol/l).

If the urinary 17-oxosteroid excretion is normal or low, with marked excretion of 17-oxogenic steroids, these findings suggest that Cushing's syndrome is caused by a cortisol-producing adenoma.

B. ECTOPIC ACTH PRODUCTION

Diagnosis is supported by the finding of plasma ACTH levels exceeding

20 ng/l when ectopic production of ACTH stimulates the adrenals maximally (although ATCH levels may be normal or fluctuate widely).

There is impaired response to the Synacthen (ACTH) test, with reduced or absent increase in plasma cortisol, and inadequate suppression by the high-dose dexamethasone suppression test of plasma cortisol and urinary excretion of 17-oxogenic steroids.

Following injections of metyrapone there is usually no rise in plasma ACTH or of urinary excretion of 17-oxogenic steroids.

C. SECONDARY TO INCREASED PRODUCTION OF ACTH BY THE PITUITARY GLAND

Diagnosis is supported by the finding of high-normal to slightly raised plasma ACTH levels (up to 250 ng/l) with no normal circadian fluctuations. Following the high-dose dexamethasone suppression test, there is at least 50 per cent suppression of plasma cortisol, and suppression of urinary 17-oxogenic steroid excretion to less than 50 per cent of the basal excretion rate. Following metyrapone injections there is an exaggerated at least 3-fold increase above basal results in plasma ACTH concentrations, and in urinary 17-oxogenic steroid excretion.

TESTS OF PROGRESS

Plasma ACTH estimations are useful in monitoring chemotherapy or replacement therapy in patients with ectopic ACTH secretion syndrome. Blood samples should be taken immediately before the morning dose.

Plasma ACTH levels are also useful in the assessment of the effectiveness of involution or ablation of the pituitary gland.

The finding of raised plasma ACTH levels after bilateral adrenalectomy for Cushing's syndrome suggests the future development of Nelson's syndrome.

Primary Hyperaldosteronism (Conn's Syndrome)

Diagnosis of this uncommon cause of hypertension with raised diastolic pressure and hypokalaemia, due to a unilateral adrenocortical adenoma secreting excess aldosterone (60 per cent) or bilateral hyperplasia or multinodular glands (40 per cent) (or very rarely carcinoma), is confirmed by the finding of:

1. Episodic hypokalaemia ($\leqslant$ 3·5 mmol/l) with increased urine potassium, plasma sodium $\geqslant$ 140 mmol/l and/or plasma bicarbonate > 30 mmol/l without respiratory trouble, the patient having had no diuretics for 3 weeks and no antihypertensives for 1 week.

2. On a diet containing about 100 mmol sodium/day and about 70 mmol potassium/day, without diuretics or antihypertensive, as in (1) above, the patient is given 80 mg furosemide orally and remains upright for the next 3 hours (quietly walking about or standing). After 3 hours, plasma renin (or angiotensin II) is low with markedly raised serum aldosterone levels.

3. On the above diet (2) without antihypertensives or diuretics for 5 days, the patient is kept in bed overnight, a 24-hour urine potassium (and 18-monoglucuronide of aldosterone) is estimated. With the patient recumbent (not having got up earlier), blood is taken for plasma aldosterone and plasma renin (or angiotensin II). The patient then gets up, and after 30 min (after

4 hours in some laboratories), plasma renin (or angiotensin II) is sampled again. Plasma potassium is low, with persistent raised urine potassium excretion, abnormally raised plasma aldosterone with low plasma renin (angiotensin II).

The sample taken after standing for 30 min (4 hours) shows an increase in plasma renin in primary nodular hyperplasia, and no rise or even a fall in plasma renin in cases of adenoma. In these latter cases, plasma aldosterone differs between adrenal venous samples taken from the two sides. Scanning investigations can follow.

USEFUL NEGATIVE RESULTS

In normal subjects after 5 days on 100 mmol sodium and 70 mmol potassium/day, urine potassium output falls to less than 20 mmol/day in normal subjects and in patients with essential hypertension without hyper-aldosteronism. Urine 17-ketosteroids and 17-hydroxycorticosteroids outputs are normal in primary hyperaldosteronism, 17-hydroxycorticosteroids excretion increasing in Cushing's syndrome.

Plasma renin (angiotensin II) is increased with increased plasma hyper-aldosterone in secondary hyperaldosteronism, and there is no reduction in raised blood pressure following treatment with spironolactone.

TESTS OF PROGRESS

Following surgical removal of an adrenal adenoma, or control of hypertension with spironolactone (or amiloride), plasma potassium rises to normal. (Spironolactone 400 mg/day causes a reduction in blood pressure in up to 20 per cent of essential hypertension cases with normal plasma aldosterone levels.)

Secondary Hyperaldosteronism

Diagnosis of the syndrome of secondary hyperaldosteronism consists of diagnosis of the primary causative condition, which may include:
1. With hypertension
   Malignant hypertension
   Renovascular hypertension
2. Without hypertension
   Nephrosis
   Cirrhosis with ascites
   Congestive cardiac failure
   Sodium-losing renal disease
   Pregnancy
   Bartter's syndrome [R]

Increased plasma renin secretion results in increased production of angiotensin II, followed by production of aldosterone.

USEFUL NEGATIVE RESULTS

Primary hyperaldosteronism is excluded by the finding of persistently raised plasma renin.

Bartter's Syndrome (Juxtaglomerular Hyperplasia) [R]

Diagnosis of this rare condition presenting in early childhood with failure to thrive, hypogonadism and delayed puberty, salt craving with polydipsia and polyuria with normal blood pressure, is supported by the finding of hypokalaemic tetany, with increased urine and plasma renin, angiotensin II, and aldosterone, with potassium wasting.

Renal biopsy shows juxtaglomerular hyperplasia (which may also be found in Addison's disease, laxative abuse and familial chloridorrhoea).

TESTS OF PROGRESS

Clinical improvement follows treatment with oral potassium supplements plus spironolactone (anti-aldosterone).

TESTS PROVIDING USEFUL NEGATIVE RESULTS

There is no evidence of adrenocortical hypofunction.

JUXTAGLOMERULAR CELL TUMOUR [R]

Renal vein renin concentrations may be used to identify the affected side.

PSEUDO-BARTTER'S SYNDROME

Results from surreptitious vomiting with chronic use of diuretics or laxatives.

Liddle's Syndrome (Pseudohyperaldosteronism) [R]

Diagnosis of this rare inherited condition, presenting clinically as primary hyperaldosteronism, is supported by the finding of hypertension with hypokalaemia, and metabolic alkalosis, but with low plasma and urine aldosterone levels.

TESTS OF PROGRESS

The abnormalities are corrected by triamterene (100 mg/day) but not by spironolactone. An abnormality of membrane transfer of sodium has been demonstrated in the red cells, and it has been suggested that the distal renal tubular cells conserve sodium and excrete potassium in the virtual absence of aldosterone.

Phaeochromocytoma

Diagnosis of phaeochromocytoma is confirmed by the finding of raised plasma noradrenaline levels, in blood taken from a supine resting patient in the morning after an overnight fast, all drugs having been discontinued for 48 hours, and no recent intake of bananas, coffee, chocolate or vanilla. Urine excretion of catecholamines, total metanephrines (metadrenaline and nor-metadrenaline) and/or 3-methoxy-4-hydroxymandelic acid (HMMA, VMA) excretions are increased significantly above normal. Collection about the time of paroxysm of hypertension is useful.

USEFUL NEGATIVE RESULTS

Plasma catecholamine levels below 1000 ng/ml exclude phaeochromocytoma. Results falling between 1000 and 2000 ng/ml are equivocal, and further tests are needed.

Provocative tests are not safe, and are no longer carried out. Normal levels of metanephrines and/or VMA in two or more 24-hour urine collections is strongly against the diagnosis of phaeochromocytoma.

TESTS OF PROGRESS

If goitre is present, serum calcitonin estimation is helpful. Serum calcium estimation should be carried out to exclude familial hyperparathyroidism.

Adrenocortical Insufficiency

Diagnosis is confirmed by the finding of abolition of the normal circadian rhythm of plasma cortisol levels with a low 0900 hrs value. Plasma cortisol concentration is less than 180 nmol/l, and fails to increase during the short 5-hour Synacthen test. In ill patients, plasma sodium $\leqslant$ 130 mmol/l, plasma potassium $\geqslant$ 5 mmol/l, plasma urea greater than 7·5 mmol/l, and plasma glucose levels are low.

Further tests are required to differentiate different causes of adrenocortical insufficiency.

A. PRIMARY ADRENOCORTICAL INSUFFICIENCY

Following demonstration of abolition of the normal plasma cortisol circadian rhythm with a low 0900 hrs level, and failure of the plasma cortisol (initially less than 180 nmol/l) to increase, to increase only inadequately, or to rise sluggishly over 5 hours, plasma ACTH levels are found to be increased. The 3-day Synacthen test is useful. Plasma cortisol fails to increase significantly, and urine excretion of 17-oxogenic steroids fails to increase.

B. ADRENOCORTICAL INSUFFICIENCY SECONDARY TO PITUITARY INSUFFICIENCY

Following results of initial tests suggesting adrenocortical insufficiency, plasma ACTH levels are found to be low.

The 3-day Synacthen test shows a marked but delayed increase in urine output of 17-oxogenic steroids and plasma cortisol. Plasma sodium concentration falls (dilutional hyponatremia) and plasma glucose concentration is low.

C. CORTICOSTEROID-INDUCED ADRENOCORTICAL INSUFFICIENCY

A short 5-hour Synacthen test carried out in the morning before any morning steroid intake can show a low basal plasma cortisol level with a blunted (or nil) response to Synacthen. It has been found that synthetic steroid analogues (e.g. prednisolone) suppress ACTH release to a greater extent than either cortisone or hydrocortisone.

Congenital Adrenal Hyperplasia

Various congenital adrenal enzyme deficiency states exist:

1. 21-HYDROXYLASE DEFICIENCY (ADRENOGENITAL SYNDROME)

This condition accounts for more than 90 per cent of all cases in this group. It occurs:

a. Mild variety — presenting with virilization in female infants, and with precocious puberty in males.

b. Severe variety — about one-third of the cases are severe, and present with severe vomiting and dehydration in newborn babies.

Diagnosis is strongly supported by the finding of markedly raised plasma 17-hydroxyprogesterone levels. Plasma androstenedione is also increased. Urine pregnanetriol and 17-oxosteroid excretion is also markedly increased. When vomiting and dehydration are severe, plasma sodium falls and plasma potassium concentration is increased. Plasma ACTH levels are high.

TESTS OF PROGRESS

Following treatment with adequate salt intake, fludrocortisone (or depot deoxycorticosterone) plus cortisol, plasma sodium, potassium and 17-hydroxy-progesterone levels return to normal.

Urine pregnanediol and 17-oxosteroids can also be used to monitor treatment.

In affected fetuses, amniotic fluid 17-hydroxyprogesterone levels have been found to be three times the upper limit of normal at 15–21 weeks.

2. C-11-HYDROXYLASE DEFICIENCY (ADRENOGENITAL SYNDROME)

This is the second most common enzyme deficiency in this group (5 per cent of all cases). The majority of cases have a partial enzyme deficiency with moderate symptoms, a minority have a severe enzyme deficiency and are hypertensive.

Diagnosis of this condition, associated with virilization and ambiguous genitalia in female infants, and normal genitalia in male infants, with sodium and water retention and hypertension in less than half the cases, is confirmed by the finding of a marked increase in plasma androstenedione, urine oxosteroids and 17-hydroxycorticosteroids.

Plasma sodium concentration is usually normal or slightly raised, with normal or slightly reduced plasma potassium levels, and normal urinary sodium output.

3. 3-BETA-HYDROXYDEHYDROGENASE DEFICIENCY [R]

There is genital ambiguity in infants of either sex, salt-losing hyponatremia and hyperkalaemia, with underproduction of cortisol, aldosterone and sex hormones.

Diagnosis is strongly supported by the finding of increased plasma dehydroepiandrosterone (DHA) and increased urinary output of 17-oxosteroids.

4. 17-HYDROXYLASE DEFICIENCY [R]

This condition is non-virilizing, with salt retention, hypertension and hypokalaemia.

Diagnosis is strongly supported by increased plasma DOC (21-hydroxy-pregn-4-ene-3,20-dione) and a markedly increased excretion of its metabolite in the urine. Plasma aldosterone is reduced.

5. 18-HYDROXYLASE/18-HYDROXYSTENOL DEHYDROGENASE DEFICIENCY [R]

This very rare condition is associated with aldosterone deficiency, with production of cortisol and sex steroids unaffected. There is salt wasting with hyponatremia and hyperkalaemia.

Diagnosis is strongly supported by the finding of increased 18-hydroxycorticosterone in the plasma, and increased excretion of its metabolites in the urine, which is not suppressed by dexamethasone.

6. 20-ALPHA-HYDROXYLASE AND 20-22-LYASE DEFICIENCY [R]

This very rare condition affecting both adrenals and gonads, presenting with very severe adrenal insufficiency, persistent vomiting and dehydration, hyponatremia, hyperkalaemia and salt loss in the urine, is usually rapidly fatal.

Isolated Hypoaldosteronism [R]

TYPE I (CORTISONE METHYLOXIDASE DEFICIENCY I) (CMO I)

Cortisone methyloxidase activity is reduced. 18-Hydroxycorticoids and aldosterone are reduced.

TYPE II (CMO II)

18-Hydroxycorticoids from the zona glomerulosa are increased with reduced aldosterone.

In both Type I and Type II there is hyperkalaemia with hyponatraemia. Neonates fail to thrive, have retarded growth and metabolic acidosis.

TESTS OF PROGRESS

Cases should be treated with mineralocorticoids and adequate salt replacement.

Thymic Tumour

Various disorders are asociated with thymoma:

1. Immunoglobulin disorders, including agammaglobulinaemia, dysgammaglobulinaemia.

2. Red-cell aplasia.
3. Myasthenia gravis.

PARATHYROID DISORDERS

Primary Hyperparathyroidism

Diagnosis of this condition, characterized by symptoms which may include symptoms from renal stones, polyuria, loss of weight, weakness and polyuria, or a feeling of malaise, is supported by the finding of an abnormally raised serum calcium level. Discriminant analysis of the raised serum calcium, low fasting plasma phosphate, raised serum chloride (more than 102 mmol/l), reduced plasma bicarbonate, plasma urea and alkaline phosphatase (raised in some cases) can be useful in diagnosis. Serial serum calcium estimations may be needed to confirm the hypercalcaemia. High serum calcium levels are also found in familial hyperparathyroidism (dominant) without overt clinical symptoms.

Urine calcium excretion, while on a low calcium intake, is increased, unless there is renal damage (> 45 mmol/24 hours on a 30 mmol/day diet, or > 100 mmol/day on a normal diet).

Plasma parathyroid hormone estimation can be useful in the localization of the tumour—multiple blood samples are taken from around the four glands, and those samples taken near the tumour give high results.

TESTS OF PROGRESS

Hydrocortisone, 40 mg 8-hourly for 10 days (followed by gradual withdrawal over the next 4–5 days), results in no change in the raised serum calcium level—in other conditions causing hypercalcaemia, hydrocortisone causes a fall towards normal of serum calcium. Urine 3′,5′-AMP (expressed as a ratio of urinary creatinine excretion) is increased during the hydrocortisone suppression test (cf. normal controls).

Following successful removal of the tumour at operation, serum calcium levels fall to normal, and may fall below, with calcium-hungry bones. Vitamin D therapy may be necessary later, if serum calcium levels remain below normal.

Schmidt's Syndrome, Multiple Adenomatosis [R]

TYPE I

Parathyroid adenoma may be associated with:

a. Pituitary adenoma—presenting with acromegaly; intracranial pressure; hypopituitarism.

b. Adenoma of pancreatic islet cells, with hypoglycaemia (Werner's syndrome).

c. Zollinger–Ellison syndrome.

TYPE II

Sipple's syndrome, pluriglandular syndrome
  a. Parathyroid tumour.
  b. Phaeochromocytoma.
  c. Medullary carcinoma of thyroid.
  d. Occasionally with Cushing's syndrome.

Multiple Endocrine Neoplasia Syndromes [AD with variable penetrance]

TYPE I

Multiple endocrine adenomatosis, which includes: hyperparathyroidism, carcinoid tumour and Zollinger–Ellison syndrome.

TYPE II

PTC syndrome, which includes: medullary thyrocalcitonin-producing thyroid carcinoma with phaeochromocytoma.

TYPE III

Multiple neuromas of mucosal surfaces with medullary carcinoma and phaeochromocytoma.

Hypoparathyroidism

Diagnosis of hypoparathyroidism, characterized by attacks of tetany, numb lips, tingling fingers, laryngeal stridor, epileptiform attacks in some, and mental confusion, with transverse grooves in the finger-nails, is confirmed by the demonstration of abnormally low serum calcium concentrations with abnormally high fasting inorganic phosphate concentrations. Serum alkaline phosphatase activity is normal or low. The output of calcium and peptide-bound hydroxyproline in the urine is extremely low, reflecting very low bone turnover.

Serum uric acid levels tend to be raised and the glucose tolerance curve is flattened.

Following injections of parathyroid hormone, there is a normal increase in urine and plasma cyclic-AMP, from subnormal levels.

TESTS OF PROGRESS

Vitamin D_2 40 000–80 000 i.u. with calcium salts are given orally each day. The serum calcium level is monitored regularly to ensure that while it increases to normal, hypercalcaemia is not induced. When the serum calcium is nearly normal the dose of oral calcium and vitamin D should be reassessed.

TESTS PROVIDING USEFUL NEGATIVE RESULTS

Blood urea and NPN levels are normal. There is no steatorrhoea.

Pseudohypoparathyroidism [R]

This rare condition is dominant with incomplete penetrance.

TYPE I

Serum calcium is abnormally low, with increased serum parathyroid hormone levels. Urine cAMP output is increased above normal, and is not affected by injections of parathyroid hormone. There is impaired secretion of prolactin into the serum after TRH or chlorpromazine injection. The receptor-cyclase coupling protein is reduced in Type I.

TYPE II

Again, serum calcium is abnormally low. Following injection of parathyroid hormone, there is a marked reduction in urine phosphate excretion, with normal or raised cAMP in the urine

TESTS OF PROGRESS

Calcium supplements and larger doses of vitamin D than in hypoparathyroidism are needed, and serum calcium levels should be monitored regularly to maintain normal values.

TESTS PROVIDING USEFUL NEGATIVE RESULTS

There is no evidence of renal disease or steatorrhoea.

Pseudopseudohypoparathyroidism (Cerebro-metacarpo-metatarsal Dystrophy)

Patients suffering from this very rare condition appear clinically similar to those suffering from pseudohypoparathyroidism, but all biochemical tests are normal. Many of the patients are mentally retarded.

Secondary Hyperparathyroidism

Secondary hyperparathyroidism occurs in many conditions which produce specific changes in laboratory tests:
Serum calcium not increased and is usually below normal:
'Renal rickets', true rickets, osteomalacia, steatorrhoea, pregnancy, lactation
Serum calcium may be slightly increased:
Myeloma, pituitary basophilism, acromegaly, osteitis imperfecta, marble bone disease, chronic hypertrophic arthritis
Serum parathyroid hormone levels are increased, but in cirucmstances in which the tendency of the serum-calcium concentration to fall leads to release of parathyroid hormone. In primary hyperparathyroidism the parathyroid gland is autonomous, and parathyroid hormone is circulating at 'inappropriate' times.

Tertiary Hyperparathyroidism

Following prolonged secondary hyperparathyroidism, if the primary condition leading to secondary hyperparathyroidism is relieved, it is found that the parathyroids have developed temporary autonomous control, leading to a situation resembling primary hyperparathyroidism.

DISEASES OF THE PANCREAS

Hyperinsulinism

Diagnosis is suggested when blood-glucose concentration falls to less than 1·7 mmol/l (30 mg/dl) after 24 hours of fasting or in an attack. There may be profound hypoglycaemia a few hours after oral glucose, having been preceded by abnormally raised blood-glucose levels. The following conditions should be considered:

Functional hypoglycaemia
Post-gastrectomy 'dumping syndrome'
Early stages of maturity-onset diabetes mellitus
Pancreatic insulinoma, *see* p. 194.

Diabetes Mellitus

Diagnosis is confirmed by the finding of impaired glucose tolerance. Glucose concentration exceeding:

1. *Fasting blood glucose*
   a. Venous whole blood >7·0 mmol/l (>120 mg/dl).
   b. Capillary whole blood >7·0 mmol/l (>120 mg/dl).
   c. Venous plasma >8·0 mmol/l (>140 mg/dl).

and

2. *After 75 g glucose in 200–500 ml fluid orally (adults) or 1·75 g/kg body weight orally in fluid (children)*
   a. Venous whole blood >10 mmol/l (>180 mg/dl).
   b. Capillary whole blood >11·0 mmol/l (>200 mg/dl).
   c. Venous plasma >11·0 mmol/l (>200 mg/dl).

Glucose tolerance is impaired (i.e. not frank diabetes mellitus)

1. *Fasting blood glucose:*
   a. Fasting venous whole blood <7·0 mmol/l (<120 mg/dl).
   b. Capillary whole blood <7·0 mmol/l (<120 mg/dl).
   c. Venous plasma <8·0 mmol/l (<140 mg/dl).

2. *After oral glucose load, as above*
   a. Venous whole blood <7 <10mmol/l (<120 <180 mg/dl).
   b. Capillary whole blood <8 <11 mmol/l (<140 <200 mg/dl).
   c. Venous plasma <8 <11 mmol/l (<140 <200 mg/dl).

INTRAVENOUS GLUCOSE TOLERANCE TEST

If the patient cannot tolerate an oral glucose tolerance test, or has had a previous gastro-enterostomy, the fasting patient is given 50 ml of 50 per cent glucose solution intravenously (or 0·5 g glucose/kg body weight). Plasma glucose concentrations are estimated every 10 min for an hour. The rate of fall of plasma glucose is slower in diabetics than in normal subjects.

(Cortisone—oral glucose tolerance test—? has been used to detect 'latent diabetes mellitus').

TESTS OF PROGRESS

Testing the patient's urine for the presence of glucose detects previous hyperglycaemia with spillover of glucose into the urine, when the renal threshold for glucose has been exceeded. Detection of ketones in the urine in insulin-dependent diabetics indicated poor inadequate control. Home monitoring of blood glucose (on portable machines), or the sending of capillary blood spots taken by the patient on filter paper is useful in showing hour-to-hour variation in blood glucose concentrations, and also encourages the patient to be careful about control of his condition. Estimation of the stable HbA_{1c} in blood taken in diabetic outpatients is very useful:

a. If HbA_{1c} concentration is high, this indicates poor control with high blood glucose concentrations during the previous few weeks.

b. If HbA_{1c} concentration is unexpectedly low, in relation to daytime blood glucose estimations by the patient, this suggests either faulty technique in estimation of blood glucose at home, or unsuspected hypoglycaemia when the patient has been asleep at night.

Acute Juvenile Diabetes Mellitus

Compared with maturity-onset diabetes mellitus, acute diabetes mellitus developing in a child, adolescent, or young adult is an acute emergency. Severe metabolic acidosis with marked ketosis and rapid depletion of liver glycogen stores is found. The glycosuric diuresis is severe, and dangerous dehydration develops rapidly.

Hyperosmolar Non-ketotic Diabetic Coma

Diagnosis of this condition, which tends to occur in older, often obese, maturity-onset diabetics, is confirmed by the finding of dehydration with increased packed cell volume, raised plasma sodium levels, very high blood-glucose levels, and abnormally increased plasma osmolality. There is a gross blood/CSF glucose difference. Complicating acute pancreatitis occurs in some cases.

It is important to distinguish those cases with raised blood lactic acid and abnormally low arterial blood P_{CO_2}, from cases with no marked increase in blood lactic acid, and only moderate depression of P_{CO_2}. Treatment of the former group with lactate-containing fluids is dangerous.

TESTS PROVIDING USEFUL NEGATIVE RESULTS

The diagnosis of this condition is supported by the finding of no, or only slight, ketosis.

DISEASES OF THE THYROID

Thyrotoxicosis, Hyperthyroidism

Diagnosis of hyperthyroidism is confirmed by the finding of raised serum T3 and T4 levels, increased T4/thyroxine-binding globulin (TBG) ratio and increased free thyroxine index (both of which reflect the level of circulating free T4), increased free T4, decreased free binding sites on TGB (T3 uptake test). Serum T3 estimation gives the best measure of the presence of hyperthyroidism. In T3 thyrotoxicosis (less than 5 per cent of all cases of thyrotoxicosis), especially in areas of iodine deficiency, the increase in serum T3 levels may be the only convincing positive laboratory test result.

Thyroid gland radio-iodine uptake tests and uptake tests after T3 or T4 suppression are no longer used in the diagnosis of hyperthyroidism. Similarly, the basal metabolic rate test, which is cumbersome and unreliable, is no longer used.

Thyroid antibodies in the serum reflects the presence of focal thyroiditis.

TESTS OF PROGRESS

Following partial thyroidectomy, antithyroid drug therapy (carbimazole or thiouracils), or radio-iodine (^{131}I) therapy, serum T4, T4/TBG ratio, and FTI all fall towards normal. During carbimazole therapy, serum T3 levels can remain raised, while during the first few weeks of treatment, serum levels of T4, T4/TBG and TSH can suggest hypothyroidism. Clinical effects of carbimazole therapy are noticeable when thyroglobulin stores in the thyroid gland are depleted. If treatment is too severe, it is found that serum TSH levels rise abnormally before the serum T4 concentration falls below normal. The order of response is: a fall in T4, then a fall in serum T3, followed by a rise in serum TSH. Serum levels should be checked after 8 weeks of maintenance therapy. If hypothyroid results are then obtained, the patient should be given 0·1 mg thyroxine daily for 1 month, followed by 0·2 mg thyroxine daily for 2 months, continuing with carbimazole dosage and checking serum T4 etc. Thyroid antibodies, if originally present, fall with treatment with carbimazole (due to methimazole, the active principle of carbimazole). In relapse, T3 levels increase months before any increase in T4 or FTI or T4/TBG ratio.

Iodide therapy before surgery suppresses release of T4 into the circulation, reduces gland vascularity and promotes colloid storage in the gland. This state of reduced activity is only temporary, and lasts 1–4 weeks. Frequently, antithyroid drugs are given for 4–8 weeks, before 7–10 days of oral iodide, and immediately prior to surgery.

Following ^{131}I therapy, a clinical response occurs in 6–10 weeks, and euthyroidism may be attained by 4 months (although an additional dose may be needed); 10–15 per cent of patients become hypothyroid within 2 years of ^{131}I therapy (50–60 per cent after 20 years). Therefore these patients must be followed up for life.

After partial thyroidectomy (removal of the bulk of the functioning gland) up to 30 per cent of all cases develop hypothyroidism during the following 10 years. Similarly these patients must be followed up for life.

If there is a positive rise in serum TSH following TRH injection, then the diagnosis of hyperthyroidism is excluded.

It is worth noting that in active hyperthyroidism, various serum enzyme estimations are affected, with increased activity in malate dehydrogenase and adenylate kinase, and reduction in creatine phosphokinase activities.

T3 Thyrotoxicosis

Diagnosis of this variety of hyperthyroidism (less than 5 per cent of all cases) is confirmed by the finding of abnormally raised serum T3 levels, with normal serum T4, thyroid hormone binding test (THBT), normal free thyroxine index, in a patient who is clinically toxic.

Following oral or intravenous TRH there is no increase in serum TSH (less than +2 mU/l).

TESTS OF PROGRESS

Sequential tests during treatment for thyrotoxicosis should show progressive fall in serum T3 levels to the upper limit of the normal range.

Endocrine Exophthalmos

It has been found that in about half of the patients with this condition, tri-iodothyronine does not completely suppress ^{131}I uptake by the thyroid gland (cf. normal controls).

The causes of this condition are not fully understood yet, the diagnosis is essentially clinical, and laboratory tests to date are not very helpful.

Peripheral Resistance to Thyroid Hormones in the Euthyroid Subject [R]

Diagnosis is confirmed by the finding of markedly raised serum T3 and T4 levels with increased levels of free hormone (free thyroxine index or T4/TBG ratio) and TSH.

USEFUL NEGATIVE RESULTS

There is a normal increase in serum TSH, following injection of 200 μg of TRH, after 20 min.

Hypothyroidism

Diagnosis of hypothyroidism is confirmed by the finding of abnormally increased serum TSH levels, with reduced serum T4 concentration, reduced free thyroxine index and T4/TBG ratio, increased free binding sites on TBG (T3 uptake test). (Serum T3 estimations are not useful in the detection of hypothyroidism.) As thyroid gland function fails, the first abnormal test result is the rise in serum TSH, followed by low serum T4, FTI and T4/TBG ratio. Following injection of TRH there is an exaggerated increase in serum TSH (two to threefold increase). Serum TSH levels should be measured, if possible, at midday. When TSH rises above 30 mU/l the normal diurnal variation is lost. In severe cases the TSH level may reach more than 100 mU/l. Microsomal and thyroglobulin antibodies are present in the serum of 80 per cent of adults with primary hypothyroidism.

USEFUL NEGATIVE RESULTS

If serum TSH levels only show a subnormal or delayed response to the injection of TRH, this suggests that the diagnosis is hypothyroidism secondary to pituitary or hypothalamic dysfunction, and other serum hormone levels should be measured.

TESTS OF PROGRESS

Thyroxine 25 µg should be given daily, as early before breakfast as possible. Dosage is increased stepwise at 4–6 weeks' intervals until maintenance dose of 150–200 µg/day is reached. Serum TSH levels should fall in 2 weeks, the ideal level should be less than 5 mU/l at noon, with a serum T4 above 100 nmol/l. If cardiovascular disease is present, then TSH should be kept above 5 mU/l. Inadequate therapy is shown by rising TSH levels. Overdose with thyroxine results in an abnormally raised serum T3.

If thyroxine therapy is stopped, or reduced, then serum T4 levels should be followed, as TSH concentration is re-established later. When treatment consists of T3 alone, it is found that the serum T3 levels fluctuate markedly (biological half-life: 22 hours), T4 levels are very low, and treatment should be guided by serum TSH levels.

If T3 and thyroxine are given, then the aim should be to maintain a steady serum T4 above 100 nmol/l, plus serum TSH below 5 mU/l. If only thyroxine is given, then serum T3 levels will continue to be subnormal without fluctuation. When TSH levels fall below 20 mU/l the normal diurnal variation returns.

Post-thyroidectomy

1. In the immediate postoperative period there may be hypocalcaemia, which may be transient or may persist.

2. Later there may develop recurrent hyperthyroidism.

3. Transient or permanent hypothyroidism may occur at 1–2 months after operation. Since thyroid hormone production often returns as a result of endogenous TSH secretion, diagnosis of permanent hypothyroidism should not be made before 6 months after the operation.

It is therefore obvious that patients, after partial or total thyroidectomy, require regular monitoring of serum T4 and TSH levels, plus T3 levels if hyperthyroidism is suspected.

Toxic Thyroid Adenoma

Diagnosis of a toxic thyroid adenoma is confirmed by thedemonstration of a 'hot nodule' on scanning of the gland after administration of radioactive iodine. In a patient who is not clinically hyperthyroid, 25 µg T3 (tri-iodo-thyronine) is given four times daily for 10 days. A repeat scan after giving radioactive iodine, shows that all functioning thyroid tissue has been suppressed, if the diagnosis is that of non-toxic nodular goitre. After injection of 5–10 u thyrotropin (TSH) a scan after radioactive iodine reveals tissue capable of stimulation (normal but suppressed para-adenomatous tissue). The presence of a confirmed 'hot nodule' is usually accompanied by a raised serum T3 level.

Familial Disorders of Thyroxine-binding Globulin [R]

1. X-LINKED DISORDER

In this variety there is increased production of thyroxine-binding globulin. Patients are euthyroid with high serum total T4 and TBG levels. Serum free T4 and T3 levels are normal.

2. X-LINKED DISORDER

In this variety the serum thyroxine-binding globulin levels are almost zero, with half-normal levels in heterozygous females. The patients have low serum total T4 levels and are euthyroid. Serum free T4 and T3 levels are normal.

Hypothyroidism due to Inherited Defect in Production of Thyroid Hormone

Diagnosis of the most common of these rare conditions, failure of organification of iodine in the thyroid gland, is confirmed by the finding of normal uptake of ^{131}I or ^{122}I by the thyroid gland when the radioactive iodine is given orally. Following subsequent oral perchlorate ^{131}I or ^{122}I is rapidly released by the thyroid gland, as the iodine has not been bound (when compared with normal results). In infants serum TSH levels are increased, and this finding is clinically valuable.

Hypothyroidism Secondary to Hypopituitarism (Pituitary Hypothyroidism)

As a result of a pituitary tumour, or of surgical or irradiation treatment of a pituitary tumour, hypothyroidism develops, with normal to low serum TSH levels, and inappropriately low serum T4 levels.

Following TRH injection there is little increase in serum TSH.

Hypothalamic Hypothyroidism

This condition occurs more commonly in children than in adults, and the diagnosis is suggested by the finding of low or normal serum TSH levels, with low serum T4 and T3 levels. Following TRH injection there is a normal increase in serum TSH, but the peak is reached more slowly than normal.

Factitious or Iatrogenic Hyperthyroidism

If T4 and T3 are taken in excess of requirement, then serum T4 levels will be inappropriately normal or low, when compared with the patient's clinical state.

Iodine Deficiency

Diagnosis is confirmed by the finding of abnormally low plasma inorganic iodide levels, with high ^{131}I uptake by the thyroid gland, and abnormally low urine iodide output.

Myxoedema

The term 'myxoedema' should be reserved for advanced hypothyroidism with undue swelling of the skin and subcutaneous tissue.

Hypothyroidism (Hypothyroidism with Autoimmune Disease)

Hypothyroidism is most commonly associated with autoimmune thyroid disease.

In addition to clinical and laboratory evidence of hypothyroidism, serum gammaglobulins are increased and serum antithyroglobulin antibodies and antithyroid-microsome antibodies are found in conditions in which variable lymphocytic infiltration occurs in the thyroid gland.

Abnormalities of Thyroid Function in the Newborn (Cretinism)

1. THYROID DYSGENESIS

(Including infants with ectopic or hypoplastic thyroid glands, or both, or total thyroid agenesis)
Diagnosis of this condition, which is the most frequent cause of permanent congenital hypothyroidism detected by screening programmes, is confirmed by the finding of raised TSH (and low T4) levels in filter paper blood spots collected at 2–5 days after birth.

2. THYROID HORMONE SYNTHESIS FAULTS

(This group comprises the second most frequent cause of permanent congenital hypothyroidism detected by screening programmes, in which congenital goitre develops in early months–years after birth)
The various defects include:
    a. Iodide trapping failure [R]
Thyroidal uptake of ^{131}I is abnormally low, in the presence of a goitre.
    b. Iodide organification defects
        i. *Pendred's syndrome [AR]*
The commonest form of dyshormonogenesis, associated with perceptual deafness.
        ii. *Peroxidase deficiency [AR]*
Both these syndromes, after radio-iodine uptake, show prompt discharge of iodide from the thyroid gland after administration of potassium perchlorate.
    c. Failure of coupling of iodotyrosines to form iodothyronine
Associated with high ^{131}I clearance and increased urinary iodide excretion.
    d. Deficiency of de-iodotyrosinase (iodotyrosine dehalogenase defect)
Large quantities of mono-iodotyrosine and di-iodotyrosine are secreted from

the gland, and detectable in the serum. There is a secondary iodide deficiency.

e. Formation of abnormal iodinated proteins

There is normal or high serum protein-bound iodine (PBI) with low serum T4 and low butanol-extractable iodine, with increased ^{131}I uptake by the thyroid gland.

3. *DEFICIENT TSH SECRETION OR EFFECT [R]*

Including:

a. TRH deficiency	Hypothalamic hypothyroidism, with low serum
b. TRH insensitivity	T4, low serum T3 and free T4. The serum TSH is low or slightly raised. There is a normal or prolonged TSH response to exogenous TRH.
c. Isolated TSH deficiency	Serum T4, T3, and free T4 all low, with low or unmeasurable TSH, with no TSH response to
d. Panhypopituitarism	TRH.

e. Thyroid gland unresponsiveness to TSH.

4. *PERIPHERAL UNRESPONSIVENESS TO THYROID HORMONE*

a. TSH-dependent hyperthyroidism late in childhood or adolescence.

b. Partial or complete unresponsiveness of all tissues, with signs of hypothyroidism. The defect is thought to be in the thyroid-hormone nuclear-receptor binding in circulating lymphocytes and defective thyroid feedback regulation of TSH secretion.

Serum T4, T3, free T4 and TSH levels are all increased.

Non-toxic Endemic Goitre (Iodine Deficiency)

Diagnosis of this condition, which occurs in areas with very low natural sources of iodide, is confirmed by the finding of increased uptake of radioactive ^{131}I by the thyroid gland (which is frequently enlarged). Serum TSH levels are normal or raised. Serum T3 levels are normal or raised, and are relatively higher than the normal serum T4 concentration. If the estimation can be carried out, urine iodine excretion is less than 50 µg/day. Following injection of TRH there is occasionally an exaggerated increase in serum TSH.

USEFUL NEGATIVE RESULTS

Serum T4 levels are normal or low.

TESTS OF PROGRESS

Normal results follow iodide supplements in the diet.

Hashimoto's Thyroiditis

Diagnosis of this autoimmune condition, characterized by a goitre which becomes increasingly firm, progressing through fibrosis to becoming impalpable, is confirmed by the demonstration of typical histological appearance, early hyperthyroidism, followed by euthyroidism and eventually hypo-thyroidism as the gland shrinks.

The tanned red cell agglutination test is positive and complement-fixation test against the thyroid is positive.

TESTS OF PROGRESS

Treatment following diagnosis involves thyroxine treatment, with regular monitoring of T4 and TSH levels for life.

Riedel's Thyroiditis (Riedel's Struma) [R]

Diagnosis of this very rare condition, characterized by progressive dense fibrosis of the thyroid gland, can be established only by histological examination of the thyroid tissue. The hard gland is clinically indistinguishable from carcinoma of the thyroid.

Laboratory tests of thyroid function are normal until late in the disease, when hypothyroidism develops.

Subacute (de Quervain's) Thyroiditis (Non-suppurative Thyroiditis) [R]

Diagnosis of this very rare condition, presenting with acute non-suppurative inflammation of the thyroid, due to viral infection, is supported by the finding of rising antibody titres or complement-fixation test titres to specific viruses (e.g. mumps). There is a sudden release of T4 and T3 into the circulation, giving a short period with very high serum thyroid hormone levels.

Radio-iodine uptake by the thyroid gland is grossly reduced, with areas of reduced uptake visible over affected parts of the gland. TSH secretion is impaired.

TESTS OF PROGRESS

The transient hyperthyroidism during the acute attack does not require specific treatment. Steroids have been given to reduce inflammation, but it is doubtful whether they affect the course of the disease.

Hypothyroidism, if it subsequently develops, requires replacement therapy.

Carcinoma of the Thyroid

1. MEDULLARY CARCINOMA OF THE THYROID

Diagnosis is confirmed by the finding of raised serum calcitonin levels, and abnormally raised serum histaminase activity. Maximum calcitonin secretion can be induced by administration of pentagastrin (0·5 µg/kg body weight i.v. as a single dose). Serum calcitonin levels peak at 5 min. This test is useful in screening of families with a high risk of medullary carcinoma (i.e. Sipple's syndrome—familial multiple endocrine neoplasia Type 2 [AD]).

TESTS OF PROGRESS

Serum histamine is useful in the detection of metastases after surgical removal of the primary tumour. Successful removal of the primary tumour is followed by a fall in serum calcitonin to normal.

2. *CARCINOMA OF THE THYROID*

A. Solitary Node

Even though less than 5 per cent of solitary nodes which fail to take up radio-iodine prove to be neoplastic on histological examination, they should all be surgically removed.

B. Differentiated Papillary and Follicular Carcinoma

There may be evidence of bony or pulmonary secondaries with leuco-erythroblastic anaemia in association with these slow-growing tumours.

TESTS OF PROGRESS

Thyroxine is given in sufficient dose to suppress TSH release and to give a flat TSH response to TRH. Then T3 is given instead of T4 for 3 weeks, followed by no treatment for 1 week, followed by a body scan using ^{131}I after TRH injection to boost TSH secretion.

Functioning metastases are detected with 100–150 mC ^{131}I.

Residual thyroid scan using ^{131}I should follow total thyroidectomy, with subsequent yearly repeats, since differentiated carcinomas can take up radio-iodine.

Pyogenic (Suppurative) Thyroiditis [R]

Diagnosis of bacterial infection of the thyroid gland is confirmed by the growth of organisms following culture of material aspirated from the affected gland.

DISEASES OF THE GONADS

Eunuchoidism, Male Hypogonadism

Diagnosis of male hypogonadism due to primary deficiency is supported by the finding of increased urinary FSH excretion.

TESTS OF PROGRESS

Following the demonstration of normal thyroid and adrenal function, treatment with chorionic gonadotrophins stimulates the Leydig cells, and spermatogenesis occurs—the so-called 'fertile eunuch'.

In secondary failure, resulting from pituitary failure, urinary FSH output is very low.

Testicular biopsy and chromosomal studies to determine chromosome pattern and nuclear sex are useful examinations, as Klinefelter's syndrome needs to be distinguished. Thyroid function tests are required to distinguish juvenile myxoedema.

Hermaphroditism

Both ovarian and testicular tissues are present.

Chromosome studies and examination for sex chromatin in buccal smears are useful.

PSEUDOHERMAPHRODITISM

a. Male

The gonads are testes. Two distinct clinical types exist.

Type 1: In the 'female' type the patient appears externally to be female, who feminizes at puberty. The condition is familial, and inherited either as a sex-linked condition or as a sex-limited autosomal dominant condition. One-half of the sibs are normal girls, one-quarter of the sibs are normal boys, and one-quarter show testicular feminization. In these latter cases, it is found that at puberty the urine contains excess pregnanediol, the testes secreting oestrogens. Sex chromatin is absent from buccal smears and the chromosomal pattern is the normal male XY.

Type 2: The external and internal genitalia appear ambiguous. These rare cases only rarely feminize at puberty.

b. Female

Due to congenital virilizing adrenal hyperplasia. *See* Adrenogenital Syndrome, p. 289.

Precocious Puberty in Girls (Puberty before 8 years)

1. Ninety per cent of such girls have idiopathic or constitutional precocious puberty, due to premature activation of the hypothalamus–pituitary axis. Hormone levels correlate with the bone age of the subject.

2. A few cases result from organic brain damage.

3. A few cases result from oestrogen-secreting tumours of either ovary or adrenal, resulting in pseudoprecocious puberty, when estimations of serum LH, FSH, oestradiol, and hCG beta-subunits are useful.

Delayed Puberty in Girls

The majority of such girls have 'physiological' or 'constitutional' delayed puberty, and are otherwise normal. A few cases result from secondary delay due to renal disease, malabsorption, liver disease, severe anaemia, infection, Turner's syndrome (chromosomal abnormality), rarely isolated deficiency of gonadotrophin secretion, hypothyroidism, or hypopituitarism.

Diagnosis depends on assessment of bone age, secondary sexual development, serum gonadotrophins, serum oestradiol, total urine oestrogens, and serum LH and FSH levels, plus detection of any secondary cause.

Precocious Puberty in Males (Onset of Puberty before 10 years)

Diagnosis is clinical.

1. True Precocity
   a. Tumour involving hypothalamus, pituitary gland, or pineal gland.
   b. Inflammation affecting hypothalamus, pituitary gland, or pineal gland.
   c. 'Constitutional' anomaly [R].
   d. Very rare
      — McCune–Albright syndrome.
      — Non-endocrine malignant tumour, e.g. hepatoblastoma secreting gonadotrophins (estimations of hCG beta-subunits and also serum alpha-fetoprotein are useful).
2. Pseudoprecocity
   Urine 17-oxosteroid excretion is abnormally raised for the patient's age. The testes are small for the size of the penis, and there is no spermatogenesis. Serum testosterone is abnormally raised, and serum LH and FSH are low. Pseudoprecocity is found in:
      Congenital adrenal hyperplasia (17-oxosteroid excretion does not fall after dexamethasone).
      Interstitial-cell tumour of the testis.

Delayed Puberty in Boys

Gonadotrophins are not detected in the urine of normal children until puberty. There is often a family history of delayed puberty in constitutional delayed puberty.

Raised serum gonadotrophins indicate a primary gonadal disorder, if serum gonadotrophins are low, serum testosterone will also be low. Later the hypothalamus–pituitary axis can be checked.

When there is growth hormone deficiency, serum levels of androstenedione, dehydroepiandrosterone, and dehydroepiandrosterone sulphate are all abnormally low. In hypogonadism, with low serum testosterone, these three substances may be present in increased concentrations.

Male Pseudohermaphroditism

TESTICULAR DIFFERENTIATION

Chromosome or gene deletion involving the Y chromosome.

TESTICULAR DYSFUNCTION

   a. Gonadotrophic unresponsiveness.
   b. Abnormalities of Müllerian inhibitory factor synthesis or action.
   c. Testosterone biosynthesis deficiencies.
   d. Cholesterol 20-alpha, 22-hydroxylase and/or 20/22-desmolase deficiency.
   e. 17-Alpha-hydroxylase deficiency.
   f. 17,20-Desmolase deficiency.
   g. 3-Beta-01-dehydrogenase: delta-5-isomerase deficiency.
   h. 17-Beta-hydroxysteroid dehydrogenase deficiency.

DISORDERS OF FUNCTION AT THE ANDROGEN-DEPENDENT TARGET AREAS:
  a. Androgen receptor defects.
  b. Enzyme deficiencies in testosterone metabolism.
  c. 5-Alpha-reductase deficiency.

Infertility

Diagnosis of infertility or subfertility needs much clinical investigation, but the following laboratory tests are useful:

1. POSTCOITAL TEST

Soon after intercourse, microscopic examination is carried out on secretions from the posterior vaginal fornix and on the cervical mucus plug.

This test should be carried out midway between menses after normal intercourse without contraceptives, preferably with the husband not having had an emission for 3 days. Spermatozoa should be found in the vagina for 18 hours, and motile spermatozoa should be found in the cervical mucus plug for 40 hours after intercourse.

2. DIRECT EXAMINATION OF SEMINAL FLUID

The volume of the fluid should average 2–5 ml (minimum 1·5 ml; maximum 6·0 ml). The pH of the specimen should be within the range 7·4–8·4. The spermatozoal count should exceed 20 million/ml, and after the gel has liquefied 60 per cent of the spermatozoa should be motile (valid only for fresh specimens within an hour of collection). Up to 10 per cent of spermatozoa from a normal adult may appears abnormal on microscopy of stained films, the maximum percentage of abnormal forms accepted as being within the normal range is up to 35 per cent. High neutrophil counts indicate underlying infection.

Samples for analysis should be obtained, preferably by masturbation, after 3 days without an emission, and the whole sample should be collected into a clean container (e.g. glass) and should be examined as soon as possible, being kept cool until examination. If this test shows low spermatozoal counts, or if a high proportion of the spermatozoa appears abnormal, microscopy of testicular biopsy material may be useful, combined with estimation of the excretion rate of urinary 17-oxosteroids, and possibly chromosomal analysis (e.g. for suspected Klinefelter syndrome). Blood or urine estimations of testosterone and gonadotrophins may be useful.

If examination of seminal fluid reveals no obvious reason for lack of fertility, then microscopical examination of smears of vaginal cells for evidence of increased or decreased oestrogenic activity can be made.

Histological examination of endometrial curettings, plus possibly culture of curettings to exclude underlying tuberculous infection, can be carried out.

Postvasectomy

Microscopy of seminal fluid obtained after surgical vasectomy (as a contraceptive measure) at 6 weeks demonstrates the presence of residual spermatozoa, and a repeat specimen later can be used to demonstrate the complete absence of spermatozoa in the seminal fluid.

Testicular Failure

Prepuberty failure—urine 17-oxosteroids output is low.
Failure at puberty—urine 17-oxosteroids output is normal.
Failure without signs of eunuchoidism—urine 17-oxosteroids output is normal.
    Plasma testosterone levels are below normal for the patient's age.

Klinefelter's Syndrome (Seminiferous Tubule Dysgenesis; XXY Syndrome)

Diagnosis of this condition, characterized by eunuchoid development in males, with intellectual impairment in some cases (least marked in 47/XXY and more marked in XXY) is confirmed by the demonstration of the chromosomal abnormality, which can include XXY, XXYY, XXXY or XXXXY. When two or more X chromosomes are present, the cell nuclei show more than one chromatin dot.
    Serum LH and gonadotrophin levels are increased. There is azoospermia in seminal fluid, and testicular biopsy reveals dysgenetic tubules lined only by Sertoli cells, clumped Leydig cells, with very few or no germ cells. Postpuberty plasma testosterone levels are low.

Reifenstein's Syndrome [R]

Diagnosis of this very rare hereditary disorder, characterized by hypospadias, postpubertal atrophy of the seminiferous tubules in the testis leading to azoospermia and eunuchoidism, is supported by the finding of low serum testosterone levels with raised serum FSH and LH levels.
    Histological examination of testicular biopsy material reveals hyalinization of tubules surrounded by elastic fibres. The Leydig cells are prominent and clumped together.

TESTS PROVIDING USEFUL NEGATIVE RESULTS

The patients have a normal 46/XY karyotype, and urine oestrogen excretion is normal.

Orchitis in Males

ACUTE ORCHITIS

Acute orchitis occurs during mumps infection, and may also very rarely be caused by other virus infections.

CHRONIC ORCHITIS

Chronic orchitis may be a complication of:
    Tertiary syphilis
    Tuberculosis

Leprosy
Brucellosis
Glanders
Filariasis
Bilharzia

Diagnosis depends on the demonstration of the primary infection.

Tumours of the Testis

1. SEMINOMA, TERATOMA, CHORIONEPITHELIOMA

Diagnosis is clinical and is supported by the finding of a marked increase in gonadotrophins in serum (or urine).

Following surgical removal of the tumour, the prognosis for chorionephithelioma is poor, and plasma gonadotrophin levels rise again with recurrence. Alpha-fetoprotein production is abnormally increased in 85 per cent of male malignant teratomas. This estimation in the serum can therefore be used as a tumour marker for evidence of successful removal of the tumour and response to treatment.

2. INTERSTITIAL-CELL TUMOUR

Diagnosis is clinical and is supported by the finding of abnormally raised urine 17-oxosteroid excretion (for the age of the boy). In adult males, very high 17-oxosteroid excretion rates are found.

Hirsutism in Females

1. IDIOPATHIC HIRSUTISM

Basal levels of LSH, FSH, serum testosterone and urine 17-oxosteroid excretion are all within normal ranges. Serial serum LH and progesterone levels in patients with regular menstrual cycles reveal no midcycle LH peak, indicating anovular cycles.

2. OVARIAN TUMOURS

Serum testosterone levels ≥ 8 nmol/l suggest ovarian tumour. Urine 17-oxosteroid excretion is also increased above normal, with suppression of gonadotrophin release.

3. ADRENOCORTICAL DISORDERS (INCLUDING TUMOUR)

There is a moderately raised serum testosterone level, with a marked increase in urine 17-oxosteroid excretion. Catheterization at operation, of blood draining from the two adrenals, can be used for differential estimation of blood samples to isolate the possible site of a tumour.

Primary Ovarian Failure

Urine 17-oxosteroids output is normal.

'Super-female' Syndrome

Diagnosis of this rare condition is confirmed by the finding of an increase in the number of chromosomes to 47, with some cell nuclei containing 2 sex chromatin bodies, 2 Barr bodies being visible, and 2 'drum-stick' bodies being found in some neutrophil nuclei.

The chromosomal pattern is XXX.

(A very few cases of XXXX and XXXXX chromosomal patterns have been found in mentally retarded patients.)

Polycystic Ovary Syndrome (Stein–Leventhal Syndrome; Hyperthecosis Ovarii)

Diagnosis of this syndrome, characterized by infertility, oligomenorrhoea progressing to amenorrhoea, often with increasing hirsutism, is confirmed by macroscopic and microscopic examination of enlarged pearly white ovaries. Wedge biopsy of the ovaries results in clinical improvement and allows exclusion of ovarian tumour.

The major circulating oestrogen in the blood is oestrone, rather than oestradiol, and this in turn results in suppression of FSH release, levels of FSH being low-normal. High oestrone levels stimulate LH levels, and LH levels exceed 20 u/l in 60–80 per cent of cases, with no midcycle surge. Serum testosterone and androstenedione levels may be increased, and urine 17-oxosteroid excretion may also be increased (in perhaps 33 per cent of cases).

TESTS OF PROGRESS

Following wedge biopsy of the ovaries, normal ovulation may follow. Ovulation can be successfully induced with clomiphene injections, but these may cause ovarian pain.

TESTS PROVIDING USEFUL NEGATIVE RESULTS

Tests for adrenal or pituitary disorders are negative. Vaginal cells show evidence of oestrogenic activity.

Turner's Syndrome (Ovarian Dysgenesis)

Diagnosis of this condition, characterized by shortness of stature, webbing of the neck, primary amenorrhoea, associated with dwarfism in the female, with congenital lymphoedema and hypogonadism noted at puberty, is confirmed by the demonstration of chromosome loss (XO), or abnormal X chromosome mosaicism. Some cases may be mentally retarded, and there is an increased incidence of colour blindness.

TESTS OF PROGRESS

It is suggested that dysgenetic gonads should be surgically removed, as they have a greater risk than normal of developing a malignancy.

The majority of XO conceptions do not survive, as the XO karyotype is the commonest form found in spontaneous abortions (about 1 in 15 of all abortions examined). Many surviving forms may be mosaics of different origin from the pure XO karyotype.

Ovarian Tumours

1. PRIMARY OVARIAN TUMOURS

Some ovarian tumours may synthesize and secrete oestrogenic or androgenic steroids, producing clinical manifestations:

A. Oestrogen excess

Precocious puberty in children, or irregular bleeding in adults (especially postmenopausal bleeding).

B. Androgen excess

Signs and symptoms include hirsutism, virilism, loss of feminine contours and oligomenorrhoea. The endocrine profile found depends on the types of androgens secreted.

Hormone assays may be useful in detection of such tumours, secondary to clinical examination, and include:
Serum oestradiol
Urine total oestrogen excretion
Serum testosterone
Urine 17-oxosteroid excretion
Serum gonadotrophin
Serum alphafetoprotein
Human chorionic gonadotrophin in serum or urine

2. SECONDARY OVARIAN TUMOURS

Detected by clinical examination.

Luteal Cyst of Ovary

It has been reported that the urinary output of pregnanediol is increased.

15 *Collagen, Bone, Joint and Muscle Diseases*

Systemic Lupus Erythematosus

Diagnosis of this episodic disease, thought to be due to a defect in suppressor T cells with B cell hyperactivity, which is characterized by variable skin rashes, joint disorders and damage to cardiovascular, respiratory, renal and nervous systems, is confirmed by clinical examination, and the demonstration of serum antinuclear factor by immunofluorescence (but about 2 per cent of the normal population give positive results). Antinuclear antibodies (ANA) predominantly IgG, against 'native' double-strand DNA are more diagnostic, and the binding power of the patient's serum can be titrated for these antibodies. Antibodies against single-strand DNA also occur, but are often present in other related diseases.

Serum complement levels fall with immune complex formation, and immune complexes are especially associated with lupus nephritis.

Serum immunoglobulins are increased with reduced serum albumin, and increased ESR and plasma viscosity. Tests for RA are positive in up to 50 per cent of cases. Direct Coombs' antihuman globulin test is positive in 10 per cent. ('Biological false-positive' tests occur in up to 50 per cent for syphilis, but the specific treponemal tests are consistently negative in the absence of syphilis.)

Antileucocyte and antiplatelet antibodies are present in up to 80 per cent of cases. LE cells may be found, but they are rarely found if antinuclear factor tests are negative, or after steroid therapy has been started.

Renal damage results in proteinuria with casts and red cells.

Rarely, circulating anticoagulants are present.

Skin biopsy (of the rash) shows a 'lupus band' of IgG immunoglobulin deposited along the basement membrane between epidermis and dermis (and this is linked with renal involvement).

TESTS OF PROGRESS

Steroid therapy with/or without plasmapheresis results in a fall in ANA-binding titre in the serum and clinical improvement.

TESTS PROVIDING USEFUL NEGATIVE RESULTS

Although the antinuclear immunofluorescence test cannot be used to screen for the presence of SLE in a population, since 2 per cent of normals give positive results, a negative result before treatment virtually excludes the diagnosis.

Drug-induced Lupus Erythematosus

Antinuclear antibody test may be positive, but tests for anti-DNA antibodies are negative, and serum complement levels are normal. LE cells may be found and the Coombs' antihuman globulin test may be positive.

The following drugs have been found to cause the syndrome:
Hydralazine
Isoniazid
Some anticonvulsants
Sulphonamides
Phenylbutazone
Procainamide (the condition developing in 12 months in slow acetylators, and in 48 months in fast acetylators).

Renal and neurological involvement is rare.

TESTS OF PROGRESS

Recovery occurs when the offending drug is discontinued.

Dermatomyositis (Polymyositis)

Diagnosis of this condition, characterized by proximal myopathy and a characteristic rash on extensor surfaces, which may be associated with malignant disease when it occurs in adults, is confirmed by clinical examination and histological examination of skin and muscle biopsy material (to exclude other collagen vascular diseases).

There is anaemia with neutrophilia and increased serum alpha- and gammaglobulins.

Tests for RA are positive in some cases.

Enzymes released from damaged muscles are increased in activity in the serum—including lactate dehydrogenase, aspartate and alanine aminotransferases and creatine phosphokinase, in the active disease.

TESTS PROVIDING USEFUL NEGATIVE RESULTS

Alanine and aspartate aminotransferase activities are not increased in rheumatoid disease.

Systemic Sclerosis (Scleroderma)

Diagnosis of this condition, characterized by hardening and thickening of the skin, with renal damage, and damage to lungs, heart and gastrointestinal tract, confirmed by clinical examination and histological examination of skin biopsy.

There is usually a mild anaemia, with raised ESR and plasma viscosity. Tests for antinuclear antibodies using fluorescence are positive in 50 per cent of cases, and to RA antibodies in 25 per cent. Occasional LE cells may be found.

The urine contains increased protein, a few red cells and casts, with an increased output of creatine.

Rarely, gastrointestinal involvement results in malabsorption.

Polyarteritis Nodosa

Diagnosis of this disease, affecting more males than females, and characterized by fever, weight loss, anaemia, hypertension, abdominal pain, renal, pulmonary or neurological damage, is confirmed by histological examination of biopsy material from affected tissues (e.g. skin, kidney, liver, muscle, etc.).

Focal necrosis of the internal elastic membrane in artery walls results in local aneurysms with neutrophilic infiltration around them.

Visceral angiography, when there are gastrointestinal symptoms, may demonstrate multiple intraparenchymal aneurysms.

There is anaemia with neutrophilia, and raised ESR and plasma viscosity, with increased serum alpha- and gammaglobulins and reduced serum albumin concentration. Haemolytic anaemia occasionally develops, and very occasionally circulating anticoagulants are found.

With renal involvement, the urine contains increased protein, red cells and casts, and renal damage progresses to uraemia without treatment.

TESTS OF PROGRESS

Steroids with azathioprine or cyclophosphamide, and possibly plasmapheresis, may result in clinical improvement.

Sjögren's Syndrome

Diagnosis of this condition, characterized by dry eyes and dry mouth, with a tendency to respiratory tract infections, and often an association with rheumatoid arthritis, is confirmed by clinical examination, and supported by histological examination of salivary gland biopsy material.

Tests for RA factor and antinuclear factor are frequently positive, and other tests for antibodies may also be positive, including thyroid auto-antibodies positive in 20 per cent of cases.

Wegener's Granuloma (Malignant Granuloma)

Diagnosis of this rare disease, characterized by granulomatous ulceration of the upper and lower respiratory tract, with generalized arteritis and glomerular damage, is confirmed by histological examination of biopsy material, which shows a necrotizing vasculitis with granuloma formation.

In the systemic stage of the disease there is anaemia, with increased ESR and plasma viscosity, neutrophilia with eosinophilia, and greatly increased serum gammaglobulins, especially IgG. When there is renal damage, the urine contains increased protein, with haematuria and granular casts. Renal damage can progress to uraemia.

TESTS OF PROGRESS

At one time, this disease was fatal. Treatment with steroids and cyclophosphamide, with suitable haematological monitoring, results in clinical improvement in many cases.

Giant-cell Arteritis and Polymyalgia Rheumatica

Diagnosis of this condition, occurring predominantly in the elderly and characterized by combinations of headache, scalp tenderness, neurological defects, 'morning stiffness' and girdle pains, with malaise and fever, is confirmed by the finding of marked increase in the ESR and plasma viscosity. Giant-cell arteritis may be seen in scalp vessel biopsy.

TESTS OF PROGRESS

Rapid improvement follows steroid therapy. The serious risk of partial or complete loss of vision in this condition, necessitates urgent treatment with steroids once the diagnosis has been considered, rather than waiting for confirmation from histological examination of artery biopsy.

Osteoarthrosis

Laboratory investigations are of value in the exclusion of other forms of joint disease. Non-specific tests of inflammatory response are negative in uncomplicated osteoarthrosis and there are no specific diagnostic laboratory tests for the condition.

Mixed Connective Tissue Disease (MCTD)

Diagnosis of this condition, affecting predominantly females, and characterized by joint pains, swollen hands with skin changes, Raynaud's phenomena and inflammatory myositis, with lymphadenopathy, is diagnosed clinically by its appearance as an 'overlap' syndrome related to SLE, scleroderma and polymyositis. Serum titres of fluorescent antinuclear antibodies (ANA) are high, and tests for RA factor are positive in 50 per cent. The characteristic finding in this condition is of a high titre of haemagglutinating antibody to extractable nuclear antigen (ENA) directed against nuclear ribonucleoprotein.

Antibodies against smooth muscle (Sm) are absent, and only 10 per cent have antibodies against 'native' DNA. Serum complement levels are not reduced.

The ESR and plasma viscosity are raised, with anaemia and leucopenia. Serum immunoglobulin levels are increased.

TESTS OF PROGRESS

There is a favourable response to steroid therapy.

Osteoporosis

Diagnosis of osteoporosis is difficult, but in *secondary osteoporosis* the diagnosis of the underlying disease can be made by means of the appropriate tests:

Cushing's disease
Thyrotoxicosis
Hyperparathyroidism
Malabsorption (low calcium intake with adequate vitamin D)

In *primary osteoporosis*, a distinct negative calcium balance is detectable in the rare variety of *idiopathic osteoporosis of children*. In *senile osteoporosis*, although 10 per cent of the skeleton and its calcium are lost between the ages 50–70 years, the average loss of 15 mg calcium/day with the normal diurnal variation is too small to be detected by balance studies. Serum calcium and inorganic phosphate levels are usually normal, but may increase during periods of immobilization. When the patient is given a low-calcium diet, the urinary calcium output remains unchanged (cf. normal reduction).

Skin biopsy material may be useful in diagnosis, as the total collagen decreases in the skin in osteoporosis, increasing following androgen therapy.

USEFUL NEGATIVE RESULTS

In the absence of complications (e.g. fractures) the serum alkaline phosphatase activity is normal.

Osteomalacia

Diagnosis is made by bone biopsy which reveals increased osteoid. Serum calcium is normal or reduced, serum phosphate is normal or decreased. Serum alkaline phosphatase activity is increased. Serum 25-hydroxychole-calciferol levels are reduced below normal. Strontium space is increased. Urine calcium output is reduced and phosphate output may be increased.

The findings vary with the specific diagnosis of the condition associated with osteomalacia:
    Vitamin D deficiency
    Malabsorption syndrome
    Renal disease
    Primary hypophosphataemia

Bone Fractures

After bone fracture, many biochemical and haematological changes occur:

Within 24 hours the total white blood-cell count rises, with neutrophilia. Plasma fibrinogen increases, and later various globulin fractions increase in the serum.

Serum calcium may increase, and urinary calcium output usually increases, especially with immobilization.

Haemorrhage always occurs around the site of a fracture, and pigment derived from this results in increased urinary and faecal urobilinogen excretion.

During healing, serum alkaline phosphatase activity rises above normal.

Prolonged Immobilization

Following prolonged immobilization various changes occur, including:
    a. Serum calcium tends to increase.
    b. Urinary calcium excretion is increased.
    c. Serum inorganic phosphate increases.
    d. Renal threshold for phosphate is increased.

e. Plasma levels of $25(OH)_2D_3$ remain normal, while levels of $1,25(OH)_2D_3$ fall.

f. Nephrogenic cyclic-AMP excretion falls, and serum immunoreactive PTH levels also fall.

(These changes accompany osteoporosis.)

Fat Embolism

Following a major long-bone fracture (especially of the femur) and less commonly after severe tissue trauma, with a latent period of hours to days, disseminated intravascular coagulation (DIC), may develop with thrombocytopenia. A petechial rash appears, and it is possible to show fat embolism in frozen sections of skin biopsy material.

Pao_2 falls dangerously, and with hyperventilation, the Pco_2 remains normal—due to impaired alveolar diffusion of oxygen, arteriovenous shunting in the lungs, and alveolar oedema, similar to the effects of multiple pulmonary emboli.

TESTS OF PROGRESS

Blood gas results may improve with pure oxygen therapy.

TESTS PROVIDING USEFUL NEGATIVE RESULTS

Examination of CSF following suspected cerebral fat embolism is disappointing, as is examination of sputum or urine for fat globules. Reports in the past of positive findings may well have resulted from contamination with lubricants.

Familial Hypophosphataemia (Phosphaturic Rickets; Vitamin-D-resistant Rickets)

Affected males suffer more severely from this condition with dominant inheritance via the X chromosome, than do hemizygous affected females.

Diagnosis is confirmed by the finding of plasma inorganic phosphate concentrations below normal, which rise less than normal after oral phosphate supplements, but which rise to normal after large doses of vitamin D. Serum calcium levels are low normal. Serum alkaline phosphatase activity is normal or raised.

Urine calcium output is markedly decreased and the urine phosphate output is grossly increased (due to impaired reabsorption of phosphate by the proximal renal tubules—the renal tubule cells have an abnormally low phosphatase content). Glycosuria occurs in some cases.

In affected symptom-free females, the low plasma inorganic phosphate concentration may be the only finding.

TESTS OF PROGRESS

The condition can be relieved by large daily doses of vitamin D (100 000–1 000 000 iu) but the dose must be controlled by regular serum calcium estimation, to maintain serum calcium levels within the normal range (i.e. not exceeding 10·5 mg/dl). The urine calcium output should not exceed

400 mg/day. Permanent treatment with vitamin D supplements is necessary or the condition relapses.

Osteitis Deformans (Paget's Disease)

Diagnosis of this condition, predominantly occurring in the elderly, which may be of X-linked intermediate inheritance, characterized by bone pain, bone deformity, pathological fracture, malignant change, or incidental detection on X-rays, is confirmed by clinical examination and radiographic appearance of the affected bone or bones.

Serum alkaline phosphatase activity may be very high (bone isoenzyme) with normal fasting serum calcium and inorganic phosphate.

Hypercalciuria follows any period of immobilization and hypercalcaemia can develop if renal function is impaired. Urine hydroxyproline output is increased, reflecting gross increase in bone turnover.

TESTS OF PROGRESS

Treatment with diphosphonate, calcitonin, actinomycin D, or mithramycin, is followed by clinical improvement, with a return to normal serum alkaline phosphatase activity by 3 months, and normal urinary output of hydroxyproline by 1 month. Prolonged treatment with disodium etidronate (diphosphonate) can result in demineralization of normal bone.

Malignant change to osteogenic sarcoma (less commonly to chondrosarcoma or malignant giant-cell tumour), is followed by a rapid rise in serum alkaline phosphatase activity.

Secondary Carcinomatous Deposits in Bone

Diagnosis of infiltration of bone marrow by carcinoma cells can be confirmed by bone-marrow aspirate examination in up to 8 per cent of cases in advanced malignant disease. Carcinoma cells in marrow are rarely found in advanced carcinoma of the gastrointestinal tract or of the genitourinary tract, or in malignancy of the head and neck.

Rapid erosion of bone results in hypercalcaemia and this hypercalcaemia can be reduced by cortisone therapy in up to 10 per cent of cases only. Urine calcium output is also increased. Serum alkaline phosphatase activity is increased if bone repair is attempting to keep pace with bone destruction, but this estimation is not reliable in the assessment of evidence of bone-marrow infiltration.

Advanced carcinomatosis with marrow invasion is often accompanied by leuco-erythroblastic anaemia, with neutropenia or, on occasions, by a leukaemoid reaction.

TESTS OF PROGRESS

Improvement in the blood count follows remission induced by chemotherapy (which may itself depress marrow function).

Osteopetrosis (Marble Bone Disease; Osteosclerosis Fragilis) [R]

This rare condition can occur in a severe form [AR] with ultimately fatal leucoerythroblastic anaemia, thrombocytopenia, or pancytopenia. There is also hepatosplenomegaly.

The milder variety [AD] is less severe.

Histological examination of bone biopsy reveals thickened closely packed trabecula and zones of osteochondroid tissue. Hypercalcification of cartilage is also found. The marrow cavities are replaced by dense structureless bone.

TESTS PROVIDING USEFUL NEGATIVE RESULTS

Serum calcium, alkaline phosphatase activity and fasting serum phosphate are normal.

Osteomyelitis

Microscopy and culture for the infecting organism (commonly staphylococcus) should be carried out on pus from the lesion. Tuberculous lesions occur and cultures for tubercle bacilli should be made. In chronic cases it may be necessary to culture biopsy material of granulation tissue or bone.

Blood cultures may be positive for the infecting organism. Otherwise, those changes associated with chronic infection are found.

Rheumatoid Arthritis (Rheumatoid Disease)

Diagnosis of this condition, characterized by morning stiffness, peripheral joint inflammation and damage, deformities (with myopathy, neuropathy and/or arteritis in severe cases) with great variation in clinical presentation, severity and duration, is confirmed by clinical examination and radiography. Tests for RA factor (IgM antibodies against altered IgG) are positive after 6 months. Ninety per cent of seropositive and 90 per cent of seronegative cases have circulating antibodies against rheumatoid arthritis-associated nuclear antigen (RANA).

There is an increased susceptibility to rheumatoid arthritis in patients with HLA DW4 or HLA DrW4.

Activity of the disease is reflected in raised ESR and plasma viscosity, plasma fibrinogen and serum C-reactive protein (CRP). Haemoglobin concentration falls (with refractory hypochromic or normochromic anaemia) and rising platelet counts (up to 600×10^9/l). Serum iron and TIBC are low, even though the bone marrow may contain stainable iron, and bone marrow aspirates show a moderate increase in plasma cells.

Histological examination of subcutaneous rheumatoid nodules and synovial material from affected joints show typical histological changes. Synovial fluid viscosity falls with increasing fibrinogen content, but examination of joint fluid is not of clinical value.

Serum albumin falls and serum globulin increases.

TESTS OF PROGRESS

Treatment with such drugs as penicillamine, gold salts, azathioprine, or cyclophosphamide, require regular haematological monitoring. Plasmapheresis has been used in cases which develop vasculitis.

TESTS PROVIDING USEFUL NEGATIVE RESULTS

Tests for the presence of lupus erythematosus are negative in most cases.

Juvenile Rheumatoid Arthritis (Still's Disease)

Diagnosis of this condition is confirmed by the finding of rheumatoid arthritic changes during the first two decades. Although the ESR and plasma viscosity are increased, and C-reactive protein is present in acute attacks, the percentage of positive tests for the presence of RA factor in the serum, such as Rose–Waaler, RA latex test and bentonite flocculation test, is lower than when rheumatoid arthritis develops in adults.

There is a normal white-cell count, with mild neutropenia often, and occasionally neutrophilia and hypochromic anaemia.

TESTS OF PROGRESS

Findings resemble those of adult rheumatoid arthritis, with response to therapy as in adults.

Felty's Syndrome

Diagnosis of this syndrome, which comprises the signs and symptoms of chronic rheumatoid arthritis with haematological evidence of hypersplenism, is supported by the demonstration of the typical laboratory results found in rheumatoid arthritis plus variable anaemia, variable neutropenia which may be cyclical, and variable thrombocytopenia. In addition to strongly positive serum Rose–Waaler and RA latex tests, LE cells may be demonstrated and serum antinuclear titres may be increased.

The bone marrow appears hyperplastic in most cases, but a few cases may show a hypoplastic marrow. Gastric achlorhydria is common.

TESTS OF PROGRESS

There is haematological improvement following administration of steroids, as well as relief of joint pains. When splenectomy is performed to eliminate active hypersplenism, the haematological findings improve, but the activity of the rheumatoid disorder is unaffected.

Ankylosing Spondylitis

Diagnosis of this condition, characterized by attacks of back pain and pain in the manubriosternal and sternoclavicular joints, with attacks of fever and weight loss, is essentially clinical and radiographic.

Ninety per cent of patients with the disease are HLA B27 positive (but not all people who are HLA B27 positive develop the disease).

TESTS OF CLINICAL PROGRESS

Laboratory evidence of activity of the disease includes mild normochromic anaemia, raised ESR and plasma viscosity, but serum C-reactive protein (CRP) is probably more useful.

TESTS PROVIDING USEFUL NEGATIVE RESULTS

Tests for RA factor are negative in most cases (cf. rheumatoid arthritis). Patients who are HLA 27 negative probably have some other condition causing their signs and symptoms.

Serum ASO titres are not raised (cf. acute rheumatic fever).

Prolapsed Intervertebral Disk

Diagnosis of prolapsed invertebral disk depends on clinical signs and symptoms and possibly X-ray myelography.

TESTS PROVIDING USEFUL NEGATIVE RESULTS

There may be a slight increase in CSF aspartate aminotransferase activity. More marked increases are found following a cerebrovascular accident or with carcinomatous metastases in the central nervous system.

Suppurative Synovitis and Tenosynovitis

Identification of the organism causing the infection may be made by microscopy and culture of fluid or pus removed by aspiration or at surgical operation. If infection with *Mycobacterium tuberculosis* is suspected, suitable cultures smould be made, and material may be injected into a guinea pig.

Such infections are secondary, either from local extension or by blood-borne organisms from an infection elsewhere, or following penetrating wounds.

Neutrophilia with increased ESR and plasma viscosity develop. If the infection is gonococcal in origin, the serum gonococcal complement-fixation test may be positive.

Gonococcal Arthritis

DIAGNOSTIC TESTS

Specific immunofluorescent staining of a deposit from synovial fluid reveals the presence of gonococci, which can be grown on culture media for more complete identification.

TESTS SUPPORTING CLINICAL DIAGNOSIS

Synovial fluid contains more than 30 000 neutrophils/100 ml, and a glucose concentration of about 30 mg/100 ml.

The GCFT may become positive.

NON-SPECIFIC TESTS

Changes associated with acute infection.

TESTS OF PROGRESS

There is a dramatic response to penicillin or other suitable antibiotic to which the organism isolated is sensitive.

Congenital Myopathies [R]

Congenital myopathies, characterized by weakness and hypotonia in infancy ('floppy babies'), delayed milestones, proximal limb weakness in a young child, myopathic abnormalities on electromyography, abnormal family history, an incidence in girls, and histological abnormalities seen on electron microscopy of muscle biopsy material, are extremely rare. They include:

1. Central core disease.
2. Nemaline myopathy, or rhabdomyopathy.
3. Myotubular myopathy (centronuclear myopathy).
4. Megaconial myopathy (mitochondrial disease).
5. Multicore disease.
6. Muscle cytochrome-b deficiency.

Conditions with later onset include:

1. McArdle's phosphorylase deficiency.
2. Paroxysmal myoglobinuria (due to various defects).
3. Familial periodic paralysis.
4. Adult glycogen storage disease.
5. Adult carnitine deficiency myopathy.

Sodium-responsive Normokalaemic Periodic Paralysis [R] [AR]

Diagnosis of this very rare recessive condition, characterized by attacks of paralysis which can last for days or weeks, and which can be provoked by oral potassium salts or salt restriction, but in which the plasma potassium levels remain normal, is confirmed by examination of muscle biopsy material. On electron microscopy, very numerous moderately enlarged mitochondria are seen in the muscle cells.

TESTS OF PROGRESS

Attacks are not provoked by exercise. Salt supplements with acetazolamide and 9-alpha-fluorohydrocortisone prevent attacks.

Hypokalaemic Periodic Paralysis [R] [AD]

Diagnosis of this dominant condition, characterized by attacks of flaccid weakness of voluntary muscles (sparing speech, swallowing and respiration usually), with onset in the second decade, occurring particularly on rising after rest following exertion, or after a large carbohydrate-rich meal, and lasting for a few hours, is strongly supported by the finding of plasma potassium levels in an attack below 3 mmol/l.

Histology of muscle biopsy taken during an attack shows vacuolation of muscle fibres following dilatation of the sarcoplasmic reticulum.

TESTS OF PROGRESS

Oral potassium supplements and spironolactone (or, paradoxically, thiazide diuretics) reduce the severity and frequency of attacks. Some permanent muscle damage may follow severe attacks.

TESTS PROVIDING USEFUL NEGATIVE RESULTS

No biochemical evidence of hyperaldosteronism is found.

Hyperkalaemic Periodic Paralysis (Hereditary Episodic Adynamnia) [R] [AD]

Diagnosis of this rare dominant disorder, characterized by attacks of paralysis precipitated by exercise or by ingestion of potassium salts, is confirmed by the finding of hyperkalaemia during attacks of paralysis (although not all patients have abnormally raised plasma potassium). The attacks occur during the daytime and last up to 30–40 min on average.

TESTS OF PROGRESS

Treatment in the past has been with acetazolamide, chlorothiazide and fludrocortisone. Severe attacks can be relieved with intravenous calcium gluconate or insulin plus glucose.

Recently, inhalation of salbutamol has been shown to be useful during attacks.

Paroxysmal Myoglobinuria

Diagnosis of this condition, characterized by acute attacks of cramp-like muscle pain and tenderness, associated with weakness or paralysis, is confirmed by the demonstration of myoglobin in the urine during or immediately after an attack.

Serum creatine phosphokinase activity is increased in proportion to the degree of muscle damage in the attack, with increased excretion of creatine in the urine. Plasma potassium may also temporarily increase and a neutrophilia may occur.

Attacks occur after prolonged exercise, fasting, a high-fat diet and/or cold weather. Electron microscopy of muscle biopsy material should be carried out. Some cases have been shown to have muscle carnityl palmityl transferase activity reduced, with raised CPK during attacks, and carbohydrates before exercise reducing the severity and incidence of attacks.

Other cases have been found to have myophosphorylase deficiency in their muscles, and yet other cases have been found with abnormally reduced muscle carnitine and attacks of episodic vomiting and acidosis.

It is therefore useful to store muscle biopsy material deep frozen, to examine muscle biopsy material by electron microscopy, pending further developments.

TESTS PROVIDING USEFUL NEGATIVE RESULTS

Exclude haemoglobinuria.

Progressive Muscular Atrophy

Clinical diagnosis of this condition is supported by the finding of increased serum phosphokinase activity and increased urinary output of creatine, reflecting progressive loss of muscle.

Progressive Muscular Dystrophy

Clinical diagnosis of this condition is supported by the finding of increased serum creatine phosphokinase activity and increased urinary output of creatine, reflecting loss of muscle. Biochemical evidence of muscle destruction is more marked in the early stages of the disease and especially in children.

TESTS OF PROGRESS

Female carriers of the condition, including the facioscapulohumeral variety of muscular dystrophy, may be detected by the finding of raised serum creatine phosphokinase activity in otherwise normal adults, and this may be helpful for genetic counselling.

X-linked (Duchenne) Muscular Dystrophy [XR]

Diagnosis of this sex-linked familial condition, characterized in males by progressive weakness, skeletal deformity, muscular contractions and cardiac damage, with death in the second or third decade, is confirmed by clinical and myographic examination.

Serum creatine phosphokinase activity is increased with muscle destruction. An increased number of echinocytes (distorted red cells) is seen in the peripheral blood.

TESTS OF PROGRESS

Female carriers may be detected by the finding of raised serum creatine phosphokinase activity in otherwise normal adults. It is important to appreciate that CPK values in the premenarchal female is the same as in the postmenopausal female, that CPK activity normally falls during menstruation, and falls even lower during pregnancy (resulting in the failure to detect carriers). Also in the Northern hemisphere, CPK activity is higher in the summer than in the winter. Screening for carriers therefore requires great care.

Pseudohypertrophic Muscular Dystrophy

Clinical diagnosis of this condition is supported by the finding of increased serum creatine phosphokinase activity and increased urinary output of creatine, reflecting loss of muscle. Biochemical evidence of muscle destruction is more marked in the early stages of the disease and especially in children.

TESTS OF PROGRESS

Female carriers of the condition may be detected by the finding of raised serum creatine phosphokinase activity in otherwise normal adults, and this may be useful for genetic counselling.

Dystrophia Myotonica [AD]

Diagnosis of this condition, characterized by myotonia, distal muscle atrophy, cataracts, gonadal atrophy, cardiomyopathy, mild endocrine anomalies and mental defect or dementia, is clinical.

The diagnosis is supported by the finding of increased serum creatine phosphokinase, lactate dehydrogenase, and alanine and aspartate aminotransferase activities in rapidly deteriorating cases.

TESTS OF PROGRESS

Myocardial infarction occurs in up to a quarter of patients, with typical ECG and laboratory findings.

TESTS PROVIDING USEFUL NEGATIVE RESULTS

In males with testicular atrophy, their karyotype is normal (cf. Klinefelter's syndrome).

Malignant Hyperpyrexia [AD]

Diagnosis of this genetic myopathy, characterized by attacks of hyperpyrexia with metabolic and respiratory acidosis and ventricular arrhythmias, chemically induced by inhalation of some anaesthetic agents (e.g. halothane, suxamethonium), or catecholamines produced by stress, is strongly suggested by the finding of marked increase in serum creatine phosphokinase, lactate dehydrogenase, and aspartate aminotransferase activities, with myoglobin excreted in the urine.

Plasma lactic acid may be increased in severe attacks.

Diagnosis can be confirmed using muscle biopsy in vitro for caffeine/suxamethonium test, with electron microscopy histological examination.

There may be brain oedema, renal failure and/or coagulopathy. Incidence is thought to be about 1 in 15 000 patients receiving general anaesthetics and can be devastatingly severe in young otherwise healthy adults (i.e. large muscle mass).

TESTS OF PROGRESS

Some patients with myotonia congenita may develop malignant hyperpyrexia following general anaesthesia.

Myositis Ossificans (Münchmeyer's Disease) [R]

Diagnosis of this rare familial condition can be confirmed by microscopy of muscle biopsy material. Affected muscle shows haemorrhages and inflammatory cells, with collagenous connective tissue, cartilage, or bone. Osseous tissue is laid down in striated muscle, bridging joints and causing serious deformities.

All biochemical analyses on blood have been found to be normal.

Idiopathic Rhabdomyolysis [R]

Diagnosis of this very rare but very dangerous condition is confirmed by the histological findings in muscle biopsy material. The biopsy shows haphazard focal necrosis of muscle fibres, with loss of cross-striation in some fibres, and poor staining of fibres. Electron microscopy is useful, if available. No muscle enzyme deficiency has been found. Following rapid destruction of muscle tissue, myoglobinuria is often found and in some cases renal damage follows with uraemia.

16 Diseases of the Central Nervous System

Anxiety State

Thyroid function tests, including serum T4 and T3, are normal in anxiety state, but may be significantly increased in thyrotoxicosis.

Idiopathic Epilepsy

After prolonged or severe convulsions there may be variable increases in the CSF of cholinesterase, aldolase and protein, probably a consequence of anoxia, otherwise no abnormality is found.

In patients who have had to be treated for long periods with large doses of anticonvulsants, folate deficiency as measured by red-cell folate activity may develop. Serum folate activity is low within 12 hours of a dose of oral anticonvulsant (especially phenytoin) and this depression is not necessarily associated with red-cell folate depression. The mean red-cell volume (MCV) is often increased in adolescent and adult patients, in the absence of anaemia. In a small proportion of cases, frank folate-deficiency anaemia develops, with megaloblastic changes in the bone marrow.

Manic-depressive Illness

Diagnosis of the disorder is clinical. Therapy with lithium carbonate is only effective in mania after 7–10 days of treatment, with plasma lithium levels about 1·3–1·4 mmol/l (i.e. near toxic levels, and other forms of treatment are preferable).

In depressive illness, after successful treatment or remission, if plasma lithium concentrations are kept at more than 0·5 mmol/l, the relapse rate is reduced.

Alzheimer's Disease

Diagnosis is supported by the finding of reduced brain choline acetyl transferase activity with age-dependent loss of 26–36 per cent of neurons from temporal lobe biopsy material (cf. non-demented elderly subjects).

Retinitis Pigmentosa

Since this clinical finding occurs in many conditions, tests relevant to those diseases should be considered according to the clinical indications:
Refsum's disease
Mucopolysaccharidoses

X-linked retinitis pigmentosa
Pigmentary changes which mimic retinitis pigmentosa:
  Following maternal infection during the first trimester of pregnancy
  Post-oedematous retinal changes after trauma
  Posterior uveitis in children
  Late stages of some cases of choroiditis

Down's Syndrome (Mongolism)

This condition is usually clinically diagnosed without difficulty. Chromosome analysis can be used to confirm the diagnosis, since two main types occur: (1) Trisomy 21; (2) Triploidy.

There are 47 chromosomes. The extra chromosome is a small acrocentric autosome with satellite bodies (therefore trisomic).

Dermatoglyphs are typical in Down's syndrome and may be useful in diagnosis. Similarly in non-anaemic adolescent and adult patients who are not being treated with anticonvulsants, the mean red cell volume (MCV) is significantly increased above normal.

Numerous conflicting reports of increases in serum enzymes have been published. It appears that neutrophil alkaline phosphatase activity is increased frequently, and serum gammaglobulin levels are also increased (roughly proportional to the patient's age). The repeated infections to which such patients are susceptible would possibly explain both these findings, or they might reflect chromosomal abnormality.

Migraine

No useful laboratory tests are known, but in cases in which initial fasting or undue hunger precedes attacks, serum free fatty acid levels (FFA) have been found to rise excessively after fasting.

Myasthenia Gravis

Diagnosis of this condition can be supported by muscle biopsy examination, showing muscle necrosis, lymphorrhages and abnormalities of nerve terminals and end-plates.

Antibodies against acetylcholine neural receptors are present in 90 per cent of adult cases, less commonly in ocular and juvenile/congenital forms. Antimuscle, antinuclear and antithyroid antibodies may occur in myasthenia gravis, but also in other diseases.

TESTS OF PROGRESS

There is a positive association with the presence of HLA-DRw3. Plasma-pheresis can be used to remove antibodies, and immunosuppressive therapy is useful if myasthenia gravis is associated with thymoma. Plasmapheresis may give relief for a few weeks while immunosuppressive therapy begins to act.

Guillain–Barré Syndrome (Acute Infective Polyneuritis)

Diagnosis of this condition, characterized by the acute development of a polyneuropathy, 1–3 weeks after an upper respiratory tract infection (usually), is clinical. The diagnosis is supported by the finding of an increase in CSF protein without a corresponding increase in cell count (any increase being of lymphocytes).

TESTS PROVIDING USEFUL NEGATIVE RESULTS

Absence of raised CSF cell count or evidence of acute poliomyelitis.

Inherited Optic Atrophy

LEBER'S HEREDITARY OPTIC ATROPHY

Serum cyanocobalamin is markedly increased above normal (e.g. 105 ± 52·5 pg/ml compared with normal 6 ± 3·4 pg/ml).

DOMINANTLY INHERITED OPTIC ATROPHY

Serum cyanocobalamin is increased above normal (e.g. 49 ± 20·5 pg/ml compared with normal 6 ± 3·4 pg/ml).

These findings suggest a new diagnostic test.

Subacute Necrotizing Encephalopathy of Leigh

Diagnosis of this condition, characterized by fatal encephalopathy developing during the first two years of life, is confirmed by demonstration of the virtual absence of pyruvate carboxylase activity in liver biopsy material. Plasma pyruvate and lactate levels are increased.

TESTS PROVIDING USEFUL NEGATIVE RESULTS

There is no evidence of vitamin B_1 deficiency.

Reye's Syndrome

Diagnosis of this condition, characterized by a febrile onset followed by progressive brain damage ending rapidly in death, is supported by the finding of fatty infiltration of the liver (biopsy material) in a child with an acute encephalopathy, with increased blood ammonia, increased serum aspartate aminotransferase activity, neutrophilia, and reduced CSF glucose concentration without any increase in CSF cell count.

TESTS PROVIDING USEFUL NEGATIVE RESULTS

Blood cultures are sterile. CSF cultures are sterile, and there is no direct evidence of virus infection of the brain.

Parkinson's Disease

As yet unexplained, the CSF homovanillic acid (HVA) is reduced below normal in many cases.

Subacute Combined Degeneration of the Spinal Cord

Diagnosis of this condition is confirmed by the finding of abnormally low serum vitamin B_{12} concentrations (usually less than 40 pg/100 ml), and megaloblastic anaemia.

TESTS OF PROGRESS

If a patient with megaloblastic anaemia due to vitamin B_{12} deficiency is given folic acid in therapeutic dosage, there is haematological remission at first, but the risk of producing subacute combined degeneration of the cord is very great. Folate accentuates the deficiency of vitamin B_{12} in the body. The Schilling test detects malabsorption of vitamin B_{12} from the gut. Vitamin B_{12} therapy results in haematological recovery and variable CNS recovery.

TESTS PROVIDING USEFUL NEGATIVE RESULTS

In this condition which is often associated with abnormal EEG readings, the CSF has a normal protein content and cell count, and tests for syphilitic infection are negative. Multiple sclerosis, intracranial tumour and syphilitic infection involving the nervous system can produce similar clinical signs and symptoms.

Disseminated (Multiple) Sclerosis

Diagnosis of this condition is clinical. There is an increased susceptibility to develop the condition in individuals with HLA-7A (5–10 × more likely). The diagnosis is supported by the finding of increased CSF IgG with oligoclonal bands. The CSF total protein is increased in 25 per cent of cases, and more than 25 per cent of the protein consists of gammaglobulin in 60 per cent of cases. The Lange gold sol test gives a 'meningitic' type of curve if there are plaques near the brain surface (e.g. 0001233210).

Platelet function tests have no place in diagnosis or prognosis as yet.

TESTS PROVIDING USEFUL NEGATIVE RESULTS

There is no evidence of infection with either pyogenic organisms or syphilis.

Sydenham's Chorea (Rheumatic Chorea)

Diagnosis of this rare condition, affecting children and adolescents and following an attack of rheumatic fever in 33 per cent of cases, characterized by irritability, agitation and inattention, is supported by the finding of increased serum ASO titres, with raised ESR, plasma viscosity and serum C-reactive protein.

TESTS PROVIDING USEFUL NEGATIVE RESULTS

CSF protein and cell counts are normal.

Schilder's Disease

Diagnosis of this rare sex-linked progressive leucodystrophy with adrenal insufficiency, dementia, cortical blindness or deafness, pyramidal damage, and ataxia, is supported by the finding of markedly increased plasma immunoreactive corticotrophin levels (which may be found long before signs of neurological damage in boys).

Intracranial Tumour Involving the CNS

Diagnosis is confirmed by air encephalography, arteriography, electro-encephalography, radio-isotope scanning of the brain, and in suitable cases by microscopy of needle-biopsy material.

LABORATORY INVESTIGATIONS SUPPORTING THE DIAGNOSIS

These include examination of samples of CSF (which may be under increased pressure), in which may be found slight to moderate increase in the protein concentration, with normal or increased numbers of cells present. Using suitable techniques and stains, malignant cells may be demonstrated. CSF glucose concentrations are normal, unless there is gross infiltration with malignant cells of the brain surfaces or of the meninges, when the glucose concentration falls. The fluid aspartate aminotransferase and lactate dehydrogenase activities may be increased above normal.

The presence of an intracranial tumour may be associated with the signs and symptoms of:

    Diabetes insipidus
    Inappropriate antidiuretic hormone syndrome
    Hypopituitarism
    Precocious puberty

and laboratory tests for these various disorders may be required.

Cerebrovascular Accident (Thrombosis; Haemorrhage; Embolism)

TESTS SUPPORTING CLINICAL DIAGNOSIS

After haemorrhage blood is found in the CSF resulting in a gross increase in the CSF red-cell count with proportional increase in the white-cell count and with the same differential count as in the peripheral blood. The CSF protein content increases in proportion to the plasma present.

After thrombosis or embolism, the red-cell count in the CSF varies, but the nearer the brain lesion to the surface, the higher is the cell count and the CSF protein.

(When local bleeding occurs at the time of lumbar puncture, consecutive samples vary in their blood content.)

CSF aspartate aminotransferase and lactate dehydrogenase are variably increased soon after the accident. When much brain has been damaged, serum creatine phosphokinase activity reaches peak values by 48 hours.

TESTS PROVIDING USEFUL NEGATIVE RESULTS

Cultures of the CSF are negative.

TESTS OF PROGRESS

Later, the red cells in the CSF are broken down and the fluid becomes tinged with yellow. When such pigment is found after a very recent cerebrovascular accident, it indicates that there has been an earlier bleed into the CSF. The raised CSF protein persists for some time.

Hyperventilation, low P_{CO_2}, and raised arterial blood pH are associated with a poor prognosis.

Subarachnoid Haemorrhage

Diagnosis is confirmed by the finding of bloodstained CSF. At first the supernatant fluid after centrifugation is colourless, and the white-cell count and protein content are in proportion to the size of the haemorrhage. By 24 hours, the supernatant fluid is coloured yellow, reaching its peak by 36–48 hours. After 12 hours, the white-cell count in the CSF rises disproportionately to the red-cell count, as a result of the inflammatory reaction to the presence of shed blood in the CSF.

TESTS PROVIDING USEFUL NEGATIVE RESULTS

When lumbar puncture is performed, two consecutive samples should be taken. If the cell count is practically identical, then the blood in the CSF is the result of subarachnoid haemorrhage and not due to bleeding at the site of the lumbar puncture produced by local trauma.

Brain Abscess

Diagnosis of brain abscess is supported by the finding of an increase in the CSF protein content and an increased lymphocyte count. If the abscess remains localized and is not near to the CSF, the fluid remains clear, but may be under increased pressure. The cell count and protein content in the CSF increase when the abscess cavity is near to CSF.

Identification of the infecting organism can be determined by microscopy and culture of pus obtained by needle biopsy or following surgical operation.

If an abscess ruptures into the CSF, then the cell count rises rapidly and there is an extremely acute meningitis, with reduced CSF chloride and glucose, and organisms may be grown on culture of CSF.

When an acute abscess is present in the brain, there is an associated neutrophilia in the blood with raised ESR and plasma viscosity.

Spinal Block

Diagnosis of a spinal block is supported by the finding of increased CSF protein concentration, with yellow tingeing and increased fibrinogen and albumin concentrations. This differs from the CSF obtained from above the block.

Cerebral Anoxia

Following cerebral anoxia, CSF protein levels and aspartate aminotransferase activity are increased.

Birth Injury of Brachial Plexus (including Erb–Duchenne Type)

Following the injury, serum aldolase, creatine phosphokinase, lactate dehydrogenase and aspartate aminotransferase activities are increased in the early stages, in proportion to the amount of muscle damage, returning to normal levels later.

INFECTIONS

Meningitis (Bacterial, Fungal and Protozoal)

Diagnosis is confirmed by microscopy of CSF, and culture of fluid as soon after collection as possible (since many anaerobic organisms die in the presence of oxygen). For the direct examination for evidence of *Mycobacterium tuberculosis*, direct microscopy followed by culture should be carried out on the centrifuged deposit from at least 10 ml of CSF.

The protein content of CSF is increased in infection, and glucose content is reduced in the presence of large numbers of neutrophils. In non-tuberculous infections, high counts of neutrophils are found at first, followed later by numbers of large mononuclear cells and lymphocytes. Blood cultures for the infecting organism are positive if the meningitis is secondary to septicaemia. Cultures should be made from local infections, if these may have caused meningitis by direct spread of infection.

In tuberculous meningitis, the cell count is variable, with predominantly lymphocytes at first, but neutrophils appearing later.

TESTS OF PROGRESS

Following successful treatment, the infecting organism disappears from the CSF, and the CSF protein concentration and cell count return to normal. If intrathecal antibiotics have been given, a slightly raised cell count may persist until this treatment is discontinued. A recurrence of infection is shown by a sudden increase in the cell count.

Mastoiditis

Identification of the infecting organism can be determined by culture of pus (usually scanty in amount) or bone fragments removed surgically. The condition is almost always secondary to otitis media, and therefore culture of pus from the middle ear will probably yield the same organism as that infecting the mastoid air-cells.

The condition is associated with neutrophilia, raised ESR, and raised plasma viscosity.

Infected Venous Sinus Thrombosis

Identification of the infecting organism can be determined by microscopy and culture of pus obtained at surgical exploration. The infection is often secondary to other infection (e.g. mastoiditis, carbuncle of face, intracranial sepsis), and therefore microscopy and culture of pus from any primary site of infection are helpful.

There is an associated neutrophilia, with increased ESR and plasma viscosity.

Huntington's Chorea [AD]

Before development of choreiform movements in an affected case, levodopa produces chorea in an asymptomatic case. No biochemical test on blood, urine, or CSF has yet been devised for the detection of cases or carriers.

In established cases, massive depletion of gamma-aminobutyric acid (GABA) has been demonstrated in the basal ganglia.

Neural Tube Defects

Neural tube defect occurs in 4–5 per 1000 births in the UK, and 5 per cent of these have encephalocele. The rate for anencephaly and spina bifida is about the same. The mother with an earlier affected child has an increased risk of bearing another affected infant.

When a fetal neural tube defect is present, the maternal serum contains an abnormally increased amount of AFP, which can be detected at 16–18 weeks, allowing time for possible amniocentesis, scan and possibly therapeutic abortion on confirmation of the abnormality.

X-linked Mental Retardation

Diagnosis of this cause of mental retardation in affected males can be confirmed by the finding of a 'fragile site' in the X-chromosome in a proportion of lymphocytes cultured in special medium.

Female carriers can also be detected in this way.

Microcephaly and Associated Infections

Blood taken from newborn microcephalic infants can be tested for evidence of infection by organisms known to cause microcephaly (TORCH screen):

T   Toxoplasmosis
O   (Other) Syphilis
R   Rubella
C   Cytomegalovirus
H   Herpes virus

17 Gynaecological Disorders

Normal Menstrual Cycle

In the normal menstrual cycle there are many biochemical and haematological changes during the various phases. Some of these are now described:

DAYS 1–5
Menstruation
There is a fall in the platelet count at menstruation, rising to normal again by the fourth day, with a slight increase in plasma fibrinogen.

About 10–40 mg of iron are lost in the shed blood. Immediately after menstruation, at 2–3 days, the urine oestrogen output is low.

After menstruation there may be a period of moderate diuresis, with increased sodium and chloride output in the urine.

DAYS 6–15
Proliferative Phase
The anterior pituitary produces follicle-stimulating hormone (FSH). The developing follicle produces more oestrogen which gradually inhibits FSH production and stimulates luteinizing hormone (LH) release. With the ripening of the ovarian follicle, the urinary oestrogen rises to the first peak.

DAY 15 (MAY BE 12–16)
Ovulation
There is a fall in urine oestrogen, with a temporary increase in the output of gonadotrophins in the urine. The urinary pregnanediol output is slightly increased for 2 days after ovulation.

DAYS 15–28
Secretory Phase
The corpus luteum develops, which produces oestrogen, and there is a second peak of urinary oestrogen output. The corpus luteum also produces progesterone, which inhibits the production of LH by the anterior pituitary gland, resulting in the degeneration of the corpus luteum from the twenty-sixth day onwards in the absence of fertilization.

DAYS 25–28
Premenstrual Phase
There is retention of water, sodium and chloride by the body, with a fall in

urine volume. There may be a trace of protein in the urine. Tension and disturbance may be associated with this premenstrual phase.

Anovulatory Cycles

There is no 'ovulatory peak' of urinary oestrogen excretion, preceded by a rise in output of pituitary gonadotrophin.

TESTS OF PROGRESS

Clomiphene citrate will induce ovulation in otherwise anovulatory amenor-rhoea, regularize ovulation in patients with irregular and prolonged intervals between ovulation, and will induce ovulation in cases of irregular anovular menstruation associated with cystic glandular hyperplasia. The 'ovulatory peak' of urine oestrogen excretion is used to indicate when fertilization can be arranged.

Post-menopause

It is found that there is a fall in urinary 17-kestosteroids output, oestrogen output, and a rise in pituitary gonadotrophin release.

Normal Pregnancy

The biochemical and haematological findings in normal pregnancy differ in many respects from those found in the normal non-pregnant adult female. It is important to remember these differences when one is dealing with a pregnant woman suffering from disease, e.g. rheumatoid arthritis or iron-deficiency anaemia. These differences vary with the stage of pregnancy, and are listed below.

FIRST TRIMESTER

The blood urea tends to fall in the first 6 months, with some reduction in urea output in relation to protein consumption. The plasma fibrinogen is moderately increased by the 16th week, and this results in a slight increase in the plasma viscosity.

Urinary output of chorionic gonadotrophin is increased from the 2nd week, to reach peak values by the 6th–12th weeks, subsequently falling approximately 10 per cent of the peak, and remaining at this level until parturition. There is an increase in urinary pregnanediol output by the 12th week from 10 mg to 35 mg/24 hours.

SECOND TRIMESTER

The urinary output of pregnanediol increases from 35 mg at the beginning of the second trimester to about 70 mg/24 hours at the end of this period. After the 3rd month there is an increase in serum alkaline phosphatase activity. Serum iron levels fall, and the iron-binding capacity is increased. During the second and third trimesters the serum albumin concentration falls by about 1 g/100 ml. There are also increases in serum alpha-globulins.

The urine oestrogen output is increased from the 6th month to term to about 10–100 μg/24 hours.

THIRD TRIMESTER

The total blood volume increases to a maximum of about 45 per cent by the 32nd week. The total plasma volume is increased by +25 to +55 per cent and the total red-cell volume is increased by +20 to +40 per cent at this time. There is an associated fall in the peripheral blood haemoglobin concentration, since the plasma volume increase is greater than the red-cell volume increase, but in normal pregnancy the haemoglobin level does not fall below 10 g/100 ml. The plasma fibrinogen levels are increased (about +33 per cent normal non-pregnant levels) and the ESR (a test originally used for the detection of normal pregnancy) and the plasma viscosity are both increased above the normal non-pregnant levels.

Plasma Factor VIII is increased markedly in late normal pregnancy, and plasma Factors II, VII, and X are increased.

Urine pregnanediol output increases from 70 mg/24 hours to 100 mg/24 hours at 36–38 weeks. The urinary human chorionic gonadotrophin output is below 20 iu/24 hours.

Serum alkaline phosphatase activity and isocitrate dehydrogenase activity are at the upper limit of normal, derived from placenta. Serum cholesterol levels are increased by about +20 per cent by the 30th week, and serum PBI levels are increased. The BMR reaches its highest readings in the third trimester of normal pregnancy, and thyroid function tests should be postponed if possible until after delivery. The blood urea tends to rise towards the normal non-pregnant level towards the end of pregnancy.

In some cases glucose tolerance is reduced, with some glycosuria. It is worth noting that in late pregnancy lactosuria is not uncommon and is harmless.

Normal Puerperium

Following delivery, with involution of the uterus, there is a marked temporary increase in urine creatine output, derived from uterine muscle. Tests of pregnancy are negative by the 9th day postpartum, and serum alkaline phosphatase levels are normal by the 3rd to 6th weeks.

In up to 20 per cent of mothers, fetal red cells may be detectable in their circulations shortly after delivery. During lactation, lactosuria, particularly in the afternoon, is not uncommon and is harmless. The serum PBI concentration returns to the normal non-pregnant level by 3–6 weeks, and plasma T3 uptake tests are normal by 12–13 weeks.

Plasma fibrinogen falls to normal in the puerperium. There is a temporary increase in fibrinolytic activity 2–4 hours after delivery. There may be a moderate increase in serum lactate dehydrogenase activity during labour, with a rapid fall to normal levels immediately afterwards.

Intrahepatic Obstructive Jaundice of Pregnancy

Diagnosis of this condition which may develop during pregnancy is supported by the finding of increased serum bilirubin and serum alkaline phosphatase activity, pale stools and excretion of bilirubin in the urine.

TESTS OF PROGRESS
Recovery follows parturition.

TESTS PROVIDING USEFUL NEGATIVE RESULTS
There is no evidence of viral hepatitis, and no signs of inflammation.

Acute Fatty Liver in Pregnancy

Diagnosis of this potentially dangerous condition is confirmed by examination of liver-biopsy material. The diagnosis is supported by the finding of increased serum alanine aminotransferase and alkaline phosphatase activities, with normal serum bilirubin levels in the early stages. With increasing liver damage, the serum bilirubin level rises excessively and both serum alanine aminotransferase and alkaline phosphatase activities fall towards normal values.

TESTS OF PROGRESS
With recovery, serum alanine aminotransferase and alkaline phosphatase activities fall to normal, with serum bilirubin concentrations remaining normal throughout.

Accidental Placental Haemorrhage

Accidental placental haemorrhage may be associated with a consumption coagulopathy, with thrombocytopenia, fibrinogenopenia, increased fibrin- and fibrinogen-degradation products, and prolonged prothrombin and activated partial thromboplastin times.

Fetal Haemorrhage into the Maternal Circulation

Diagnosis is confirmed by the demonstration of red cells containing fetal haemoglobin (HbF) in the peripheral circulation in significant numbers.

Pre-eclamptic Toxaemia (Toxaemia of Pregnancy)

Diagnosis is supported by the finding of increasing proteinuria in late pregnancy associated with sudden gain in weight, oedema, hypertension, headache, with or without vomiting. Plasma-fibrinogen levels are increased with cryofibrinogen present, and serum alanine and aspartate aminotransferase activities increase with coexisting liver damage, with a rising serum-bilirubin concentration. Plasma fibrinopeptide A and beta-thromboglobulin levels are increased, indicating early intravascular clotting and platelet activation. Within 48 hours of the onset of placental degeneration, serum isocitrate dehydrogenase activity is increased above normal. The urine contains increased amounts of protein.

TESTS OF PROGRESS

If convulsions occur, the case has developed into frank eclampsia.

Eclampsia

Diagnosis of eclampsia is supported by the finding of oliguria with protein concentrations of 10–40 g/l (a trace of protein in the urine being normal in normal pregnancy), with reduced urine-urea concentration, haematuria, with hyaline, cellular and granular casts. The urine may contain ketones.

Plasma-fibrinogen levels are increased, with neutrophilia. The plasma-activated partial thromboplastin time is reduced below normal. Thrombocytopenia may occur, and later the plasma-fibrinogen level may fall with the appearance of fibrin- and fibrinogen-degradation products in the plasma.

Ectopic Pregnancy

It is worth noting that tests of pregnancy often give negative results.

Fetal Distress

1. ASSESSMENT OF PLACENTAL INTEGRITY

Urine oestriol excretion can be useful, as a low and falling output indicates that the fetus is in danger.

Human placental lactogen (chorionomammotropin) is present in the maternal plasma from early pregnancy onwards, reaching peak values at 35 weeks. Low results for dates indicate fetal distress. Plasma heat-stable alkaline phosphatase activity has also been used.

2. ASSESSMENT OF FETAL LUNG MATURITY

Amniotic fluid lecithin/sphingomyelin ratio and lamellar body phospholipid in amniotic fluid are related to fetal lung surfactant factors. Low levels are used to predict respiratory distress syndrome in the newborn infant after birth.

Abortion

Diagnosis is supported by the finding of low output or urinary chorionic gonadotrophins, oestriol and pregnanediol. When the urinary output of pregnanediol falls below 5 mg/24 hours, abortion is inevitable.

Retention in Utero of Dead Fetus

Diagnosis is supported by the finding of low urinary output of chorionic gonadotrophins, pregnanediol and oestriol. In addition, plasma-fibrinogen levels may fall, with thrombocytopenia, plus prolongation of both the prothrombin time and the activated partial thromboplastin time (i.e. a consumption coagulopathy may develop after a few weeks of retention of a dead fetus).

Amniotic Fluid Embolism

Diagnosis is supported by the finding of a sudden fall in plasma fibrinogen, with thrombocytopenia, prolonged prothrombin times and activated partial thromboplastin times, and increasing fibrin- and fibrinogen-degradation products in the plasma.

Hydatidiform Mole

Diagnosis of hydatidiform mole is supported by the finding of strongly positive pregnancy test results with increased human chorionic gonadotrophin excretion in the urine, with a rising titre at the end of the third month of pregnancy. Plasma-fibrinogen levels may fall dramatically following release of placental tissue thromboplastin into the circulation.

TESTS OF PROGRESS

Following successful removal of a mole, the pregnancy tests become negative and the urinary excretion of human chorionic gonadotrophin falls to very low levels by the end of the first week after operation.

Subsequently, a rising titre occurring a few weeks after operation for the removal of a mole suggests involvement of deeper uterine tissues.

Chorionepithelioma, Chorioncarcinoma

Diagnosis of either invasive mole or chorioncarcinoma is supported by the finding of persistently raised serum and/or urine human chorionic gonado-trophin levels for several months after termination of pregnancy.

TESTS OF PROGRESS

Following successful surgical removal of the tumour, the urinary output of chorionic gonadotrophin falls to negligible amounts, but following recurrence the output rises again.

TESTS PROVIDING USEFUL NEGATIVE RESULTS

Oestrogen and progesterone are excreted in amounts less than are found in normal pregnancy.

Puerperal Sepsis

Diagnosis of puerperal sepsis can be confirmed and identification of the infecting organism carried out by aerobic and anaerobic cultures of high vaginal swabs. Blood cultures should be taken during a rise in body temperature and should be incubated: (*a*) anaerobically; (*b*) in CO_2-rich atmosphere; (*c*) in air, at 37 °C. From these cultures it may be possible to isolate and identify infecting strict anaerobes, which die rapidly on exposure to air.

Examination and culture of midstream urine specimens should be carried out.

If the infection is due to organisms of the type disseminated by respiratory carriers (e.g. staphylococci or *Streptococcus pyogenes*) nose and throat swabs should be cultured. Umbilical stumps may be reservoirs for pathogens and cultures should be taken from them in a nursery.

Phage-typing and antibiotic sensitivity patterns of isolate staphylococci, and Griffiths typing of isolated Group A streptococci, are useful in epidemio-logical studies, since carriers must be detected and cleared.

Female Breast Carcinoma

Diagnosis: There are no biochemical or haematological tests which can be used for diagnosis. Diagnosis is made by histological examination of surgically removed material.

TESTS OF PROGRESS

Various markers have been used in assessing the prognosis of proven cases. Patients with no detectable CEA in their serum survive longer than those with positive tests. Following surgical removal, serum CEA, alkaline phosphatase activity and gamma-glutamyl transferase activity, estimated every 3 months, show increases in patients developing metastases.

CEA, C-reactive protein, ferritin, alpha-1-antitrypsin in serum and the urine hydroxyproline : creatinine ratio have been used also to detect the development of metastases.

Endometritis and Salpingitis

Identification of the infecting organism is made by microscopy and culture of pus removed during surgery, or occasionally appearing as cervical discharge. Microscopy of biopsy material may be useful, especially if the nature of the lesion is obscure, or if it is due to tuberculosis, when animal inoculation is useful.

The gonococcal fixation test (GCFT) may be positive in cases due to gonococcal infection.

Neutrophilia with raised ESR and plasma viscosity are found.

18 *Newborn Infant*

Normal Newborn Infant

The major differences which are found when the normal newborn infant is compared with the normal adult include:

BLOOD

The haemoglobin concentration, haematocrit, white blood-cell count, and red-cell count are increased immediately after birth, with increased total white-cell count falling to less than 15 000/cmm by the fourth day, and the haemoglobin, haematocrit and red-cell count falling to their lowest levels by the end of the first week, and slowly rising to adult levels again over the next few years. The MCV and MCD are greater than in normal adults, falling during the next 6 weeks, and both the nucleated red-cell count and the reticulocyte count are increased at birth, falling to normal levels during the first few days. Fetal haemoglobin F comprises about 70 per cent of the total haemoglobin present in the blood. The red cells are mechanically more fragile, are more sensitive to Heinz-body-inducing agents, and are more sensitive to methaemoglobin-inducing agents than are adult red cells. The siderocyte count is raised for a few days after birth. Haptoglobins remain low after birth.

Fibrinolytic activity is increased in the plasma, and the antithrombin titre is increased. Plasma Factor II is reduced in activity (25–40 per cent of normal adult values), plasma Factor V is reduced (60–130 per cent), plasma Factor VII (25–45 per cent), plasma Factor IX (10–15 per cent), plasma Factor X (3–35 per cent), plasma Factor XI are reduced during the first 5 days, and the prothrombin time, Thrombotest, and activated partial thromboplastin times may be prolonged. The platelet count rises to normal adult value by 3 months.

Serum total protein values are increased at birth, but fall during the first few weeks, rising to adult values again by the fifth year. Serum gammaglobulins are above normal at birth, but fall below normal adult values within a few days, and rise slowly to adult levels by 5–11 years, the various immunoglobulins rising at different rates. Both alpha- and betaglobulins are above normal adult values at birth and fall slowly. Plasma-fibrinogen levels are lower than in the adult. The ESR is less than 5 mm and the plasma viscosity is at or below the normal lower limit for adult values.

The blood urea and NPN are low and fasting blood-glucose levels are low, and dangerous hypoglycaemia may develop in some infants if intervals between feeds are prolonged. Serum-cholesterol values are increased at birth, fall rapidly, and then climb slowly until middle age. Serum PBI is raised for a few days, then falls to normal slowly. Serum iron, raised at birth, rapidly falls to low levels, and the adult normal range is reached by 7–10 years. The TIBC is low after birth and rises slowly to 400 μg/100 ml by 2 years. Serum copper, caeruloplasmin and copper oxidase activities are low and rise slowly after birth.

Serum inorganic phosphate is increased, and serum bilirubin and pyruvate levels are increased for a few days after birth. Plasma alkaline phosphatase, aspartate aminotransferase, lactate dehydrogenase, isocitrate dehydrogenase and aldolase activities are increased immediately after birth. Serum cholinesterase and red-cell cholinesterase activities are low after birth, and serum amylase activity is not detectable for the first 2 months.

URINE UREA

Urine urea output is low, the GFR is low, and the renal ability to concentrate or dilute urine is much less than in the adult. 17-Oxosteroid, 17-oxogenic steroids and 17-hydroxycorticosteroid outputs are all very low.

STOOLS

The stools are yellow at birth, and the output of faecal stercobilinogen (urobilinogen) is very low. During the first year, faecal trypsin activity is parallel to the duodenal juice trypsin activity. The faecal fat comprises less than 50 per cent of the dry weight of the stools, and two-thirds of the fat is split.

CSF

The upper limit of the CSF protein concentration during the first year of life is 80 mg/100 ml.

BILE

The bile contains only taurine conjugates. Glycine conjugates only appear later.

PANCREATIC JUICE

The pancreatic juice contains very little amylase in the newborn infant.

Physiological Jaundice of the Newborn (Icterus Neonatorum)

Diagnosis is supported by the finding of jaundice developing by the second day after birth, with peak serum bilirubin results by the second to third day, serum bilirubin being predominantly in the unconjugated form and rarely exceeding 7 mg/100 ml. This condition is probably due to immaturity of the liver, with reduced activity of glucuronyl transferase.

TESTS OF PROGRESS

Serum bilirubin levels return to normal by 2–3 weeks.

TESTS PROVIDING USEFUL NEGATIVE RESULTS

Bilirubin is absent from the urine. No evidence of haemolytic disease of the newborn is found.

Low Birth-weight Infant (Premature Infant)

The expected date of delivery, and hence the degree of prematurity, may be calculated, if the date of the last menstrual period is known. The weight at birth may be well below the expected weight for the length of the pregnancy. The consequences are:

The infant is often anaemic, with an increased reticulocyte count. (In a third-month fetus the reticulocyte count = 90 per cent, sixth-month fetus reticulocyte count = 15–30 per cent, and at normal term the reticulocyte count = 4–6 per cent.) The red cells have an increased MCV and MCD and there is an increased nucleated red-cell count. (Full-term newborn count = 3–10 per 100 white blood cells. Premature infant count = 10–20 per 100 white blood cells.) The siderocyte count is increased, and there is an increased tendency to develop Heinz bodies, especially if certain drugs are given, since the red-cell reduced glutathione content is low. In addition to anaemia, there is a greater proportion of the haemoglobin in the form of haemoglobin F (more than 75 per cent).

Various clotting factors are reduced in activity, and the prothrombin time, activated partial thromboplastin time and Thrombotest result are all prolonged. The plasma-fibrinogen concentration is at the lower limit of normal. The capillary fragility is increased. Fibrinolytic activity is lower than normal, with an increased risk of hyaline membrane disease.

Protein reserves are low, and the serum proteins are reduced with low serum albumin and gammaglobulins, with reduced rate of synthesis of immunoglobulins and the associated risk of infection. Glycogen stores in the liver are low and these infants have an increased liability to develop severe hypoglycaemia, with an increased tendency to ketosis. Liver glucuronyl transferase activity is lower than normal and the conjugation of bilirubin is impaired, with associated jaundice. The urine contains both bilirubin and an excess of urobilinogen.

Renal function is less effective than in more mature infants. The blood urea clearance and urine concentrating and diluting powers are below normal, a dilute urine being passed. Renal tubular function, including ability to excrete increased amounts of ammonia, and acid–base-regulating mechanisms are all functioning below normal.

The significance of all these reductions in function is that the low birth-weight baby has very much less reserve function than a full-term baby and any illness and its treatment are therefore that much more potentially dangerous.

Pemphigus Neonatorum

Identification of the infecting organism can be made by microscopy and culture of blister fluid or of swab of skin under a recently ruptured blister. This infection is usually due to *Staphylococcus pyogenes*, and if this organism is isolated, it may be important for epidemiological purposes to phage-type the organism and to establish its sensitivity pattern to a battery of antibiotics.

Neonatal Umbilical Sepsis

Identification of an infecting organism can be made by microscopy and microscopy of swabs taken from the stump. The umbilicus may form an important reservoir of pathogenic organisms without showing gross signs of sepsis. The infecting organism is usually a staphylococcus or streptococcus; neonatal tetanus can occur.

Breast Milk Jaundice

Diagnosis is supported by the finding of peak serum bilirubin increases at 1 week after birth, mainly due to unconjugated bilirubin, with recovery following change from mother's milk to some other milk (whether human or cow's).

Postmature Infant

The normal newborn infant has about 70 per cent of haemoglobin in the form of HGF. In postmature infants the HbF content may be as low as 55 per cent.

Haemolytic Disease of the Newborn (Erythroblastosis Fetalis)

Diagnosis is confirmed by the finding of antibodies to the infant's blood group in the maternal circulation during pregnancy, or in the infant's blood (cord blood) at birth. When the blood group difference is in the Rhesus blood group system, the infant's blood group make-up includes C, and/or D, and/or E, the most frequent maternal antibody against fetal cells being anti-D, less frequently anti-C or anti-E. Rhesus incompatibility develops more frequently when the fetal and maternal ABO groups are compatible. When the blood group difference is in the ABO system, the infant's blood group make-up includes A, whereas the maternal blood group is O, the mother developing haemolytic anti-A antibodies against the fetal cells. Other group incompatibilities are rare.

Fetal red cells may be demonstrated in the maternal circulation, and these cells may immunize the mother against a fetal blood group or boost an already existing blood group incompatibility. With the development of Rhesus-group antibodies, the Coombs' antihuman globulin test (either direct or indirect) is positive using the infant's blood.

In an affected newborn infant, serum unconjugated bilirubin concentrations are increased, and haemoglobin levels fall with progressive destruction of the infant's red cells by intravascular haemolysis. There is an accompanying leuco-erythroblastic anaemia, with increasing numbers of nucleated red cells and myelocytes in the peripheral blood. The white-cell count is raised (15 000–30 000/cmm). The reticulocyte count is also raised above 5–6 per cent.

In ABO incompatibility, the Coombs' test is usually negative, but many of the red cells are spherocytic, and the saline osmotic fragility is increased above normal, as the maternal haemolysin damages the infant's red cells.

The platelet count may be normal or reduced. Following red-cell destruction, the serum lactate dehydrogenase activity is increased.

TESTS OF PROGRESS

During pregnancy, in which the paternal and maternal blood groups make it possible that incompatibility develops between fetal red cells and the maternal circulation (e.g. Rhesus-positive male and Rhesus-negative female), it is important to estimate the titre of antibodies in the mother's serum (*a*) for predicting the condition and (*b*) for deciding when to induce labour since the pregnancy should not be allowed to proceed to full term if the fetus is being damaged.

Amniotic fluid withdrawn during pregnancy can be useful in assessing fetal damage, as the bile pigment derivatives in the amniotic fluid increase abnormally when the fetal red cells are being damaged.

Immediately after delivery of a mother who is Rhesus-negative with a Rhesus-positive baby, the maternal peripheral blood should be examined for the presence of infant red cells (high HbF content). If such cells are present, it has been found that inoculation with anti-D serum can be used to destroy the circulating fetal cells, before there is time for the mother to be immunized against the paternal Rhesus factor, reducing the risk of Rh-incompatibility and haemolysis during a subsequent pregnancy.

Index